Nu
poc

M000078045

A
B
C
D
E
F
G
H
I
J
K
L
M
N
O
P
Q
R
S
T
U
V
W
X
Y
Z

Börm
Bruckmeier
Publishing

Authors: Suzanne Bowden, RN, MSN, RNP (Nursing Instructor, Pulaski Technical College, Little Rock, AR), Marc Deschka
Editor: Andrea Rauneker, M.D.
Production: Natascha Choffat
Cover Illustration: Bastian Börm
Publisher: Börm Bruckmeier Publishing, LLC, www.media4u.com

IMPORTANT NOTICE—PLEASE READ!
This book is based on information from sources believed to be reliable, and every effort has been made to make the book as complete and accurate as possible and to describe generally accepted practices based on information available as of the printing date, but its accuracy and completeness cannot be guaranteed. Despite the best efforts of authors and publisher, the book may contain errors, and the reader should use the book only as a general guide and not as the ultimate source of information about the subject matter.
This book is not intended to reprint all of the information available to the authors or publisher on the subject, but rather to simplify, complement and supplement other available sources. The reader is encouraged to read all available material and to consult the package insert and other references to learn as much as possible about the subject.
This book is sold without warranties of any kind, expressed or implied, and the publisher and authors disclaim any liability, loss or damage caused by the content of this book.
IF YOU DO NOT WISH TO BE BOUND BY THE FOREGOING CAUTIONS AND CONDITIONS , YOU MAY RETURN THIS BOOK TO THE PUBLISHER FOR A FULL REFUND.

Printed in China through Colorcraft Ltd., Hong Kong
ISBN 978-1-59103-237-3

Preface to the first edition

Advances in medical science always bring about an expansion in medical terminology. Until now, only large and comprehensive dictionaries have been available for looking up medical terms. Also, these large competitor books can barely stay abreast of the new information available on the Internet, and therefore the detailed medical information provided in such publications is often out of date.

The Nursing Dictionary pocket addresses these issues by providing 10,000 up-to-date basic medical terms, with many illustrations and tables, all presented in a practical pocket format. It focuses primarily on terms, prefixes and suffixes essential to daily medical practice, and its lexical structure offers users quick access to information required for academic study and medical practice environments.

The user also has the option to update this information with the latest Internet-based knowledge. With additional useful information provided in the appendix, as well as a listing of abbreviations, signs and symbols relevant to daily medical practice, this book is an indispensable companion for nurses, nursing students, healthcare teachers and healthcare professionals alike.

From the author and the publisher   El Segundo, CA, August 2008

Additional titles in this series:

Acupuncture pocket
Anatomy pocket
Canadian Drug pocket 2009
Differential Diagnosis pocket
Drug pocket 2008
Drug pocket plus 2008
ECG pocket
ECG Cases pocket
EMS pocket
Homeopathy pocket
Medical Abbreviations pocket
Medical Classifications pocket
Medical Spanish Dictionary pocket
Medical Spanish pocket plus
Medical Translator pocket
Normal Values pocket
Respiratory pocket
Wards 101 pocket

Börm Bruckmeier Publishing, LLC on the Internet:
www.media4u.com

A

abasia inability to walk

abdomen belly; the portion of the trunk between the *diaphragm* and *pelvis*; abbr. *abd*

abdominal pert. to the *abdomen*

abdominal aortic aneurysm *aneurysm* in the abdominal *aorta*; abbr. *AAA*

abdominal pregnancy pregnancy located in the abdominal cavity; see *extrauterine pregnancy*

abdominal reflex *physiological* multisynaptic *reflex* in which stimulating the skin of the abdomen from the side toward the middle causes a contraction of the abdominal muscles on that side; mapping T6T12 *dermatome*

abdominal retractor *surgical* instrument used to hold the abdominal wall open without damaging the *tissues*

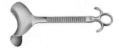

Fig. 1: abdominal retractor [A]

abducens nerve (nervus abducens) *6*ᵗʰ *cranial nerve;* contains motor fibers; together with the *oculomotor* and *trochlear nerves*, it controls eye movement

abduct to move away from the median plane; opp. *adduct*

abduction movement of a body part away from the medial plane; opp. *adduction*

abductor a muscle that enables abduction; opp. *adductor*

aberrant adj. of *aberration*

aberration deviation from the norm

abiosis absence of life

abiotic without life

ablactate to wean

ablactation weaning an infant off breast milk

ablate to remove

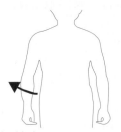

Fig. 2: abduction

ablatio retinae retinal detachment

ablation removal, detachment or eradication by surgery, laser or freezing; also due to injury or disease, e.g. ablatio retinae (detached retina), ablatio placentae

abort to terminate a pregnancy intentionally

abortion miscarriage before 24 full weeks of gestation with birth weight below 500 g; early abortion (first trimester abortion) is miscarriage before the 12ᵗʰ week; late abortion is miscarriage between the 13ᵗʰ and completed 24ᵗʰ week. Other terms include **a) complete abortion:** *abortion* in which all the products of conception are expelled; opp. *incomplete abortion;* **b) habitual abortion:** repeated occurrence of *abortion;* **c) imminent abortion:** impending abortion; **d) inevitable abortion:** *abortion* in initial stages where sonography does not show an intact pregnancy and the *cervix* is slightly dilated; **e) incomplete abortion:** *abortion* in which only a portion of the products of conception is expelled; opp. *complete abortion;* **f) induced abortion:** (therapeutic abortion) intentional termination of pregnancy

abrasion *superficial injury or scraping of the skin*

abruptio placentae (ablatio placentae) premature detachment of the placenta

abruption detachment, tearing away
absence seizure (petit mal) brief loss of consciousness (2–20 seconds) without aura or postictal symptoms
abscess circumscribed accumulation of pus
abscessing abscess-forming
absorb to take in by *absorption*
absorber absorbent substance
absorption taking in; incorporation of matter by multiple actions in multiple body sites, e.g. intestines
abstinence refraining from consumption of drugs, alcohol, etc.; refraining from sexual activity
abstinent adj. of *abstinence*
abulia lack of willpower or initiative
abuse misuse, wrong use
acarodermatitis skin disease caused by *mites,* e.g. *scabies*
acceleration increase in speed
accessory nerve *11th cranial nerve;* contains motor fibers; provides the *innervation* of the *sternocleidomastoid* and *trapezius muscles*
accidental unforeseen, unintentional
acclimatization adaptation to a climate
accommodate to adjust or adapt

accommodation adaptation, adjustment, e.g. change in the refractive power of the lens of the *eye* for near vision
accumulate to build up or collect
accumulation buildup, collection
ACE inhibitor drug used to inhibit *angiotensinconverting enzyme;* used to treat hypertension, etc.
acetabular fracture *fracture* of the *acetabulum,* usually due to a *dashboard injury* or falling from a considerable height; usually occurs in combination with *dislocation* of the hip joint

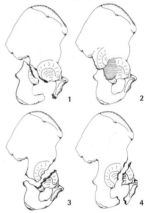

Fig. 4: acetabular fracture
1 Posterior column fracture 2 Acetabular roof fracture 3 Transverse fracture 4 Anterior column fracture

acetabulum socket of the hip joint; articulates with the head of the femur
acetone simple organic compound found in blood and urine when fats are not oxidized
acetonemia increased *acetone* in the blood
acetonuria excretion of *acetone* in the urine

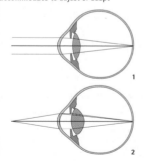

Fig. 3: accommodation
1 Far accommodation 2 Near accommodation

achalasia spasmodic closure of a *sphincter* muscle, e.g. the lower esophageal sphincter

Achilles tendon tendon extending from the calf muscle to the heelbone

Achilles tendon reflex contraction of the calf muscles with flexion toward the sole of the foot when the slightly tensed *Achilles tendon* is tapped; absence or exaggeration of the reflex is usually associated with *central nervous system (CNS)* damage

achlorhydria failure to produce gastric acid, e.g. as a consequence of *chronic gastritis*

acholia suppressed secretion of *bile* into the intestine, usually due to severe liver disease

achromatopsia complete colorblindness

achylia (apepsia) absence of gastric juices

acid chem. substance that releases hydrogen ions in an aqueous solution; see also *base*

acid burn (acid corrosion) chemical burn *wound* caused by *acids*; usually leads to *coagulation necrosis*

acid phosphatase important *tumor marker* for *prostatic carcinoma*

acidity acid content of a solution

acidosis acid-base imbalance with the blood *pH* falling below 7.36; metabolic and respiratory types are distinguished; opp. *alkalosis*

acidosis, compensated pH is WNR because of repiratory and metabolic actions; however, blood bicarbonate and CO2 may not be within normal range (WNR)

acidosis, metabolic *metabolic acids* (excluding H_2CO_3) accumulate and bicarbonate is lost in *extracellular* fluids

acidosis, respiratory failure to eliminate CO_2 in the blood, usually from respiratory problems

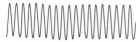

Fig. 5: acidotic breathing

acidotic breathing (Kussmaul's breathing) regular deep breathing with increased release of *carbon dioxide* in order to compensate for *metabolic acidosis*

acne (vulgaris) skin disease occurring mainly during *puberty* marked by purulent inflammation of the *sebaceous glands*; can cause scarring in the affected areas

acoustic neuroma benign auditory canal tumor involving the 8th cranial nerve

acrocyanosis blue discoloration of the extremities due to lack of *oxygen*

acromegaly disproportionate enlargement of the extremities due to overproduction of *growth hormone*, usually caused by *adenoma* of the *adenohypophysis*

acromioclavicular joint shoulder joint between the *acromion* and *clavicle*; abbr. *ACJ*

acromioclavicular joint dislocation (shoulder dislocation) *dislocation* of the shoulder; see *Tossy classification*

acromion (acromial process) outer end of the spine of the scapula

actin endogenous *protein* important for contraction of muscles; combines with *myosin* to form *actomyosin*

Actinobacillus genus of rod-shaped *gramnegative bacteria*. mallei can cause *glanders*

actinomycosis infection caused by *Actinomyces israelii* leading to bluish (livid) swelling with *abscess* formation; usually occurs after *tooth extraction* or *lesions* of the oral mucosa; however, bicarbonate may not be within normal range (WNR)

active 1) ongoing, in progress, in effect; 2) functioning or acting independently; opp. *inactive; passive*

active immunization administration of killed or weakened pathogens for *immunization*

actomyosin endogenous *protein* important for contraction of muscles; consists of *actin* and *myosin*

acupressure Chinese healing method in which pressure is applied to specified points on the body in order to reduce/minimize pain

acupuncture Chinese healing method in which needles are inserted into specified points on the skin in order to reduce/minimize pain

acute abdomen life-threatening abdominal disease with sudden onset, from a variety of causes; requires immediate examination and decision on further treatment, see Fig. 7

acute having a sudden onset progressing quickly; opp. *chronic*

acute hearing loss *acute* unilateral hearing loss with no dizziness or accompanying *neurological* or *ophthalmological* symptoms

Adam's apple *thyroid cartilage*

addiction physical and mental dependency that adversely affects the patient and his/her environment and leads to increased tolerance

addiction potential an individual's *predisposition* to develop an *addiction*

Addison's disease a disease in which the *adrenal cortex* fails to produce or produces insufficient *hormones*, leading to bronze discoloration of the skin

Addisonian crisis acute *decompensation* of *adrenal cortex insufficiency*

adduct to move toward the median plane; opp. *abduct*

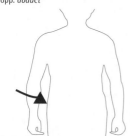

Fig. 6: adduction

adduction movement of a body part toward the median plane; opp. *abduction*

adductor muscle that enables *adduction*; opp. *abductor*

adductor muscle of the thumb muscle that draws the thumb toward the center of the palm; *innervation: ulnar nerve*

adenitis *inflammation* of a gland

adenocarcinoma malignant tumor of glandular *tissue*, usually occurring in the *stomach*, *pancreas* or intestine

adenofibroma benign mixed tumor consisting of fibrous and glandular *tissue*, usually occurring in the *ovaries* or *uterus*

adenohypophysis anterior lobe of the *pituitary gland*; produces *hormones* such as *FSH*, *LH*, *prolactin*, *TSH*, *ACTH* and *STH*

adenoid glandlike

adenoidectomy *surgical* removal of the adenoids (*pharyngeal tonsils*)

adenoids *pharyngeal tonsils*

adenoma benign tumor occurring in epithelial tissue

adenomatosis disease characterized by formation of multiple *adenomas*

adenomectomy surgical removal of an *adenoma*

adenomyoma tumor consisting of *adenoma* and *myoma* tissue

adenosarcoma tumor consisting of *adenoma* and *sarcoma* tissue

adenosclerosis hardening of a *gland*

adenose glandlike

adenovirus common type of *virus* that causes *inflammations* of the pharyngeal mucosa or *bronchitis*, among other things

adhesion binding or sticking together; fibrous structure binding normally separate parts together

adhesive bandage (band-aid) adhesive bandage with a small gauze pad for covering minor cuts and other wounds

adipose refers to fatal

adipsia absence of thirst; opp. *polydipsia*

adjuvant a drug that enhances the effect of another drug; supportive additional therapy

ADL abbr. activities of daily living

adnexa appendages to an organ, e.g. the *fallopian tubes* and *ovaries* in relation to the *uterus*; sing. adnexum

adnexectomy removal of adnexa

adnexitis inflammation of the *fallopian tube* and *ovary*

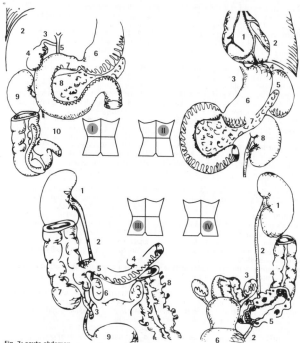

Fig. 7: acute abdomen
1) Right upper quadrant: 1 Pneumonia, pleuritis **2** Hepatic abscess **3** Acute cystic duct occlusion
4 Cholecystitis **5** Cholelithiasis **6** Gastric ulcer **7** Duodenal ulcer **8** Pancreatitis **9** Kidney stone
10 Appendicitis
II) Left upper quadrant: 1 Myocardial infarction **2** Pneumonia **3** Hiatal hernia **4** Pleuritis
5 Splenic infarction **6** Gastric ulcer **7** Pancreatitis **8** Pyelonephritis
III) Right lower quadrant: 1 Kidney stone **2** Ureter stone **3** Acute appendicitis **4** Diverticulitis
5 Inflammatory bowel disease **6** Adnexitis **7** Cecal carcinoma **8** Diverticulitis **9** Cystitis
IV) Left lower quadrant: 1 Kidney stone **2** Ureter stone **3** Acute adnexitis **4** Colon cance **5** Diverticulitis
6 Urinary retention, cystitis

adolescence period of development from puberty to adulthood

adrenal pert. to the *adrenal glands*

adrenal cortex inner part of the *adrenal gland* that produces *hormones*, including aldosterone, glucocorticoids and mineralocorticoids

adrenal gland endocrine gland located on top of the *kidney*, consisting of the inner *adrenal medulla* and outer *adrenal cortex*

adrenal medulla inner part of the *adrenal gland* that produces *hormones*, including epinephrine and norepinephrine

adrenalectomy surgical removal of the *adrenal glands*

adrenaline see *epinephrine*

adrenocorticotropic hormone *hormone* produced by the *adenohyophysis* that mainly stimulates production and release of glucocorticoids from the *adrenal cortex*; abbr. ACTH

adrenogenital syndrome hereditary *enzyme* defect leading to reduced production of *cortisol* and thus to excessive production of *ACTH*; abbr. AGS

Adson's maneuver test for *thoracic outlet syndrome* in which *reclination* and *rotation* of the head leads to diminished *radial pulse* on the affected side

adsorption binding to a surface

adult respiratory distress syndrome (shock lung) acute respiratory failure in adults; abbr. ARDS

advanced life support extensive lifesaving interventions (IV line, defibrillation, intubation) to prevent death; certification course is required; abbr. ALS; opp. *basic life support*

adventitia outermost layer of *organs* and vessels

adventitious breath sounds abnormal breath sounds heard upon auscultation

adynamia not dynamic; opp. *hyperdynamic*

aerobe *bacterium* requiring oxygen; opp. *anaerobe*

aerobic requiring oxygen; opp. *anaerobic*

aerogenic forming gas

aerophagy swallowing of air

aerosol drug nebulized into the finest possible particles; abbr. *aer*

afebrile having no fever; opp. *febrile*

affect observable physical signs of emotional state or lack of same, e.g. facial expressions that lack emotion (flat effect)

affected stricken by or involved in a disease process

affection emotional state of fondness

afferent leading toward, climbing, rising, e.g. nerves leading from the *spinal cord* to the *brain*; opp. *efferent*

affidavit written declaration under oath made before an authorized official

affinity relationship, attraction; tendency to create chemical bonds

African trypanosomiasis *sleeping sickness*

afterload resistance against which the left ventricle must work to pump blood out of the heart

afterloading procedure used in radiation therapy of tumors; technique: the radioactive source is inserted into the tumor area via a *catheter* in order to irradiate the affected *tissue* from the shortest possible distance

agalactia lack of milk secretion during nursing period, e.g. due to infant's sucking weakness

agenesia absence of or failure of a body part to develop or to grow normally

agent active substance

ageusia (ageustia) absence or impairment of the sense of taste; involves sensory pathways to the brain; found when assessing 12th cranial nerve (hypoglossal)

agglutinate to clump together

agglutination clumping of *cells*, e.g. *thrombocytes* or *bacteria*

aggregation inhibitor anticoagulant drug that inhibits the clumping of *thrombocytes*

agitated adj. of *agitation*

agitation state of excitement

agnosia impaired perception of sensory stimuli despite intact function of sense organs e.g. *optic agnosia*

agonadism absence of *gonads*

agonist counterpart to the *antagonist* in the interplay of chemical substances or *muscles* (e.g. *extensors* and *flexors*)

agony death struggle; phase immediately prior to death; extreme suffering

agoraphobia fear of open spaces

agranulocytosis drastic reduction in *granulocytes* in the blood, e.g. due to reaction to a drug

agraphia (logographia) loss of ability to write

air embolism obstruction of a blood vessel by an air bubble

air–fluid level horizontal boundary line of an accumulation of fluid as seen in an x-ray image, e.g. in *ileus*

air sac see *alveoli*

Aitken 0 damage to the *epiphyseal growth plate* due to shearing force marked by epiphyseolysis with no accompanying fracture or destruction of the growth zone

Aitken I partial *epiphyseolysis* with breakage of the *metaphysis* caused by shearing force and torsion

Aitken II partial *epiphyseolysis* with *epiphyseal* fragmentation caused by shearing force and impaction

Aitken III *fracture* of the *epiphysis* and *metaphysis* caused by shearing force and impaction

Aitken IV *axial* impaction of the *epiphyseal* plate with irreversible damage to the growth plate; corresponds to Salter-Harris V

Aitken fracture classification classification of *epiphyseal growth plate* injuries

akathisia (acathisia) severe restlessness with nagging urge to move around; may present as a side effect of a *neuroleptic* drug

akinesia lack of movement, e.g. in *Parkinson's disease*; opp. *hyperkinesia*

akinetic adj. of *akinesia*; opp. *hyperkinetic*

albinism congenital lack of pigmentation in the skin, hair and eyes

albumin blood *protein* formed in the *liver* that functions as a reserve *protein*; maintains fluid distribution in the body and transports chemical substances

albuminuria presence of *albumin* in the urine, e.g. in kidney disease

alcoholism alcohol dependence

aldosterone *hormone (mineralocorticoid)* formed in the *adrenal cortex* that regulates water and *electrolyte* balance

aldosteronism pathological increase in production of *aldosterone*

alexia inability to read

algometer instrument for measuring sensitivity to pain

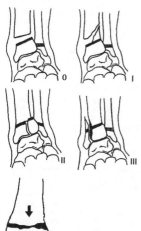

Fig. 8: Aitken 0 – Aitken IV

Fig. 9: algometer [H]

algophobia morbid fear of pain
alimentary pert. to *nutrition*
alimentation *nutrition*
alkali burn chemical *wound* caused by *lye* that can lead to *colliquative necrosis*

Fig. 10: alkali burn

alkaline phosphatase *enzyme* present in all body cells that cleaves *phosphate* from phosphate-containing compounds; important as a *tumor marker* for *osteosarcoma* and pancreatic cancer; abbr. AP
alkalosis disturbance of acid–base balance with blood *pH* rising above 7.44; opp. *acidosis*
alkalosis, metabolic see *metabolic alkalosis*
alkalosis, respiratory *respiratory alkalosis*
alkylating agent *cytostatic* drug for treatment of malignant neoplastic diseases
allegation assertion made by a party that must be proved or supported with evidence

Allen test test to assess circulatory disturbances in the arm or to test collateral circulation prior to *arterial puncture*, e.g. for invasive *blood pressure* measurement; procedure: patient raises the arm and makes a fist repeatedly while pressure is applied at the wrist to compress the *radial* and *ulnar arteries*, both together at first and then one at a time; if collateral circulation is insufficient in the noncompressed artery, there will be loss of color and pain in the hand
allergen substance that causes an *allergic* reaction
allergenic causing an *allergic* reaction
allergic pert. to *allergy*; hypersensitive
allergy extreme reaction to *allergens* by the *immune system*
Allgöwer suture (interrupted single button suture) special *surgical* suturing technique for *wound* closure

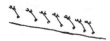

Fig. 12: Allgöwer suture

allodynia condition in which repeated brief touches cause pain while constant pressure causes none
allogeneic belonging to the same species but genetically different; see also *syngeneic, xenogeneic*
allogenic graft (allogeneic) *homologous graft*
allogenic stem cell transplant a transplant from a human donor who is not an identical genetic match, in which bone marrow or peripheral blood stem cells from a donor (usually related) are collected, stored and infused into a patient following high-dose chemotherapy and/or radiation therapy
allograft (*homograft*) *transplantation* of tissue or organs from a donor to a recipient; opp. *xenogeneic graft*
alloplastic graft *transplantation* of artificial organs

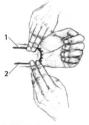

Fig. 11: Allen test
1 Radial artery **2** Ulnar artery

alloplasty plastic surgery in which body tissues are replaced with foreign material

alopecia absence/loss of hair esp. on head

alpha1-antitrypsin a blood test to identify a deficiency known to be present in those prone to emphysema and liver disease

alpha-amylase *enzyme* vital to starch digestion

alpha-fetoprotein important *tumor marker* for *hepatocellular carcinoma*; abbr. AFP

alpha-interferon leukocyte interferon; used in a nasal spray intended to stop the spread of the common cold

alternating occurring in turn

alveolar pert. to the *alveoli*

alveoli 1) tiny sacs in the lungs where gas exchange takes place (*oxygen* and *carbon dioxide*); 2) tooth cavity in the jawbone; sing. alveolus

alveolitis *inflammation* of the pulmonary *alveoli,* usually due to inhalation of *allergens*

Alzheimer's Association a national network of chapters dedicated to advancing research and providing education and support for Alzheimer's patients and their families

Alzheimer's disease progressive *dementia* with memory loss and other cognitive disorders, without additional *neurological* symptoms or altered mental state; a common cause of dementia abbr. AD

amalgam mercury alloy used as a filling material in dentistry

amaurosis complete blindness

amaurosis fugax temporary blindness in one eye

ambivalence simultaneous presence of contradictory feelings, e.g. in *schizophrenia*

amblyopia weak vision

Ambu bag trade name for a *manual* ventilation device for patients with inadequate or arrested breathing; ventilation is achieved by use of a mask held in place using a *C-grip* or via an *endotracheal tube*

ameba (amoeba) unicellular microorganism that can cause *dysentery* (*amebic dysentery*)

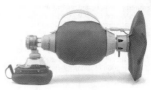

Fig. 13: Ambu bag [B]

amebiasis *amebic dysentery*

amebic dysentery (amebiasis) *dysentery* caused by *amebas*, which can lead to *abscesses* in various *organs,* e.g. the *liver*

amelia disorder of skeletal development marked by absence of one or more limbs

amenorrhea absence of *menstruation* for more than 3 months; *endocrine* or *organic* causes

amenorrhea–galactorrhea syndrome *syndrome* that includes *amenorrhea* and *galactorrhea*, caused by elevated *prolactin* in the blood, e.g. due to *prolactinoma*

ametropia imperfect vision due to incorrect ratio of axis length to refractive power

amines chemical compounds that can be derived from *ammonia*

amino acid building block for *proteins*

ammonia substance formed by the breakdown of *protein* by the intestinal *bacteria*; it is converted in the liver to *urea* and then excreted in the urine via the kidneys; in disorders of liver function increased ammonia levels in the blood can lead to *hepatic coma*; chemical abbr. NH_3

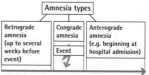

Fig. 14: amnesia

amnesia memory gap, quantitative memory
disturbance, e.g. following accidents,
epileptic seizures or other *traumas*
amnion inner fetal membrane, which
contains the *fetus* and *amniotic fluid*
amniocentesis puncture of the *amnion*
after the 14th week of gestation for
examination of *amniotic fluid* to diagnose
potential chromosomal defects

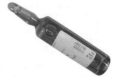

Fig. 16: ampule

ampulla dilated section of a hollow *organ*
amputate to remove a body part *surgically*
amputation *surgical* removal of a body part
e.g. a limb
amputation knife extremely sharp *surgical*
knife, e.g. according to Liston, used as a
cutting instrument for *amputations*

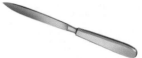

Fig. 17: amputation knife [A]

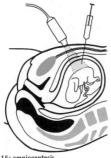

Fig. 15: amniocentesis

amnioscopy examination of *amniotic fluid*
amniotic fluid fluid inside the *amniotic sac*
that surrounds and protects the cells of the
amnion; amount: approx. 1000 ml in the
38th week of gestation
amniotic fluid embolism lifethreatening
embolism caused by entry of *amniotic fluid*
into the mother's bloodstream
amniotic sac commonly called the bag of
waters; amniotic fluid within the sac
protects the fetus
amniotomy *surgical* opening of the *amnion*
performed if rupture of fetal membranes
does not occur spontaneously during birth
amorphous formless, lacking sharp boundaries
amplitude magnitude or extent of
movement, e.g. of *QRS complexes* in an *ECG*
ampule single-dose glass container of a
drug; abbr. amp.

amputation saw *surgical operating*
instrument, e.g. according to Rust, for
cutting through bones during *amputations*

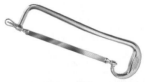

Fig. 18: amputation saw [A]

amylase (diastase) *enzyme* for digestion of
starches and *glycogen*, produced in the
parotid glands and *pancreas*
amyotrophia (amyotrophy) muscular *atrophy*
anabolic pert. to *anabolism*; opp. *catabolic*

anabolic agent drug used to promote anabolism, e.g. anabolic steroids for *doping*

anabolism constructive phase of *metabolism*; conversion of nutrients into body tissues; opp. *catabolism*

anacidity insufficient production of hydrochloric acid by the *stomach*; opp. *hyperacidity*

anaerobe *bacterium* that is able to live without *oxygen* or can only live without oxygen; opp. *aerobe*

anaerobic surviving without air or oxygen; opp. *aerobic*

anaerobic glycolysis metabolism of *glucose* in the absence of *oxygen* e.g. due to reduced blood flow to regions of the body shock or *hypoxia*; the resulting end product is *lactate*

anal pert. to the *anus*

anal carcinoma malignant tumor of the *anus*

anal fissure painful linear tear in the skin near the *anal* canal

anal prolapse prolapse of the *anal* mucosa, usually due to *pelvic floor* insufficiency; cf. *rectal prolapse*

Fig. 19: anal prolapse

anal reflex (anal wink) *physiological* polysynaptic *reflex* in which stimulation of the *perianal* skin causes *contraction* of the anal sphincter; mapping: S3–S5 *dermatome*

anal vein thrombosis (perianal vein thrombosis) *thrombosis* caused by *rupture* of the *perianal veins*, usually due to intense straining to pass bowel movements

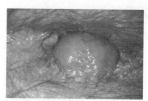

Fig. 20: anal vein thrombosis

analeptic drug with stimulating or invigorating qualities

analgesia absence or suspension of ability to feel pain

analgesic 1) drug used to treat pain; 2) having an analgesic effect

analogous functionally equivalent; similar

analysis separation of a whole into its component parts

anancasm (compulsion) impulsively occurring thoughts or actions, usually against the patient's will, which are felt to be senseless and subjectively disturbing but cannot be suppressed

anaphylactic pert. to *anaphylaxis*

anaphylactic shock *shock* triggered by *anaphylaxis*

anaphylaxis most severe form of *allergy*, which can lead to life-threatening *shock*

anarthria inability to speak

anasarca (dropsy) generalized positional *edema* (e.g. on the back when supine); usually occurs with *heart* or *renal failure*

anaspadias (epispadias) atypical opening of the *urethra* on the dorsal surface of the *penis*

anastomose to create an *anastomosis*

anastomosis natural or artificial connection between two hollow *organs, nerves* or blood vessels; pl. anastomoses

anatomic(al) pert. to *anatomy*

anatomy study of the structure of the body

androgen male sex hormone

androgyny pseudohermaphroditism

andrology study of male diseases

andros (viri) males

anectodal based upon one's experience, usually in story form

anemia reduced *hemoglobin, hematocrit* and/or *erythrocyte* count in the blood; other types include: a) **autoimmune hemolytic,** abbr. **AIHA:** antibodies that are produced by the patient's own body destroy red blood cells (abbr. RBC); b) **hyperchromic:** mean corpuscular *hemoglobin* concentration and MCHC are greater than normal; opp. hypochromic; c) **iron deficiency:** decreased hemoglobin (abbr. Hb), caused by abnormalities in iron intake; d) **megaloblastic:** sometimes called milk anemia; abnormal amounts of megaloblasts are found in blood samples; e) **pernicious:** cells in stomach lining fail to secrete enough intrinsic factor to absorb vitamin B12, which is an extrinsic factor; f) **posthemorrhagic:** anemia due to acute or chronic blood loss

anemic pert. to *anemia*

anesthesia numbing, lack of sensation

anesthesia system ventilation and tubing system of an *anesthesia ventilator,* which controls the flow direction and separation of *inspiration* and *expiration* mixture; see also *rebreathing system*

anesthesia ventilator apparatus for mechanical artificial ventilation with the ability to mix in anesthetic gas

anesthesiological pert. to *anesthesiology*

anesthesiologist medical doctor who is a specialist in *anesthesiology*

anesthesiology study of *anesthetic* methods

anesthetic 1) drug used to cause *anesthesia;* 2) pert. to *anesthesia*

anesthetist *licensed healthcare provider who administers anesthesia*

aneurine thiamine

aneurysm localized dilation in the wall of the heart or an *artery;* types include: a) **dissecting aneurysm:** aneurysm caused by a tear in the *intima* of a blood vessel, resulting in bleeding into the vascular wall that does not reenter the vascular lumen; b) **false aneurysm** (aneurysma spurium):

injury to the vascular wall with formation of a *hematoma* next to the vessel; subsequent organization and covering with *epithelial* tissue without creation of a true vascular wall c) **true aneurysm** (aneurysma verum): aneurysm involving all three layers of the *arterial* wall; d) berry: small congenital aneurysm of a cerebral vessel, found in Circle of Willis; e) cerebral: found in a blood vessel in the brain

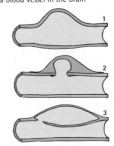

Fig. 21: aneurysm
1 True aneurysm 2 Sacculated aneurysm
3 Dissecting aneurysm

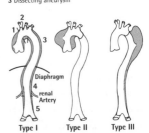

Fig. 22: dissecting aortic aneurysm
(DeBakey classifications)
1–5 Sections of the aorta

aneurysmectomy surgical removal of an *aneurysm*

angiectasis pathological dilation of blood vessels

angiitis *inflammation* of a blood vessel

angina pectoris chest pain due to inadequate circulation in the *coronary arteries*; degree of severity is classified using CCS classification; abbr. AP

anginose pert. to *angina pectoris*

angiocardiogram *angiocardiography*

angiocardiographic pert. to *angio-cardiography*

angiocardiography (angiocardiogram) *radiography* of the *heart* and its blood vessels following injection of a *contrast medium*

angiodysplasia malformation of blood vessels

angiodysplastic pert. to *angiodysplasia*

angioedema (angioneurotic edema, Quincke's disease) swelling of the skin and mucosa, mainly in the facial area, associated with *allergies*; danger of asphyxia due to laryngeal swelling

angiogenesis formation of new blood vessels

angiogram *angiography*

angiographic pert. to *angiography*

angiography radiography by blood-filled structures, e.g. blood vessels

angiology study of the blood vessels

angioma tumor consisting of newly formed vessels

angiopathy (angiosis) nonspecific collective term for diseases of the blood or lymph vessels

angiospasm spasmodic contraction of one or more blood vessels

angiotensin blood *protein* derived from angiotensinogen through the action of *renin*, which raises *blood pressure* and stimulates release of *aldosterone* and *norepinephrine* by the *adrenal cortex*

angiotensin–converting enzyme *enzyme* present in the vascular endothelial cells that converts *angiotensin I* to *angiotensin II* and thus increases *blood pressure*; abbr. ACE

angular dislocation (dislocatio ad axim) simple dislocation of a *fracture* with bending of the bone

angularis, V. *vena angularis*

angulus angle

anhidrosis lack of sweat secretion

anima soul, spirit

anion negatively charged *ion*

anion gap difference between measured *cations* and *anions*

aniridia absence of the *iris* of the eye

aniseikonia (anisoiconia) condition in which the retinal images differ in size between the left and right eyes

anisochromia variance in coloration of *erythrocytes* caused by variance in *hemoglobin* content

anisocoria inequality in *pupil* size with a difference in diameter of > 1 mm; opp. *isocoria*

anisocoric adj. of *anisocoria*; opp. *isocoric*

anisotropia impaired vision

ankle collective term for the *joints* that connect the lower leg with the foot; divided into the talocrural joint (the articulation below the *tibia* and *fibula*) and the subtalar joint (articulation of the *talus*, *calcaneus* and *navicular* bones)

ankle bones *ossa tarsi*

ankylosing spondylitis *Bechterew's disease*

ankylosis complete immobility and consolidation of a joint due to a disease process within the interior of the joint

anode *electrode* with its positive pole connected to a power source; opp. *cathode*

anomaly condition that deviates from the norm

anomia inability to find words or name objects

Anopheles genus of mosquito that transmits *malaria*

Anoplura order of insects comprising the sucking lice

anorectal pert. to the *rectum* and *anus*

anorexia lack of appetite

anorexia nervosa psychologically based eating disorder seen most often in young girls

A

anosmia absence of the sense of smell

anosognosia failure to recognize one's own illness

anotia congenital absence of the auricle of the ear

anoxia lack of oxygen in the *tissues*

antacid agent that binds or neutralizes stomach acid

antagonist counterpart of the *agonist* in the interplay of chemical substances or muscles (e.g. *flexors* and *extensors*)

antagonize to work against

antebrachium forearm

anteflexion bending forward; opp. *retroflexion*

antegrade (anterograde) moving or extending forward; opp. *retrograde*

antegrade amnesia *amnesia* in which the loss of memory relates to events that occur after a traumatic event

anterior pert. to the front surface of the body; opp. *posterior*

anterior deep temporal artery *arteria temporalis profunda anterior*

anterior interventricular artery (ramus interventricularis anterior, LAD) part of the left *coronary artery* (LCA); supplies the anterior wall of the left ventricle and 2/3 of the anterior septum; abbr. RIVA, LAD

anterior jugular vein *vein* that transports blood from the chin and neck area to the *external jugular* or *subclavian vein*

anterior perineum see *perineum*

anterior serratus muscle muscle that extends the arm forward; *innervation* long thoracic nerve

anterior tibial artery arteria tibialis anterior

anterior tibial muscle muscle along the front of the shin that raises the foot; innervation: deep peroneal nerve

anterior wall infarct *myocardial infarction* affecting the anterior wall of the heart; abbr. AWI

anterolateral infarction *myocardial infarction* affecting the anterior and lateral walls of the heart

anteroposterior reaching from the front to the back of a structure

anteroseptal infarction *myocardial infarction* affecting the anterior part of the intraventricular septum

anteversion tipping forward (e.g. of the arm in its socket) in the *sagittal* plane; opp. *retroversion*

anthelmint(h)ic drug used to treat infection with parasitic worms

anthrax *infectious disease* caused by *Bacillus anthracis*, affecting the *lungs*, *spleen* and skin; transmitted to humans by animals (cattle, horses, sheep, goats), usually via skin contact, consumption of meat, or inhalation of animal dust

anthropology study of humans

anthropos (homo*)* human being

antiandrogen drug used to block the effect of *androgens*

antianemic drug used to treat *anemia*

antiangiogenesis measures taken to block formation of new blood vessels; used in treatment of malignant neoplastic diseases to cut off blood supply to the tumors

antiarrhythmic drug used to treat cardiac *arrhythmias*

antiasthmatic drug used to treat *asthma*

antibiotic drug used to kill disease-causing *microorganisms* or to prevent their proliferation; see attack sites

antibodies, antimitochondrial see *antimitochondrial antibodies*

antibodies, antinuclear see antinuclear antibodies

antibody *protein* body produced by the *immune system* to defend against *antigens*; abbr. AB

antibody, antineutrophil cytoplasmic *antineutrophil cytoplasmic antibody*

anticholinergic drug used to inhibit *acetylcholine*

anticipate to occur in advance of a given event; to expect or act in expectation

anticipation acting in advance, expecting

anticipatory occurring in advance, in expectation

anticoagulant drug used to inhibit clotting of blood

anticoagulated treated with *anticoagulants*

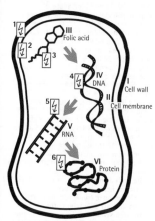

Fig. 23: attack sites of various antibiotics
I Cell wall synthesis II Cell membrane synthesis
III Folic acid synthesis IV DNA synthesis
V RNA synthesis VI Protein synthesis
1 Penicillins, cephalosporins, bacitracin, vancomycin 2 Polymyxins 3 Sulfonamide, trimethoprim
4 Gyrase inhibitors, metronidazole 5 Rifampicin, ethambutol 6 Tetracycline, aminoglycoside, chloramphenicol, erythromycin, clindamycin

anticoagulation therapy physician-ordered treatment with *anticoagulation* drugs, such as *heparin* and/or *coumadin*
anticonvulsive drug used to prevent convulsions
antidementia drug drug used to treat *dementia*
antidepressant psychotropic drug used to treat *depression*
antidiarrheal drug used to treat *diarrhea*
antidiuretic hormone (vasopressin) *hormone* produced in the *hypothalamus* that decreases fluid excretion by the *kidneys*; abbr. ADH

antidote substance that neutralizes poisons or other toxins
antiemetic 1) preventing or relieving vomiting; 2) drug used to prevent vomiting; 3)drug used to treat vomiting
antiepileptic drug used to treat *epilepsy*
antiepileptic drug level lab test to determine subtherapeutic levels in patients taking antiepileptic drugs, e.g. Dilantin; levels should be taken at trough (shortly before the next dose)
antiestrogen drug used to block the effects of *estrogens*
antigen substance recognized by the body as foreign, which triggers an immune response by the *antibodies*
antigen–antibody reaction reaction between an *antigen* and its *antibody*, resulting in formation of an *immune complex*; abbr. AAR
antihelix (anthelix) ridge on the external ear running parallel to the *helix*
antihemophilic globulin A important blood coagulation factor (*Factor VIII*); deficiency leads to *hemophilia A*
antihemophilic globulin B important blood coagulation factor (*Factor IX*); deficiency leads to *hemophilia B*
antihemorrhagic drug used to stop bleeding
antihidrotic drug used to inhibit secretion of sweat
antihistamine drug used to inhibit the release of *histamine* due to *allergies*
antihypertensive drug used to treat high *blood pressure*
antihypotensive drug used to treat low *blood pressure*
antimetabolite drug with metabolisminhibiting properties for treatment of malignant neoplastic diseases
antimitochondrial antibodies *antibodies* produced by the body that attack an *antigen* located on the membrane of the body's own *mitochondria*; abbr. AMA
antimycotic drug used to treat fungal infections
antineoplastic preventing malignant neoplastic diseases

antineutrophil cytoplasmic antibody *antibody* produced by the body that attacks a given *antigen* in the cytoplasm of its own *neutrophil granulocytes*; abbr. ANCA

antinuclear antibodies collective term for antibodies produced by the body that attack a given *antigen* in the nucleus of its own *cells*; abbr. ANA

antioxidant substance that breaks down oxygen products harmful to human cells; this substance can be added to or found in sweet potatoes, carrots, squash, cantaloupe, pumpkin, spinach, apricots, tomatoes, oranges, broccoli, green peppers, strawberries, almonds and artichokes

antipruritic drug used to treat *pruritus (itching)*

antipsoriatic drug used to treat *psoriasis*

antipyretic drug used to treat fever

antirheumatic drug used to treat *rheumatism*

antiscabietic drug used to treat *scabies*

antisepsis measures taken to achieve sterile or near-sterile conditions

antiseptic 1) substance for reduction or elimination of pathogens; 2) pert. to *antisepsis*

antistreptolysin *antibody* that counteracts the toxin *streptolysin* that is formed by *streptococci*; abbr. ASL

antistreptolysin titer laboratory test for the presence of an *acute* or previous *streptococcal* infection; abbr. AST

antithrombosis stockings *medical elastic stockings;* often called TED hose; used post surgery to prevent blood clots in the legs

antitoxin *antibody* produced by the human *organism* that counteracts a biological *toxin*

antitussive drug used to relieve coughing

antivertiginous drug drug used to treat disequilibrium

antrocele collection of fluid in the maxillary sinus

antroscope rigid *endoscope* for *antroscopy*

antroscopy *endoscopy* of a cavity, esp. the *sinuses*

antrum cavity or chamber inside the body e.g. in the stomach, maxilla, etc.

antrum, pyloric portion of the *stomach* before the *pylorus*

anulus fibrosus outer layer of fibrous cartilage around an *intervertebral disk*

anuria decrease of urine volume to less than 200 ml per 24 hours

anus lower opening of the digestive tract

anus praeter *artificial anus*

anvil (incus) one of the three bones in the middle ear

anxiety feeling of dread, apprehension, uneasiness

anxiolytic drug used to relieve anxiety

aorta body's main artery; originates in the left ventricle of the heart

aortic pert. to the aorta

aortic aneurysm *aneurysm* in the wall of the *aorta* more than 56 cm in size; see also *aortic dissection*

aortic arch arch of the *aorta* located slightly above the heart, from which the *brachiocephalic trunk, common carotid artery* and left *subclavian artery* branch off

aortic arch syndrome (Takayasu's arteritis, pulseless disease) *stenosis* or occlusion of at least one of the *arteries* branching off the *aortic arch,* usually caused by *arteritis*

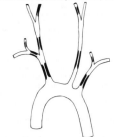

Fig. 24: aortic arch syndrome

aortic bifurcation point where the *aorta* forks near the pelvis

aortic dissection formation of an *aortic aneurysm* due to spontaneous tearing of the intima of the *aorta*

aortic insufficiency (aortic valve insufficiency) inability of the *aortic valve* to close fully, usually acquired in connection with a *rheumatic* disease or *endocarditis*; causes ventricle to enlarge and become ineffective in pumping blood

aortic isthmus stenosis congenital *stenosis* of the *aorta distal* to the branching of the *left subclavian artery*; usually occurs in combination with other defects

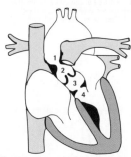

Fig. 27: aortic stenosis (narrowing of left ventricular outflow tract)
1 Supravalvular aortic stenosis 2 Valvular aortic stenosis 3 Membranous subvalvular aortic stenosis 4 Idiopathic hypertrophic subaortic stenosis (IHSS) = hypertrophic obstructive cardiomyopathy

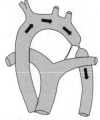

Fig. 25: aortic isthmus stenosis

aortic sclerosis *arteriosclerosis* (hardening) of the *aorta*

aortic stenosis narrowing of the outflow tract of the left ventricle, see Fig. 27

aortic valve heart valve between the left ventricle and *aorta*

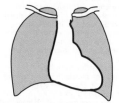

Fig. 28: aortic valve insufficiency (cardiac silhouette)

apathogenic not diseasecausing; opp. *pathogenic*

apathy pathological indifference or lack of interest

ape hand typical hand position in patients with damage to the *median nerve*

apepsia lack of digestive juices

aperiodic irregular

aperture opening, entrance

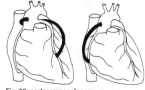

Fig. 26: aortocoronary bypass

aortocoronary bypass see *bypass*; abbr. ACB

apex beat tremor caused by the heart's *contractions*, palpable on the chest at the 5th *ICS* on the *medioclavicular line*

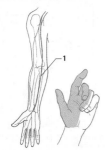

Fig. 29: ape hand
1 Median nerve

apex top of the head, tip, pointed or outermost end

Apgar score system for assessing the general condition of an infant immediately after birth (at 1, 5 and 10 minutes); < 4 points = critical condition; 5-6 = fair; 7-8 = low normal; 9-10 = normal

aphacia (aphakia) absence of the *lens* of the eye

aphagia inability to swallow

aphasia central speech impairment with disorder of production and/or reproduction of speech

apheresis procedure in which blood is taken from a donor, after which WBCs (white blood cells), RBCs and/or plasma are separated out and remainder of components returned to donor

aphonia loss of voice

aphrodisiac drug used to increase sex drive

aphtha rounded ulceration of the oral mucosa; pl. aphthae

apical pert. to the *apex*

apicotomy *resection* of the *apex* of the *dental root*

aplasia lack of development or formation of new *cells* or *tissues*

aplastic adj. of *aplasia*

aplastic anemia (Ehrlich anemia) decrease in *erythrocytes*, *granulocytes* and *thrombocytes* in the blood due to damage to the blood-forming *stem cells* of the *bone marrow*

apnea cessation of breathing

apneic adj. of *apnea*

aponeurosis broad flat sheet of connective tissue

apophyseal avulsion avulsion of a *tendon* at its origin under excessive muscular strain

apophysis projection or process of a bone, usually serving as the attachment point of a muscle or tendon; pl. apophyses

apoplexy *stroke*

appeal an application or proceeding for review by a higher court

appendectomy removal of the vermiform appendix at the *cecum*

appendicitis inflammation of the vermiform *appendix*

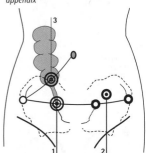

Fig. 30: test points and tender points in appendicitis
1 Lanz's point 2 Pressure point with rebound pain 3 McBurney's point

appendix (vermiformis) (processus vermiformis, vermiform appendix) worm shaped process at the end of the *cecum*

appendix testis small vesicular structure at the upper end of the *testis*

apply to administer

approximate bringing the edges of a wound together to stimulate cell growth in order to promote healing

apraxia inability to perform voluntary purposive ordered movements and/or to use tools despite intact primary *motor* function; main types are a) **ideomotor**: inability to perform normal activities on request; b) **ideational**: inability to handle objects correctly; c) **constructional**: inability to perform activities involving copying a pattern, e.g. drawing

apudoma tumor originating in the *neuroendocrine* system

aqueous humor fluid in the chambers of the eye, produced by the ciliary body

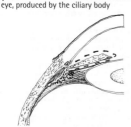

Fig. 31: aqueous humor circulation

arachnodactyly (acromacria) long spidery fingers; typical of *Marfan's syndrome*

arachnoidea arachnoid membrane; part of the brain and spinal cord membranes

arbovirus *virus* that causes *dengue fever*

areflexia absence of reflexes; opp. *hyperreflexia*

arm *brachium*

arm deviation test test in which patient is asked to hold the arms parallel with eyes closed; in *latent pareses*, one arm drops or drifts

aromatase inhibitor drug used to treat malignant neoplastic diseases; inhibits production of *estrogen* outside the ovaries

arrhythmia irregularity, usually in reference to heartbeat; seen in atrial fibrillation

arrhythmic absence of regular rhythm

arteria axillaris (axillary artery) *artery* that connects the *subclavian* with the *brachial artery*

arteria basilaris (basilar artery) *artery* that arises from the *vertebral* arteries and supplies the *brain* in the *cranial base* area

arteria brachialis (brachial artery) artery in the upper arm that arises from the *axillary artery*

arteria carotis ... major *artery* of the head and neck area

arteria carotis communis (common carotid artery) *artery* that arises from the *aorta* and *brachiocephalic trunk*

arteria carotis externa (external carotid artery) external branch of the *common carotid artery*

arteria carotis interna (internal carotid artery) internal branch of the *common carotid artery*

arteria centralis retinae (central retinal artery) *artery* that supplies the *retina*, arising from the *ophthalmic artery*

arteria colica dextra (right colic artery) *artery* that supplies the *ascending colon*, arising from the *superior mesenteric artery*

arteria colica media (middle colic artery) *artery* that supplies the *transverse colon* arising from the *superior mesenteric artery*

arteria colica sinistra (left colic artery) *artery* that supplies the *descending colon*, arising from the *inferior mesenteric artery*

arteria coronaris see *coronary artery*

arteria cystica (cystic artery) *artery* of the gallbladder, arising from the *hepatic artery proper*

arteria dorsalis pedis (dorsal pedis artery) *artery* of the top of the foot, arising from the *anterior tibial artery*

arteria epigastrica inferior (inferior epigastric artery) inferior *artery* of the abdominal wall, arising from the *external iliac artery*

arteria epigastrica superficialis (superficial epigastric artery) superficial *artery* of the abdominal wall, arising from the *femoral artery* and supplying the umbilical region

arteria epigastrica superior (superior epigastric artery) superior *artery* of the abdominal wall arising from the *internal thoracic artery*

arteria facialis (facial artery) *artery* of the facial area, arising from the *internal carotid artery*

arteria femoralis (femoral artery) *artery* of the thigh, arising from the *external iliac artery*, in which the *femoral pulse* is palpable at the groin

arteria gastrica dextra (left gastric artery) right *artery* of the stomach, arising from the *common hepatic artery*

arteria gastrica sinistra (right gastric artery) left *artery* of the stomach arising from the *celiac trunk*

arteria hemorrhoidalis media *arteria rectalis media*

arteria hemorrhoidalis superior *arteria rectalis superior*

arteria hepatica artery of the liver

arteria hepatica communis (common hepatic artery) *artery* of the liver arising from the *celiac trunk*

arteria hepatica propria (hepatic artery proper) *artery* that supplies the left and right lobes of the liver arising from the *common hepatic artery*

arteria hepatica artery of the liver

arteria iliaca communis (common iliac artery) right and left branches starting at the *bifurcation* of the *aorta* in the pelvic area, dividing into the *internal* and *external iliac artery*

arteria iliaca externa (external iliac artery) *artery* that supplies the inguinal area, parts of the iliac region and the abdominal wall, arising from the *common iliac artery*

arteria iliaca interna (internal iliac artery) *artery* arising from the *common iliac artery* that subdivides in the minor pelvis

arteria lienalis (arteria splenica, splenic artery) *artery* of the *spleen*, arising from the *celiac trunk*

arteria lingualis (lingual artery) *artery* of the *tongue*, arising from the *external carotid artery*

arteria maxillaris (maxillary artery) *artery* of the upper jaw, arising from the *external carotid artery*

arteria mesenterica inferior (inferior mesenteric artery) *artery* that supplies mainly the *descending colon*, *sigmoid colon* and rectum, arising from the *aorta*

arteria mesenterica superior (superior mesenteric artery) *artery* that supplies mainly large segments of the large and small intestine, arising from the *aorta*

arteria ophthalmica (ophthalmic artery) *artery* of the eye, arising from the *internal carotid artery*

arteria ovarica (ovarian artery) *artery* that supplies the *ovary* arising from the *uterine artery*

arteria poplitea (popliteal artery) *artery* of the hollow of the knee, arising from the *femoral artery*, in which the popliteal pulse is palpable

arteria profunda femoris (deep femoral artery) *artery* in the thigh, arising from the *femoral artery*

arteria pudenda interna (internal pudendal artery) internal *artery* of the genital area that supplies the *anal* area, *scrotum* or *labia*, and clitoris or *penis*, arising from the *internal iliac artery*

arteria pulmonalis dextra (right pulmonary artery) *artery* of the right *lung*, arising from the *pulmonary trunk*

arteria pulmonalis sinistra (left pulmonary artery) *artery* of the left *lung*, arising from the *pulmonary trunk*

arteria radialis (radial artery) *artery* of the forearm, arising from the brachial artery; *radial pulse* is palpable at the radial end of the forearm

arteria rectalis inferior (inferior rectal artery) *rectal artery*, arising from the *internal pudendal artery*

arteria rectalis media (*arteria hemorrhoidalis media*) middle *rectal artery*, arising from the *internal iliac artery*

arteria rectalis superior (*arteria hemorrhoidalis superior*) superior *rectal artery*, arising from the *inferior mesenteric artery*

arteria renalis (renal *artery*) *artery* of the *kidney*, arising from the *abdominal aorta*

arteria splenica *arteria lienalis*

arteria subclavia (subclavian artery) *artery* of the *clavicle*, flowing into the axillary artery, arising from the *brachiocephalic trunk* on the right and the *aortic arch* on the left

arteria sublingualis (sublingual artery) *artery* beneath the tongue, arising from the *lingual artery*

arteria temporalis media (middle temporal artery) middle *artery* of the *temporal* area, arising from the *superficial temporal artery*

arteria temporalis profunda anterior (anterior deep temporal artery) anterior deep *artery* of the *temporal* area, arising from the *maxillary artery*

arteria temporalis profunda posterior (posterior deep temporal artery) posterior deep *artery* of the *temporal* area, arising from the *maxillary artery*

arteria temporalis superficialis (superficial temporal artery) superficial *artery* of the *temporal* area, arising from the *maxillary artery*

arteria thoracica interna (internal thoracic artery) *artery* of the *thorax*, arising from the *subclavian artery*

arteria thoracica lateralis (lateral thoracic artery) lateral *artery* of the *thorax*, arising from the *axillary artery*

arteria tibialis anterior (anterior tibial artery) anterior *artery* of the shin, arising from the *popliteal artery*

arteria tibialis posterior (posterior tibial artery) posterior *artery* of the shin, arising from the *popliteal artery*

arteria ulnaris (ulnar artery) *artery* of the forearm, arising from the *brachial artery*

arteria uterina (uterine artery) *artery* of the *uterus*, arising from the *internal iliac artery*

arteriae cerebrales (cerebral arteries) collective term for *arteries* that supply the brain

arteriae digitales (digital arteries) collective term for *arteries* of the fingers and toes

arteriae intestinales (intestinal arteries) collective term for *arteries* in the small and large intestine

arteriae umbilicales (umbilical arteries) *arteries* in the *umbilicus* that connect the *fetus* with the *placenta*

arteriae vertebrales (vertebral arteries) arteries of the vertebrae, arising from the *subclavian artery*

arterial pert. to an *artery*; opp. *venous*

arterial catheter *catheter* inserted into an *artery*, usually for direct *invasive blood pressure* measurement; abbr. AC

arterial pulses palpable reflection of heartbeat see palpation points for assessment

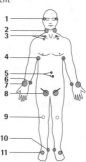

Fig. 32: palpation points for arterial pulses
1 Temporal 2 +C652 Carotid 3 Subclavian 4 Axillary 5 Aorta 6 Ulnar 7 Radial 8 Femoral 9 Popliteal (back of knee) 10 Posterior tibial 11 Dorsalis pedis

arteries, digital *arteriae digitales*

arteries, intestinal *arteriae intestinales*

arteries, umbilical *arteriae umbilicales*

arteries, vertebral *arteriae vertebrales*

arteriitis inflammation of an *artery*

arteriole smallest type of *artery*, continuous with *capillaries*; opp. *venole*

arteriosclerosis (atherosclerosis) chronic metaplastic processes in the *arteries* with hardening, thickening, loss of elasticity and luminal narrowing

arteriovenous fistula (arteriovenous shunt) pathological shunt between the *arterial* and *venous* systems, usually congenital or caused by injury; abbr. AV fistula, AV shunt

arteriovenous hemofiltration (continuous arteriovenous hemofiltration) procedure for removing urinary excreted substances and fluids from blood in *renal failure*; technique a membrane with a specific pore size is inserted between an *artery* and a *vein* and filters out a urinelike liquid by hydrostatic pressure; depending on electrolyte balance status and need this fluid is substituted by an electrolyte solution; abbr. *CAVH*

arteriovenous shunt *arteriovenous fistula*

artery anterior tibial artery *arteria tibialis anterior*

artery blood vessel leading away from the heart; abbr. A.; opp. *vein*

artery, basilar *arteria basilaris*

artery, brachial *arteria brachialis*

artery, carotid *arteria carotis*

artery, central retinal *arteria centralis retinae*

artery, common carotid *arteria carotis communis*

artery, common hepatic *arteria hepatica communis*

artery, common iliac *arteria iliaca communis*

artery, cystic *arteria cystica*

artery, deep femoral *arteria profunda femoris*

artery, dorsal pedis *arteria dorsalis pedis*

artery, external carotid *arteria carotis externa*

artery, external iliac *arteria iliaca externa*

artery, facial *arteria facialis*

artery, femoral *arteria femoralis*

artery, hepatic proper *arteria hepatica propria*

artery, inferior epigastric arteria epigastrica

artery, inferior mesenteric *arteria mesenterica inferior*

artery, inferior rectal *arteria rectalis inferior*

artery, internal carotid *arteria carotis interna*

artery, internal iliac *arteria iliaca interna*

artery, internal pudendal *arteria pudenda interna*

artery, internal thoracic *arteria thoracica interna*

artery, lateral thoracic *arteria thoracica lateralis*

artery, left colic *arteria colica sinistra*

artery, left gastric arteria gastrica sinistra

artery, left pulmonary arteria pulmonalis sinistra

artery, lingual arteria lingualis

artery, maxillary arteria maxillaris

artery, middle colic arteria colica media

artery, middle rectal arteria rectalis media

artery, middle temporal *arteria temporalis media*

artery, ophthalmic *arteria ophthalmica*

artery, ovarian *arteria ovarica*

artery, popliteal *arteria poplitea*

artery, posterior deep temporal *arteria temporalis profunda posterior*

artery, posterior tibial *arteria tibialis posterior*

artery, radial *arteria radialis*

artery, renal *arteria renalis*

artery, right pulmonary *arteria pulmonalis dextra*

artery, right colic *arteria colica dextra*

artery, right gastric arteria gastrica dextra

artery, splenic *arteria lienalis*

artery, subclavian *arteria subclavia*

artery, sublingual *arteria sublingualis*

artery, superior epigastric *arteria epigastrica superior*

artery, superior mesenteric *arteria mesenterica superior*

artery, superficial temporal *arteria temporalis superficialis*

artery, superior rectal *arteria rectalis superior*

artery, supreme thoracic *arteria thoracica suprema*

artery, ulnar *arteria ulnaris*

artery, uterine *arteria uterina*
arthralgia pain in a *joint*; see also *polyarthralgia*
arthrectomy *surgical* removal of a joint
arthritis joint *inflammation*; see also *polyarthritis*
arthrodesis artificial *surgical* immobilization of a joint
arthropathia psoriatica *psoriatic arthritis*
arthropathy nonspecific collective term for joint diseases
arthroscope instrument used to visualize the mechanisms of a joint

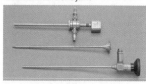

Fig. 33: arthroscope [F]

arthrotomy *surgical* opening of a *joint*
articular pert. to a joint
arthroscopic pert. to *arthroscopy*
arthrosis joint deterioration due to cartilage wear often occurring in the knee (*gonarthrosis*) or hip (*coxarthrosis*)
articulation joint; mobile connection between two bones
artifact abnormal or erratic signal seen on an ECG monitor e.g. due to patient movement during ECG or loose electrode placement
artificial anus (anus praeter) artificially created *anus* in the abdominal wall
asbestosis lung disease caused by asbestos dust
ascendens rising, climbing; opp. *descendens*
ascending rising, climbing; opp. *descending*
asceticism strict, austere lifestyle
ascites accumulation of fluid in the abdominal cavity, e.g. due to *cirrhosis* of the liver

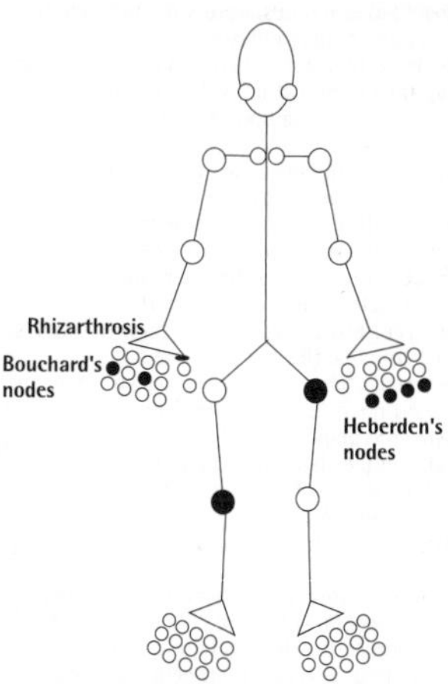

Rhizarthrosis
Bouchard's nodes
Heberden's nodes

Fig. 34: joints affected by arthrosis

ascorbic acid (vitamin C) water-soluble *vitamin* with an important role in many metabolic processes; vitamin C deficiency can lead to *scurvy*, among other things
asepsis sterile conditions
aseptic adj. of *asepsis*
aseptic fever fever caused by reabsorption of *tissue* debris
asexual without sex
aspergilloma typical *granulomas* caused by *Aspergillus*
aspergillosis *mycosis* caused by *Aspergillus*, which can affect the skin, mucosa, ears and lungs, among others; *aspergilloma* is also typical of these infections
Aspergillus genus of fungi that causes *aspergillosis*
aspermia lack of *sperm* production or ejaculate; see also *azoospermia*

asphyxia severe respiratory disturbance that can endanger cardiovascular function

aspirate to suction fluid or air with a syringe

aspiration inhalation of foreign substances (e.g. vomit); suction of fluid or air with a syringe

aspiration pneumonia form of *pneumonia* caused by *aspiration*

assimilation uptake and conversion of nutrients into body substance

association coming together, uniting, connection; opp. *dissociation*

astereognosis inability to recognize objects by touch with the eyes closed

asterixis (flapping tremor) jerking tremor in the fingers, often due to liver disease

asthenic debilitated

astheno(zoo)spermia *ejaculate* with less than 50% motile *sperm* as measured by *spermiogram*

asthma severe respiratory distress occurring in the form of attacks; chronic *inflammation* of the airways, which leads to *bronchial* hypersensitivity and to attacks of respiratory distress with difficulty in exhaling; also called bronchial asthma

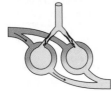

Fig. 35: bronchial asthma

asthmatic pert. to *asthma*

astigmatism defective curvature of the *cornea*, leading to distorted images of objects viewed

astringe to constrict or contract

astringent agent causing contraction of *tissues*, e.g. to arrest bleeding; having astringent qualities

astrocytoma tumor originating in the supporting *cells* of the *central nervous system*

Astrup method laboratory assessment for measuring acid–base balance; pH and pCO_2 readings are calculated using a grid, see Fig. 37

asymmetrical lacking symmetry; opp. *symmetrical*

asymptomatic showing no signs of disease; opp. *symptomatic*

asystole complete cardiac standstill with a flat *electrocardiogram*

asystolic adj. of *asystole*

ataxia impaired coordination in voluntary movements, manifested by inability to judge distances in purposive movements, with disordered interaction of individual muscles and of rapid sequences of *antagonistic* movements e.g. in diseases affecting the *cerebellum*

atelectasis collapse of a portion of the lung due to loss of air in the *alveoli*

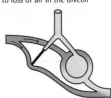

Fig. 36: atelectasis

atheroma (epidermoid cyst, sebaceous cyst) fatty cyst in the skin due to obstruction of a sebaceous gland

atherosclerosis *arteriosclerosis*

athetosis involuntary slow twisting or undulating movements of the *extremities*, mainly *distal*, e.g. in *neurological* diseases

athymhormia lack of drive or motivation

atlas the first cervical vertebra, supporting the skull

atony lack of muscle tone, limpness

atopic dermatitis/eczema (neurodermatitis) itchy, red skin; can be caused by emotional stress

atopy type I *allergic* reaction; mediated by *IgE*

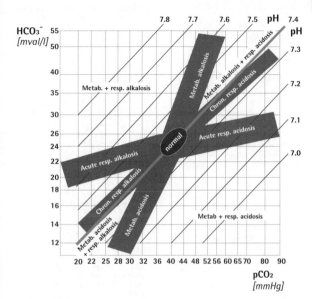

Fig. 37: astrup method

atresia absence or closure of a natural body orifice, e.g. the *anus*

atrial pert. to the atrium

atrial fibrillation atrial *dysrhythmia* visible in an *ECG* that leads to continuous arrhythmia; usually caused by atrial *reentry* with an atrial *frequency* of 230 to 380 beats per minute usually with normal heart rate; identifiable by fine atrial fibrillation waves with no identifiable *P waves* in the ECG, see Fig. 38

atrial flutter atrial *dysrhythmia* visible in an *ECG* marked by an atrial *frequency* of 290 to 310 beats per minute usually with normal heart rate; usually caused by atrial *reentry*, identifiable by the sawtooth deflections in the ECG, see Fig. 39

atrial septal defect congenital heart defect in which an opening between the right and left atria leads to a left-to-right shunt; abbr. ASD, see Fig. 40

atrial veins *veins* that arise from an atrium of the *heart*

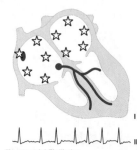

Fig. 38: atrial fibrillation
1 Schematic 2 ECG

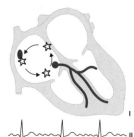

Fig. 39: atrial flutter
1 Schematic 2 ECG

atrioventricular pert. to the area between the *atrium* and *ventricle* of the heart

atrioventricular block conduction defect between the atrium and ventricle of the heart, visible in an *ECG*; abbr. *AV block*; see also *1st degree AV block, 2nd degree AV block, 3rd degree AV block*

atrioventricular node structure located between the atrium and the ventricles that conducts impulses from the *sinus node* and carries them from the atrium to the ventricles; takes over impulse generation if sinus node fails; see also *excitation and conduction system*; abbr. *AV node*

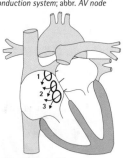

Fig. 40: atrial septal defect
1 Ostium primum defect 2 Ostium secundum defect 3 Sinus venosus defect

atrioventricular veins *veins* that arise from the area between the atrium and ventricle

atrium upper chamber of the heart

atrophic adj. of *atrophy*; opp. *hypertrophic*

atrophy shrinkage or wasting of *tissue* or *organs*; opp. *hypertrophy*

attack sudden onset or episode of illness or symptoms

audimutitas mutism lasting beyond the 3rd year of age despite normal ability to hear, intact *peripheral* speech organs and normal intelligence

audiometer device used to test hearing

auditory pert. to hearing

auditory tube sometimes called the *eustachian tube;* extends from middle ear to nasopharynx

Auer bodies (Auer rods) cell type associated with *acute myelogenous leukemia* with thin rod-shaped *leukocyte* inclusions

augment to enlarge

augmentation enlargement

augmented enlarged

aura *acoustic* or *optical* sensations that precede an *epileptic seizure*

auricular pert. to the ear

auris *ear*

auscult(ate) to examine by *auscultation*

auscultation examination by listening to body sounds with a *stethoscope*

autism exclusion of the outside world due to preoccupation with one's own thoughts

autoantibody *antibody* to autologous substances or *tissues*

autoclave 1) apparatus for *sterilization* of thermostable objects with steam pressure; 2) to sterilize using an autoclave

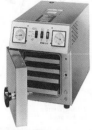

Fig. 41: autoclave [H]

autogenic training concentrated self-relaxation technique that works via inner visualization

autograft *autogeneic graft*

autoimmune disorder condition caused by the formation of *autoantibodies* directed against the body's own constituents or *tissues*

autoimmune hemolytic anemia *anemia* due to *hemolysis*; caused by *IgG-type autoantibodies*

autologous (homologous) belonging to or originating with the same individual; opp. *heterologous*

autologous graft (autograft) *transplantation* of tissue from one site to another in the same person, e.g. a skin graft; *autogeneic graft*

autologous stem cell transplant/rescue procedure where patient's own stem cells from the bone marrow or peripheral blood are collected, stored and reinfused following high-dose chemotherapy and/or radiation therapy; sometimes referred to as stem cell rescue because the patient's stem cells "rescue" the patient from the effects of the cancer therapy

autolysis self destruction

automutilation self-injuring behavior

autonomic not directed voluntarily, independent

autonomic nervous system part of the nervous system not directed voluntarily; directs body functions like circulation, digestion, sweating, etc.; opp. *motor nervous system*

autopsy (postmortem examination) 1) dissection of a cadaver; 2) to perform an autopsy

auxiliary supplemental, providing back-up

auxiliary transplantation *transplantation* performed to support a weakened *organ*; see also *substitutive transplantation*

AV (atrioventricular) blocks electrical conduction abnormalitiesdisturbances involving the AV node; types include: a) **1s- degree AV block:** AV block visible in an ECG with a PQ interval prolonged to more than 0.2 seconds; b) **2nd-degree AV block:** AV block visible in an ECG with periodic prolongation of the PQ interval to the point that ventricular action is lost (Wenckebach type) or an intermittent AV block in which only every n^{th} P wave is conducted to the ventricles (Mobitz type); c) **3rd-degree AV block** (complete AV block)**:** visible in an ECG with P waves that are regular but are not conducted to the ventricles, and escape rhythm from the AV node or the ventricles, see Fig. 42

AV fistula abnormal passageway between an artery and a vein, see Fig.43

AV node abbr. *atrioventricular node*

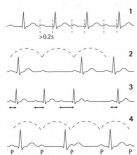

Fig. 42: AV block
1 1st-degree AV block **2** 2nd-degree AV block
(Mobitz type) **3** 2nd-degree AV block (Wenckebach
type) **4** 3rd-degree AV block

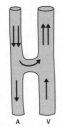

Fig. 43: AV fistula

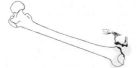

Fig. 44: avulsion fracture

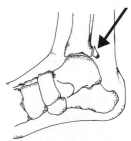

**Fig. 45: avulsion fracture
of Volkmann's triangle**

axial 1) pert. to the second cervical vertebra;
2) pert. to any body organ or joint axis
axilla armpit
axillaris, A. *arteria axillaris*
axillaris, N. *axillary nerve*
axillaris, V. *vena axillaris*
axillary pert. to the *axilla*
axillary artery *arteria axillaris*
axillary line imaginary line for orientation
on the lateral surface of the thorax;
anterior axillary line (A) runs along the
prolongation of the anterior border of the
deltoid muscle; posterior axillary line (B)
runs along the prolongation of the
posterior border of the deltoid muscle
axillary nerve nerve arising from the
brachial plexus that innervates the deltoid
muscle

avascular necrosis of the femoral head
osteonecrosis of the head of the *femur,*
associated with *ischemia* from various
causes
avitaminosis disease caused by *vitamin*
deficiency
avulsion fracture *fracture* caused by
traction with tearing away of a bone
fragment

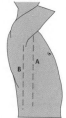

Fig. 46: axillary line

axillary vein *vena axillaris*
axiom fundamental principle not requiring proof
axis 1) the second cervical vertebra;
2) center line of a body *organ* or joint
axis dens *dens axis*
axon extended process of a nerve cell through which the impulses are conducted
azoospermia absence of *sperm* in the semen
azotemia increased amounts of nitrogen in the urine; see *uremia*
azygos, V. *vena azygos*

B

Babinski's reflex *reflex* in which stimulation of the lateral aspect of the sole of the foot results in slow *dorsiflexion* of the great toe and spreading of the other toes; *physiological reflex* up to age 2, thereafter *pathological*
BAC abbr. blood alcohol concentration
bacillary dysentery *shigellosis*
bacillus usually motile rod-shaped *gram-positive microorganism* that can form *spores*
Bacillus anthracis type of *bacillus* that forms extremely resistant *spores* and causes *anthrax*

Backhaus towel clamp (towel clamp) sharp clamp used during *surgery* for fastening or fixation

Fig. 47: Backhaus towel clamp [A]

bacteri– combining form: bacteria
bacteria pl. of *bacterium*
bacterial pert. to *bacteria*
bacteremia presence of *bacteria* in the blood
bactericide *bacteria*-killing substance
bacteriological pert. to *bacteriology*
bacteriology study of *bacteria*
bacteriostatic inhibiting the growth and proliferation of *bacteria*
bacterium unicellular *microorganism* lacking a *nucleus* occurring in numerous forms, many of which can cause *infectious diseases* in humans; pl. bacteria
bacteriuria presence of *bacteria* in the urine
bag of waters *amniotic sac*
Baker's cyst *cyst* appearing in the popliteal space; usually occurs with *chronic inflammation* of the knee joint
BAL abbr. blood alcohol level; bronchoalveolar lavage
balan(o)– combining form: glans
balanitis *inflammation* of the *glans penis*, usually associated with inflammation of the *foreskin*
ballism (paralysis agitans) involuntary violent jerking movements of the *extremities*, mainly from *vascular* causes
balloon angioplasty (percutaneous transluminal angioplasty) dilatation of blood vessels by threading a *balloon catheter* through the vascular system, which is then inflated at the stenosis point in order to widen it; abbr. PTA
balloon catheter *catheter* with an inflatable balloon at one end, e.g. *indwelling catheter*
balneology healing with medicinal baths

B

balneotherapeutic drug used in preparation of a medicinal bath

balsam resinous plant-based remedy for topical application

Band Aid® brand name for an *adhesive bandage*

bandage strip of gauze or other material used to stop bleeding, as a supportive binding, etc.

bandage scissors (Lister scissors) scissors with blunt tips to prevent injury to tissue (skin) when cutting through bandages

Bandl's ring ring-shaped indentation forming the boundary between the *uterine corpus* and *cervix*

Bang's disease *brucellosis* caused by *Brucella abortus* marked by fluctuating fever *hepatosplenomegaly* and organ involvement with *granuloma* formation

Bárány's (pointing) test pointing test to assess coordination and function of the cerebellum

barbiturate drug used as a sedative

barium swallow *radiography* of the *esophagus* using a *contrast medium*

baroreceptors *receptors* that react to pressure or tension; these sensory nerves are found in the atrial walls of the heart and carotid sinus, and are affected by drugs

barotrauma *trauma* caused by sudden change in barometric pressure, e.g. *caisson disease*

Bartholin's glands glands located on either side of the *vagina* that secrete mucus upon sexual stimulation

bartholinitis inflammation of *Bartholin's glands*, which can lead to *abscess* formation

bas(i)– combining form: base, foundation

basal pert. to a base or foundation

basal cell carcinoma *basalioma*

basal ganglia cluster of *neurons* that play an important part in movement

basal temperature body temperature measured before getting up in the morning; used to calculate when *ovulation* occurs

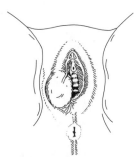

Fig. 48: bartholinitis

basalioma (basal cell carcinoma) malignant tumor originating in the *basal cells* of the epidermis

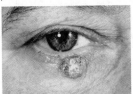

Fig. 49: basalioma on lower lid

base (lye, alkali) chemical substance that reacts with *acid* in water and forms salts

base excess in *blood gas analysis*, base excess is a calculated value that specifies the amount of base or acid required to restore a normal blood *pH* value; normal value is – 2 to + 2; abbr. BE; formula: BE = SBC – 24

Basedow's disease (*Graves' disease*) *autoimmune* disease of the *thyroid* gland associated with *hyperthyroidism*; can lead to *goiter* and *exophthalmos*

basic life cardiac support basic life-saving measures taken in the context of resuscitation, e.g. *chest compressions and rebreathing; healthcare personnel must earn certification* every 2 years; abbr. BCLS; opp. *advanced cardiac life support*

basilar bone cranial base, consisting of the *occipital* and *sphenoid bones*

basilaris, A. *arteria basilaris*

basilic vein *vein* on the *ulnar* side of the forearm that empties into the *axillary vein*

basilica, V. *vena basilica*

basophilic 1) staining readily with basic dyes; 2) consisting of structures or *cells* with this property

bathmotropic influencing the cardiac excitation threshold; positive bathmotropic: increasing excitability by decreasing the excitation threshold; negative bathmotropic: decreasing excitability by increasing the excitation threshold; cf. *inotropic, dromotropic, chronotropic*

Bauhin's valve *ileocecal valve*

bayonet deformity *radial* deviation of the hand e.g. in *distal fracture* of the radius

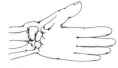

Fig. 50: bayonet deformity

B-cell lymphoma (non-Hodgkins lymphoma) group of B or T lymphocytes, usually malignant

bead fracture impaction *fracture* seen in children, with impaction of the cortical substance

Bechterew's disease (ankylosing spondylitis) *chronic inflammatory* disease of the axial skeleton, usually with involvement of the limb joints and tendon insertions

beef tapeworm (Taenia saginata) *parasite* measuring 4 to 30 feet in length that can infest the human intestine

Bellocq's tamponade *packing* for the posterior nares, most often to arrest bleeding in *epistaxis*

Bell's palsy one-sided facial paralysis; onset is sudden; involves upper and lower part of the face

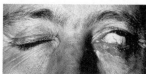

Fig. 51: Bell's phenomenon

Bence–Jones proteinuria *pathological* excretion of light chains of immunoglobulins, usually occurring in *plasmacytoma*

bending fracture *fracture* caused by direct or indirect-force traction; leads to a break on the *convex* side, and pressure of the bone on the *concave* side leads to formation of a wedge-shaped gap

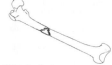

Fig. 52: bending fracture

benign harmless; opp. *malignant*

benign prostatic hypertrophy (benign prostatic hyperplasia) benign enlargement of the *prostate gland*, usually causing constriction of the *urethra*; abbr. BPH

Bennett fracture *fracture* occurring in the midhand area (1st *metacarpal bone*) with joint involvement; see also *Winterstein fracture, Rolando fracture*

benzodiazepine anti-anxiety drug

beriberi disease caused by a lack of *vitamin B_1*, characterized by myocardial insufficiency, nerve paralysis, mental impairments and muscle atrophy

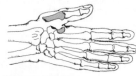

Fig. 53: Bennett fracture

Berlin's edema swelling of the *retina* following blunt-force trauma

beta-adrenergic receptor receptor in the sympathetic nervous system that reacts to epinephrine, et al.

beta-adrenergics drugs that inhibit the sympathetic nervous system; used to treat high blood pressure, heart attacks, angina, dysrhythmias and glaucoma

beta-blockers drugs that block the effects of beta-adrenergic drugs

beta-carotene *provitamin* of vitamin A, found in fruits and vegetables; supplements should not be used by smokers

Beta interferons drugs that reduce frequency, severity and duration of exacerbations in *multiple sclerosis, e.g.*

betatron apparatus used in irradiation of tumors

bezoar solid bolus composed of swallowed hairs

bi– combining form two

biceps two-headed upper arm muscle that raises the upper arm and enables flexion and external rotation of the arm; innerv.: *musculocutaneous nerve*; see also *triceps*

biceps (tendon) reflex monosynaptic *reflex* in which percussion against the *biceps* tendon triggers flexion of the forearm; mapping: see C5-C6 *dermatome*

biceps brachii, M. *biceps*

biceps femoris, M. *(musculus biceps femoris) biceps muscle of the thigh*

biceps muscle of the thigh two-headed thigh muscle that flexes the knee and extends the hip joint; innervation: *tibial* and *peroneal nerve*

biconcave *concave* on both sides, e.g. an optical lens; opp. *biconvex*

biconvex convex on both sides, e.g. an optical lens; opp. *biconcave*

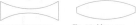

Fig. 54: biconcave   Fig. 55: biconvex

bicuspid valve (mitral valve) two-cusp valve between the left atrium and left ventricle

Biermer's disease *pernicious anemia; see anemias*

bifurcation forking e.g. the branching of the trachea into two main *bronchi carina tracheae* or of the *aorta* in the pelvic region

bigeminy cardiac *dysrhythmia* visible in an *ECG* in which every normal heartbeat is followed by a *ventricular extrasystole*; bigeminy is usually palpable as a doubled pulse

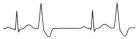

Fig. 56: bigeminus

bilateral on both sides; opp. *unilateral*

bilateral periorbital hematoma (black eye) bilateral *hematoma* of the upper and lower eyelids; classic sign of *fracture* of the *cranial base*; see also *monocular periorbital hematoma*

bile fluid produced by the *liver*, which gets its green color from *biliverdin*; it is secreted into the *duodenum* either directly or after storage and thickening in the *gallbladder*; aids in the digestion of *fats* in the *intestine*

bilharziasis *schistosomiasis*

bili– combining form: bile

biliary pert. to *bile*

biliary atresia disorder of the flow of bile from the liver due to congenital absence or malformation of the bile ducts

biliary colic *colic* originating in the *gallbladder*, usually due to incarcerated gallstones

bilirubin yellowish *bile* pigment that is produced primarily in the liver through the breakdown of *hemoglobin*; it flows into the intestine along with *bile*; increased bilirubin in the blood leads to *icterus*

bilirubin encephalopathy see *kernicterus*

bilirubinemia (hyperbilirubinemia) increased *bilirubin* in the blood, e.g. due to liver disease

bilirubinuria increased *bilirubin* in the urine, which can give it a "beer-brown" color

bilis *gallbladder*

biliverdin greenish *bile* pigment produced by breakdown of *hemoglobin*

Billroth operation *surgery* to shorten the stomach via *anastomosis* of the pylorus to the *duodenum* (Billroth I or gastroduodenostomy) or to the *jejunum* (Billroth II or gastrojejunostomy)

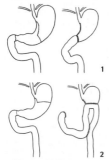

Fig. 57: Billroth operation
1 Billroth I 2 Billroth II

bimanual with both hands

Binswanger's dementia (vascular dementia, subcortical arteriosclerotic encephalopathy, multiinfarct dementia) *dementia* resulting from *ischemic* brain damage

bio- combining form: life

biochemistry study of the chemical processes in living *organisms*

biology study of life processes

biopsy 1) tissue sample taken for examination; 2) to take a biopsy

bios life

Biot's breathing pathological breathing pattern marked by periods of *apnea*; caused by injuries and/or diseases of the brain or an increase in *intracranial* pressure

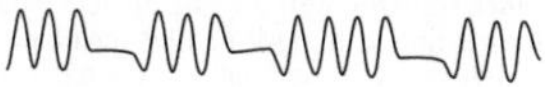

Fig. 58: Biot's breathing

biotin (vitamin H) water-soluble *vitamin* with an important role in hair and skin formation; lack of vitamin H can lead to hair loss and skin *inflammations*, et al.

bipolar having two poles

birth *partus*

birth control pill *oral contraceptive*

birthmark *nevus*

bite wound combination of *puncture*, *crushing* and *laceration wound* from animal or human teeth

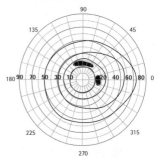

Fig. 59: Bjerrum's sign in glaucoma

Bjerrum's sign (Bjerrum's scotoma) typical *visual field* deficit in *glaucoma*; sickle-shaped blind spot originating on the nasal side

BKA abbr. below-the-knee amputation

black lung *silicosis;* found in coal miners
blackwater fever complication of *malaria* marked by *hemolysis* and *hemoglobinuria*
bladder bilharziasis see *schistosomiasis*
bladder catheter *urinary catheter* inserted into the bladder via the urethra
bladder scanning instrument used to detect residual urine in the bladder
Blalock–Taussig method *surgical* technique for treating *tetralogy of Fallot*, including *anastomosis* of the *pulmonary artery* and *subclavian artery*

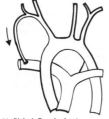

Fig. 60: Blalock–Taussig shunt

-blast, blast- combining form: immature cell
blastocyst (blastodermic vesicle) stage of embryonic development following the morula

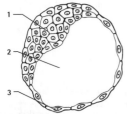

Fig. 61: blastocyst
1 Embryoblast (inner cells) 2 Blastocyst cavity
3 Trophoblast (outer cells)

bleaching dental procedure for whitening the teeth
bleeder slang expression for person suffering from *hemophilia*
bleeding time initial exploratory blood coagulation test measuring the length of time that bleeding continues after an approx. 3-mm deep puncture is made in the earlobe; normal range: 2 to 5 minutes
blenn(o)- combining form: mucus
blennorrhea discharge from a mucous membrane, e.g. due to infection in the *conjunctiva*
blephar(o)- combining form: eyelid
blepharitis *inflammation* of the eyelid
blepharon (palpebra) *eyelid*
blepharorrhaphy (tarsorrhaphy) temporary closure of the eyelid with a *suture*
blepharospasm twitching of the eyelid
blind spot *optic papilla*
block anesthesia (conduction anesthesia, neural anesthesia) local anesthesia achieved by *injection* of a *local anesthetic* in the immediate vicinity of the *nerves* supplying the surgical site; results in *sensory* and *motor nerve* conduction block; e.g. *spinal anesthesia, epidural anesthesia* or *Oberst's method*
blood chemistries laboratory tests
blood count measurement of the number, type and composition of blood *cells;* abbr. BC
blood culture incubation of pathogens in a blood sample using a growth medium for diagnosis of *infectious diseases*
blood gas analysis test that measures the amounts of gases dissolved in arterial blood (pO_2, pCO_2, SO_2) as well as important acid-base balance values (*pH* value, *standard bicarbonate base excess*); abbr. BGA
blood glucose profile series of blood sugar measurements taken throughout the day to detect deviations from the normal range
blood group surface properties of *erythrocytes* that are determined along with the *Rh factor* prior to a *transfusion;* according to the presence or absence of the *antigens* A and B on the erythrocytes, the main blood groups A, B, AB and O are

distinguished; A = antigen A, B = antigen B, AB = A + B, O = neither A nor B

blood level concentration of a given substance in the blood, e.g. a drug

blood plasma *plasma*

blood pressure measurable pressure in the *arteries* dependent on blood volume, cardiac output and vascular resistance; abbr. RR, BP

blood sedimentation rate (erythrocyte sedimentation rate) rate at which blood settles in the bottom of a test tube filled with saline; used to monitor severity of inflammation, infection and/or cancer; abbr. ESR, BSR

blood serum watery portion of blood remaining after coagulation; contains antibodies

blood sludge clumping of *erythrocytes* due to changes in the viscosity of the blood

blood substitute plasma dextran solution used in place of a blood transfusion

blood sugar (blood glucose) *glucose* (sugar) present in the blood

blood–brain barrier barrier between the bloodstream and the brain tissues, which protects the *nerve cells* from harmful substances

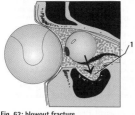

Fig. 62: blowout fracture
1 Herniation of orbital fat and part of the inf. rectus muscle into the fissure

blowout fracture *fracture* of the floor of the *orbit* with displacement of the *eyeball*, usually due to a blow to the eye

BLS abbr. *basic life support*

Blumberg's sign (rebound tenderness) pain occurring on release of pressure on the left lower abdomen, e.g. due to *appendicitis*

BMI abbr. *body mass index*

BMT abbr. *bone marrow transplant*

Bobath's method form of physical therapy exercise for facilitation of movements, e.g. for patients with *spasticity*

body corpus, soma

body mass index index for classifying body weight; abbr. BMI; formula: (body weight in kilograms) ÷ (height in meters)^2; optimal values based on age 19-24 years = BMI19-24; 20-34 years = BMI 20-25; 35-44 years = BMI 21-26; 45-54 years = BMI 22-27; 55-64 years = BMI 23-28; > 65 years = BMI 24-29

body surface area calculated surface area of the body expressed in square meters; formula: (weight in kg)^{0425} x (height in cm)^{0725} x 139.32; abbr. BSA

Boeck's sarcoid *sarcoidosis*

Boerhaave syndrome long tear in the *esophagus* with *rupture* of all wall layers due to violent vomiting and previous damage to the mucosa, e.g. from alcohol consumption

Böhler cast circumferential lower-arm cast enclosing the metacarpophalangeal joints of the thumb and index finger, e.g. for wrist fracture

Bolivian hemorrhagic fever (Machupo) *hemorrhagic fever* caused by the Machupo virus

bolus 1) mass of chewed food; 2) large foreign object

bolus death death by asphyxiation caused by obstruction of the airways by a foreign body

bolus injection rapid injection of the total amount or a major part of a drug dose

bone conduction conduction of sound waves through bone; tested as part of the *Rinne test* or *Weber test*

bone curette spoon-shaped *surgical* instrument with sharp edges, used for scraping bone or tissue

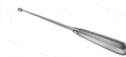

Fig. 63: bone curette [A]

bone marrow tissue inside the bones where blood cells are formed

bone marrow aspiration removal of bone marrow using a needle

bone marrow transplant transfer of donated *bone marrow* into a recipient following high-dose chemo- and/or radiotherapy; abbr. BMT

bone phosphatase bone-specific isoform of *alkaline phosphatase*

bone scan a diagnostic test for diagnosing infection and/or spinal metastasis

booster effect increase in immune protection against *infections*, acquired through an additional dose of a vaccine

borderline hypertension see *hypertension*

borderline personality disorder (borderline syndrome) *psychic* disorder marked by multiple *neurotic* and *near-psychotic symptoms* (borderline between *schizophrenia* and *neurosis*)

borderline syndrome *borderline personality disorder*

Bordetella genus of nonmotile short rod-shaped *gram-negative bacteria*

Bordetella pertussis *bacterium* of the genus *Bordetella* that can cause *pertussis*

Borrelia genus of motile spiral *bacteria* that can cause *infectious diseases*, such as *relapsing fevers* or *Lyme disease*

borreliosis collective term for *infectious diseases* caused by *Borrelias*, e.g. *relapsing fevers* or *Lyme disease*

Borrmann's classification classification system for advanced *gastric carcinomas*: 1) *polypoid*; 2) *ulcerating*; 3) *ulcerating-infiltrating*; 4) *diffuse infiltrating*

Botalli's duct (ductus Botalli, ductus arteriosus) *physiological fetal shunt* between the *aortic arch* and the *pulmonary artery trunk*, occurring while the lungs are still underdeveloped

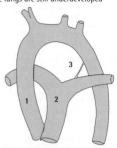

Fig. 64: Botalli's duct
1 Aorta 2 Pulmonary trunk 3 Ligamentum arteriosum (vestige of Botalli's duct)

Botox (botulinum toxin type A) potent neurotoxin produced by *Clostridium botulinum*, a bacteria that causes food poisoning (botulism); safely used to treat torticollis

bottle sign sign of *paresis* of the *musculus abductor pollicis brevis*; when patient grasps a bottle, no fold appears in the skin between the thumb and forefinger due to insufficient abduction of the thumb

botulin (botulinum toxin) neurotoxin produced by *Clostridium botulinum* in *anaerobic* conditions (e.g. in improperly processed canned foods), which can lead to *botulism*

botulism form of food poisoning leading to paralysis, caused by the neurotoxin *botulin*

bougienage stretching of a constricted opening using a bougie

Boutonnière deformity classic malposition of the middle finger due to extensor tendon rupture or *rheumatoid arthritis*, see Fig. 66

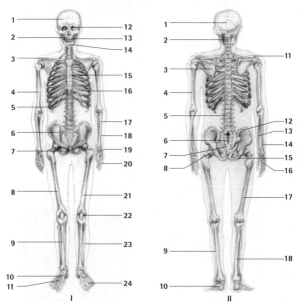

Fig. 65: bones
I Human skeleton, anterior view 1 Skull (cranium) **2** Upper jaw (maxilla) **3** Collarbone (clavicle)
4 Upper arm (humerus) **5** Ribs (costae) **6** Pelvis **7** Pubic bone **8** Thighbone (femur) **9** Shin (tibia)
10 Ankle (tarsals) **11** Foot (metatarsals) **12** Eye socket (orbit) **13** Teeth (dentes) **14** Lower jaw (mandible)
15 Breastbone (sternum) **16** Rib (costa) **17** Forearm (ulna) **18** Forearm (radius) **19** Wrist (carpals)
20 Fingers (phalanges) **21** General: Bones (ossa) **22** Kneecap (patella) **23** Calf (fibula) **24** Toes (phalanges)
I Human skeleton, posterior view 1 Skull (occiput) **2** Neck (cervical vertebrae) **3** Shoulder blade (scapula)
4 Upper arm (humerus) **5** Spinal column (vertebrae) **6** Sacrum **7** Tailbone (coccyx) **8** Greater trochanter
9 Calf (fibula) **10** Heelbone (calcaneus) **11** Collarbone (clavicle) **12** Ilium **13** Forearm (radius)
14 Forearm (ulna) **15** Ischium **16** Hand (metacarpals) **17** Thighbone (femur) **18** Shin (tibia)

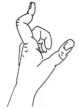

Fig. 66: boutonnière deformity

bowing fracture bending fracture occurring in children, with small fissures in the cortical substance

bowleg *genu varum*

brachi– combining form arm

brachial pert. to the arm

brachial muscle muscle between the *humerus* and *ulna* that flexes the elbow joint; innervation: *musculocutaneous nerve*

brachial plexus nerve *plexus* comprising the branches of the 5th–8th cervical nerves and the 1st thoracic nerve, which contains the *nervus axillaris, nervus musculocutaneus, nervus radialis, nervus thoracicus longus* and *nervus thoracodorsalis*, et al.

brachialis, A. *arteria brachialis*

brachialis, M. *musculus brachialis*

brachiocephalic trunk (truncus brachiocephalicus) common trunk of the right *subclavian* and *carotid arteries,* arising from the *aortic arch*

brachiocephalic vein (vena anonyma) common branch from the *internal jugular* and *subclavian veins,* joining the *superior vena cava*

brachiocephalica, V. *vena brachiocephalica*

brachioradial muscle upper arm muscle that flexes the forearm at the elbow; innervation: *radial nerve*

brachioradialis, M. *musculus brachioradialis*

brachium upper arm

Bracht's maneuver obstetrical maneuver for *vaginal* delivery of a *breech presentation*

brachy– combining form: short, small

brachytherapy radiation treatment at close range for treatment of neoplastic diseases

Braden's scale assessment tool to determine a patient's risk for a pressure ulcer

brady– combining form: slow, sluggish

bradycardia *dysrhythmia* with a heart rate below 60 bpm; opp. *tachycardia*

bradykinesia general slowness of movements

bradypnea respiratory rate slowed down to less then 10 breaths per minute in adults; usually caused by disorders of the *CNS*, increased *intracranial pressure*, drugs or medications; opp. *tachypnea*

brain cerebrum, encephalon, enkephalos

brain attack stroke

brain death irreversible brain damage, but cardiac and respiratory function are preserved; criteria and protocol for diagnosis vary by institution and state laws

brain edema (cerebral edema) *edematous* swelling of the brain, e.g. after a *trauma* or due to *ischemia*; leads to increased *intracranial pressure* as a rule

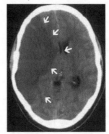

Fig. 67: brain edema (CT)

brain scan identifies brain hemorrhage

brain stem section of the brain consisting of the *mesencephalon* (midbrain), *pons* and *medulla oblongata*; sends information to and receives information from spinal and peripheral nerves; controls respiration and heart rhythm

breakbone fever *dengue fever* caused by one of the flaviviruses; transmitted to humans by the bite of the Aedes aegypti mosquito

breastbone *sternum*

breath sounds obtained by auscultation of anterior and posterior chest

breech presentation (pelvic presentation) abnormal position of the fetus during birth in which the pelvis precedes the head

brevis short; noun: brevity

bridge permanent denture for bridging a gap created by missing teeth

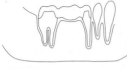

Fig. 68: bridge

broad spectrum antibiotic *antibiotic* that is effective against multiple types of *bacteria*

Broca's area region of the brain located in the frontal lobe of the left hemisphere; important for speech

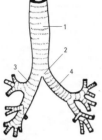

Fig. 69: bronchi
1 Trachea 2 Bifurcation 3 Right primary bronchus 4 Left primary bronchus

bronchi main branches of the *trachea* extending from its *bifurcation*; sing. bronchus

bronchial pert. to the *bronchi*

bronchial asthma see *asthma*

bronchial carcinoma malignant tumor of the *bronchi*

bronchiectasis pathological saclike or cylindrical dilation of a *bronchus*

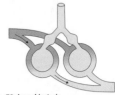

Fig. 70: bronchiectasis

bronchiolitis (obliterans) acute *inflammation* of the smallest *bronchi*

bronchitis *acute* or *chronic inflammation* of the *bronchial* mucosa

bronchoalveolar lavage irrigation of the lungs using a *bronchoscope*; the lavage fluid can be used for microbiological tests; abbr. BAL

bronchodilator drug used to dilate the *bronchi*

bronchophony increase in vocal resonance due to solidified lung tissue, audible on *auscultation*

bronchopneumonia common in the elderly; one or more lobes of the lungs are inflamed

bronchoscope rigid or flexible *endoscope* for *bronchoscopy*

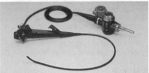

Fig. 71: flexible bronchoscope [I]

bronchoscopic pert. to *bronchoscopy*

bronchoscopy involves the use of a flexible endoscope to examine the larynx, trachea and bronchial tree

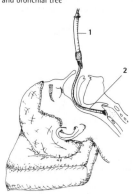

Fig. 72: bronchoscopic intubation
1 Tube 2 Bronchoscope

bronchosecretolytic drug used to loosen mucus in the *bronchi*

bronchospasm spasmodic contraction of the *bronchial* muscles, e.g. in *bronchial asthma*

bronchospasmolytic agent drug used to relieve *bronchospasm*

bronchus sing. of *bronchi*

Brown–Sequard syndrome neurological disorder producing paralysis on the same side as the lesion; on the side opposite of the lesion, the patient has loss of pain sensation and temperature

Brucella genus of rod-shaped *gram-negative bacteria* that can cause various types of *brucellosis* such as *Malta fever* (B. melitensis) or *Bang's disease* (B. abortus)

brucellosis *infectious disease* caused by *Brucellas* that can affect various *organs*;

transmitted through contact with contaminated material, diseased animals and consumption of contaminated milk products

Brudzinski sign expansion pain in the *meninges* caused by irritation from *inflammatory* processes, *neoplastic* processes or a *subarachnoid bleed*; test: with patient supine and relaxed with legs extended, flexion of the neck causes reflexive flexion of the hips and knees

bruxism involuntary tooth grinding

BS abbr. *blood sugar*

BSA abbr. *body surface area*

BSR abbr. *blood sedimentation rate*

bubonic plague *plague* transmitted by the bite of a rat flea that has fed on an infected rat

bucc(o)– combining form: cheek

bucca cheek

buccal pert. to the mucous membrane inside the cheek

Buerger's disease *(thromboangiitis obliterans)* chronic, inflammatory disease of peripheral arteries and veins of fingers and toes; seen mostly in men who smoke.

buffy coat layer of *leukocytes* resting on top of the *erythrocyte* layer in centrifuged blood

bulbar paralysis *paralysis* originating in the medulla oblongata

bulbar pert. to the eyeball (*bulbus oculi*)

bulemia eating disorder marked by binge eating followed by self-induced vomiting (purging)

bulla blister; one of the *primary efflorescences;* skin eruption with a cavity measuring more than 0.5 cm; see also *vesicle*

bulldog clamp *arterial* clamp with a self-closing spring mechanism

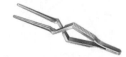

Fig. 73: bulldog clamp [A]

bullous like a blister

BUN abbr. for blood urea nitrogen; lab test on blood to determine the level of urea in the blood, which may affect kidney function

bundle branch block *(intraventricular block)* failure to conduct electrical impulses down the bundle of His or the left or right bundle branch; abbr. BBB

bundle of His structure consisting of bundled fibers located below the *atrioventricular node* of the *heart*, which conducts its impulses; it separates into the left and right *Tawara branches*; see also *excitation and conduction system*

buphthalmia (buphthalmos, hydrophthalmia, infantile glaucoma) congenital enlargement of the eyeball due to elevated intraocular pressure

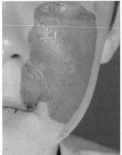

Fig. 74: burn

burns wounds with various causes, including heat, chemicals, electricity and radioactivity; 1st-degree burn (combustio erythematosa): burn involving only the *epidermis* with redness and pain in the burned area; 2nd-degree burn (combustio bullosa): burn involving the *epidermis* and *dermis* with redness, blistering and pain in the burned area; classified as superficial or deep depending on whether only the upper

dermis is involved or the deeper layer as well; 3rd-degree burn (combustio escharotica): burn involving the *epidermis*, *dermis* and *subcutaneous layers* with charred skin and no sensation in the burned area

burs- combining form: synovial sac

bursa (synovialis) sac filled with synovial fluid located at a joint

bursectomy *surgical* removal of a *bursa*

bursitis *inflammation* of a *bursa*

bursotomy *surgical* incision of a *bursa*

butterfly fracture bilateral anterior *pelvic ring fracture*

butterfly needle small, fine needle with wings used for *intravenous infusion* or drawing blood from fragile veins

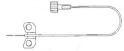

Fig. 75: butterfly [C]

butterfly rash butterfly-shaped facial *rash* that classically occurs as a result of *systemic lupus erythematosus*

buttocks prominences posterior to the hips and below the waist

button cannula *needle* with a blunt tip for rinsing *wounds*

bypass 1) surgical circumvention; 2) to create such a circumvention, e.g. coronary or gastric bypass

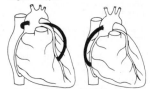

Fig. 76: aortocoronary bypass

C

C-section (cesarean section) obstetrical
surgery in which the *uterus* is opened via
an *incision* in the lower mid-abdomen,
e.g. when the life of mother or child is
endangered

C abbr. *Celsius; cervical* portion (of the spine)

c symbol: hundredth (10^{-2}); prefix: *centi-*

C1, C2, ...C7 abbr. *cervical* vertebra; there are
7 cervical vertebrae in the human skeleton

Ca abbr. *calcium; carcinoma*

CABG abbr. *coronary artery bypass graft;*
surgical intervention to improve blood
supply to the muscles of the heart; veins
(often saphenous) are grafted onto
occluded coronary arteries; blood supply to
the muscle is improved, thereby reducing
pain and abnormal heartbeats

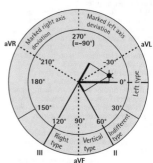

Fig. 78: Cabrera's circle

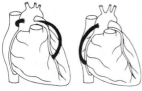

Fig. 77: aortocoronary bypass

Cabrera´s circle theoretical model to
describe the axis deviation of the heart in
an electrocardiogram

cachectic pert. to *cachexia;* opp. *obese*

cachexia wasting; emaciation

cadaveric rigidity *rigor mortis*

cal abbr. *calorie*

calcan– combining form: heelbone

calcaneal fracture (duckbill deformity)
avulsion fracture of the upper posterior
part of the *calcaneus,* which is displaced
upward due to traction from the *Achilles
tendon*

calcaneal spur bone spur beneath the
calcaneus, which can cause intense pain
when walking

calcaneal tendon *Achilles tendon*

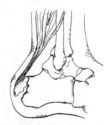

Fig. 79: calcaneal avulsion fracture

calcaneus heelbone; hindmost of the *tarsal
bones*

calciferol (vitamin D2) dietary supplement
that is used to treat rickets

calcification hardening due to deposition of
calcium salts

calcinosis abnormal deposition of *calcium*

calcitonin *hormone* made by the thyroid
gland that reduces *calcium* and *phosphate*
levels in the blood and incorporates
minerals into bone tissue; antagonist:
parathyroid hormone

calcium electrolyte with particular importance for bone building, blood clotting (*Factor IV*), muscle and nerve function; total amount in the body is 12 kg, of which > 98% is bound in the skeleton; chemical symbol: Ca

calcium antagonist drug used to inhibit the uptake of *calcium* into the *cells*; used for cardiac arrhythmias et al.

calculus dentis *dental calculus*

calf bone *fibula*

calibration precise adjustment of a device

calix renalis *renal calyx*

callous ulcer (ulcus callosum) *gastric ulcer* with heavy scar tissue formation

callus proliferation of *connective tissue* at the site of a bone fracture

calor heat; see also *signs of inflammation*

calorie (kilocalorie) outdated unit of heat; 1 kilocalorie will heat 1 kg of pure water by 1°C; the more modern unit is the *joule*: 1 joule equals 0.239 calories while 1 calorie equals 4.187 joules; abbr. cal, Cal, kcal

calvaria skullcap dome of the skull

calx heel

canal of Schlemm (scleral venous sinus) vessel at the anterior margin of the *sclera* which takes up the *aqueous humor*

canalis carpi *carpal tunnel*

cancellous bone screw device for *osteosynthesis* of a *fracture* using tensioning screws to create inter*fragmentary compression*, e.g. in a *calcaneal fracture*

cancer generic term for malignant neoplastic diseases

cancerogenic *carcinogenic*

Candida a genus of fungus with yeastlike qualities

Candida albicans fungus that can cause *thrush* et al.

candidiasis (candidosis) fungal *infection* of the skin or mucosa, usually with *Candida albicans*, which usually begins in the oral cavity and can then spread through the whole body, e.g. as candida pneumonia, with the danger of *sepsis*; usually occurs in persons in weakened general condition

candidosis *candidiasis*

cannula sharp hollow needle for *injection*, *puncture* or blood drawing

capacity potential ability to perform; ability to hold or contain

Capgras' syndrome delusion occurring in *schizophrenia* in which the patient believes that a given person has been replaced by a double

capitatum os *os capitatum*

capillary smallest blood vessel in the body; enables transfer of substances between the bloodstream and *tissues*

capillary resistance test in which the resistance of *capillaries* is measured by constriction

capillus (thrix, pili) hair

capitate bone one of the *carpal bones*

capitellum fracture *fracture* of the head of the humerus (capitulum humeri); see *Neer* classification

capnometry measurement of *carbon dioxide* in expired breath using a capnometer

capsule endoscopy outpatient procedure to examine the small intestine (duodenum, jejunum and ileum)

capsulorrhexis circular *surgical* incision to open the anterior lens capsule, e.g. for *cataracts*

caput head

caput–collum–diaphysis angle angle between the *femoral* neck and shaft; abbr. CCD angle

caput medusae descriptive term for the dilated and meandering veins of the abdominal wall in patients with *portal hypertension*; resembles head of Medusa from Greek mythology

carb abbr. *carbohydrate*

CARB abbr. *carbohydrate*

carboanhydrase inhibitor drug that inhibits the *enzyme* carboanhydrase, which leads to increased excretion of water and *carbon dioxide*

carbohydrate chemical compound containing carbon and water, e.g. the nutrients *glucose* or *starch*; important nutritional substance with 4.1 kcal / 17.1 KJ per gram; abbr. carb

carbohydrate antigen 125 / 125 important *tumor marker* for *ovarian cancer* and others; abbr. *CA 125 / 125*

carbohydrate antigen 153 important *tumor marker* for *breast cancer*; abbr. *CA 153*

carbohydrate antigen 199 important *tumor marker* for *colorectal cancer* and *pancreatic cancer*; abbr. *CA 199*

carbohydrate antigen 724 important *tumor marker* for *gastric carcinoma*; abbr. *CA 724*

carbon dioxide a gas produced in the body as part of most metabolic processes, which is carried to the lungs via the *venous* blood and then exhaled; chemical symbol: CO_2

carbonic acid weak acid resulting from solution of *carbon dioxide* in water; chemical symbol: H_2CO_3

carbuncle several *furuncles* clustered together

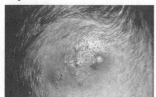

Fig. 80: carbuncle

carcinoembryonic antigen important *tumor marker* for *colorectal, hepatocellular* and *pancreatic carcinomas*; abbr. CEA

carcinogenic causing malignant neoplastic diseases

carcinoid semimalignant tumor of the *neuroendocrine system*, usually occurring in the *small intestine*, which is capable of producing *hormones*, e.g. *serotonin*

carcinoma malignant tumor of glandular or *epithelial* tissue; abbr. Ca

carcinoma in situ malignant but localized tumor of the skin or mucous membranes that has not penetrated the basement membrane; abbr. CIS

carcinomatosis (carcinosis) widespread metastasis of malignant tumors through the body

carcinosis carcinomatosis

card(io)- combining form: heart

cardia opening of the *esophagus* into the *stomach*

cardiac pert. to the heart

cardiac asthma respiratory distress due to left heart insufficiency with subsequent pulmonary congestion

cardiac catheterization insertion of a *catheter* into the central vessels or chambers of the *heart* for purposes of examination or treatment; catheters are differentiated into left-heart and right-heart types

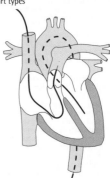

Fig. 81: left- and right-heart catheterization (via femoral or brachial vein and femoral artery)

cardiac glycoside drug that increases the *contractile* strength of the *heart*

cardiac index index of heart performance that is calculated based on *body surface area*; can be measured with a *pulmonary artery catheter*; formula: *cardiac output per minute* divided by *body surface area*; normal value: 2.5–3.6 l/min/m²; abbr CI

cardiac insufficiency left or right *heart failure*; see also *respiratory insufficiency*; opp. *global insufficiency*

cardiac massage resuscitation technique used in cardiac arrest

cardiac output (per minute) amount of blood that the heart pumps per minute; can be determined using a *pulmonary artery catheter*, among other methods; formula<. stroke volume x beats per minute; normal value: 58 l/min; elevated in *anemia*, *sepsis* and *hyperthyroidism*; decreased in *hypovolemia*, *cardiogenic shock* and *heart failure*; abbr. CO

cardiac silhouette shadow cast by the heart and great vessels in a chest x-ray

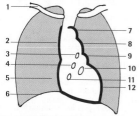

Fig. 82: cardiac silhouette
1 Clavicle 2 Pulmonary valve 3 Superior vena cava 4 Aortic valve 5 Right atrium 6 Diaphragm 7 Aorta 8 Pulmonary trunk 9 Left atrium 10 Mitral valve 11 Tricuspid valve 12 Left ventricle

cardiac tamponade compression of the heart due to an accumulation of blood in the pericardium

cardinal symptom principal characteristic *symptom* in a disease or injury

cardioactive agent drug used to treat *heart* disease

cardiogenic shock *shock* triggered by *heart failure*

cardiologic(al) pert. to *cardiology*

cardiologist specialist in *cardiology*

cardiology study of diseases of the heart

cardiolysis separation of *adhesions* in the *pericardium*

cardiomyopathy disease of the heart muscle associated with impaired cardiac function

cardiomyotomy *surgical* longitudinal separation of the *cardia* muscles to treat *achalasia*

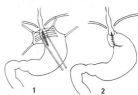

Fig. 83: cardiomyotomy
1 Heller/Gottstein cardiomyotomy
2 Nissen fundoplication

cardiopathy congenital or acquired heart disease

cardioplegia cardiac arrest induced by instilling a special chilled solution into the *coronary arteries*; protects the *myocardium* during *heart* surgery

cardioselective affecting only the *heart*, e.g. a drug

cardiospasm cramping at the entrance to the *stomach*

cardiotocogram simultaneous recording of the *fetal* heart rate (normal 120–160/minute) and maternal *labor* activity to monitor the pregnancy; abbr. CTG

cardiovascular pert. to the *heart* and blood vessels

cardioversion treatment of *cardiac arrhythmias*, usually with electroshocks from a *defibrillator* (R-wave synchronized defibrillation), but also done mechanically or with drugs

cardiovert to perform *cardioversion*

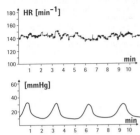

Fig. 84: normal cardiotocogram

or spontaneously by turning the head sharply

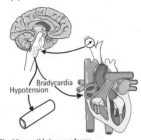

Fig. 85: carotid sinus syndrome

caries (tooth decay) destruction of the *enamel* and *dentin* of the *tooth* caused by external factors, e.g. by lactic acid-forming *bacteria*

carina (tracheae) *bifurcation* of the *trachea* into the two primary *bronchi*, located at approximately the level of the 4th *thoracic vertebra*

cariogenic causing *caries*

carious pert. to or affected with *caries*

carminative drug used to treat abdominal gas

Caroli syndrome congenital dilation of the bile ducts inside the liver

carotene *provitamin* of *vitamin A*

carotid artery located on either side of the neck

carotid bruits abnormal sounds heard when auscultating carotid arteries

carotid pulse *pulse* in the *carotid artery*, *palpable* next to the *larynx*

carotid sinus receptors that cause reflex changes in vessel diameter and heart rate when stimulated

carotid sinus syndrome attack of *bradycardic dysrhythmia* and reduced *blood pressure* leading to *syncope* due to hypersensitive *carotid sinus reflex*; triggered by pressure on a sensitive point in the *carotid artery* in the throat area,

carotis, A. *arteria carotis ...*

carp mouth fishlike distortion of the lips in *tetany* due to *hypocalcemia*

carpal pert. to the wrist

carpal joints *joints* between the carpal bones

carpal tunnel (canalis carpi) channel for the long flexor tendons and *median nerve* to pass through the wrist joint

carpal tunnel syndrome weakness in the thenar muscles (*thenar atrophy*) and loss of sensation in digits 1–3 due to nerve damage in the *carpal tunnel*

carpopedal spasms cramps in the hands and feet due to *tetany*

carpus wrist

cartilage type of dense *connective tissue* found mainly in joints, as well as the nose, external ear, *larynx, trachea* and *bronchi*

caruncle small fleshy growth; see also *lacrimal caruncle*

castration removal of the testes

casuistics description of clinical cases

cata– combining form: down, after, against

catabolic pert. to *catabolism*; opp. *anabolic*

catabolism destructive phase of *metabolism*; opp. *anabolism*

catalepsy postural rigidity; condition in which the patient stiffly maintains a posture once he has assumed it

cataplasm poultice

cataract clouding of the lens of the eye, which causes decreased vision; a) **hypermature type** (overripe cataract): *cataract* with dissolution of the lens fibers and collapse of the nucleus; b) **immature type**: *cataract* with *peripheral* clouding of the lens; c) **mature type**: *cataract* with complete clouding of the lens, where only light can be perceived; d) **premature type**: *cataract* with cortical clouding extending to the center of the lens and reduction of visual acuity; e) **senile**: *cataract* with increasing *sclerosis* of the lens due to reduced metabolism and exposure to ultraviolet light

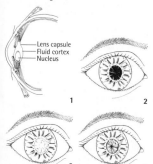

Lens capsule
Fluid cortex
Nucleus

Fig. 86: cataracts
1 Hypermature cataract 2 Immature cataract
3 Mature cataract 4 Premature cataract

cataract surgery *surgical* treatment of cataracts. usually by posterior lens *implantation*

catarrh *inflammation* of the mucosa, usually associated with *infections* of the respiratory or intestinal tract

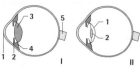

Fig. 87: cataract surgery with posterior lens implantation
I Before surgery 1 Cornea 2 Iris 3 Cataract (clouded lens) 4 Ciliary body 5 Optic nerve
II After surgery 1 Lens capsule 2 Artificial lens

catatonia phase of *schizophrenia* with pronounced impairment of voluntary *motor function*

catecholamine collective term for substances such as *adrenaline*, *norepinephrine* and *dopamine*

catgut *surgical* suture material that can be *resorbed* by the body

catheter tube for moving fluids into or out of the body, e.g. *urinary catheter*

catheter urine urine collected for testing via a bladder catheter

catheterize to insert a *catheter*

cathode *electrode* with its negative pole connected to a power source; opp. *anode*

cation positively charged *ion*

cauda final portion or tail of an *organ*

cauda equina pointed end of the *spinal cord* with the spinal nerve roots

cauda equina syndrome *radicular compression syndrome* with damage to various nerve roots below the second lumbar vertebra due to pressure on the *cauda equina*; usually associated with urinary and bowel *incontinence*, *saddle block anesthesia* and absence of the *Achilles tendon reflex* (in contrast to medullary cone syndrome)

caudal toward the lower end of the body or downward; opp. *cranial*

caudalis (inferior), V. *inferior vena cava*

caudate lobe (of the liver) small lobe on the visceral surface of the *liver*

causal pert. to a cause

causal treatment treatment of the cause of a disease

causalgia burning skin pain

cauterization see *electrocautery*

cautery see *electrocautery*

cav(it)- combining form: cavity

cava, V. *vena cava*

cave caution! (Latin)

cavern pathological encapsulated cavity

CAVH abbr. *continuous arteriovenous hemofiltration*

cavity hollow space, e.g. hole in a *tooth* caused by *caries*

cavum cavity

cavum tympani *tympanum*

CCD angle abbr. *caput-collum-diaphysis angle*

CCRN abbr. Critical Care Registered Nurse

CCSC abbr. (Canadian Cardiovascular Society Classification) system for rating the severity of *angina pectoris*

CCT abbr. *cranial computed tomography*

CCU abbr. coronary care unit

cecum saccular structure at the beginning of the *ascending colon*

CDC abbr. Centers for Disease Control and Prevention

CEE abbr. *Central European encephalitis*

CEE virus *virus* that causes *CEE*

celiac disease form of nontropical *sprue* marked by inability to tolerate the *gluten* present in grains

celiac trunk common trunk of the common hepatic, splenic and left gastric arteries, arising from the abdominal *aorta*

celiocentesis *puncture* of the abdomen

cell smallest independently existing unit in the human *organism*

cell membrane outer covering of the *cell*

cell nucleus the central body of a *cell* which contains the *cytoplasm* and *chromosomes*

cellula *cell*

cellulitis *inflammation* of skin and soft tissues that spreads rapidly

cementum (periodontium) substance that covers the *dentin* of the *dental root*

-centesis combining form: puncture

centi- combining form: hundredth (10^{-2}); abbr. c

central on the inside, in the center of the body; *peripheral*

central hepatic veins central veins of the liver, into which the capillaries of the liver's lobes flow

central nervous system part of the *nervous system* comprising the *spinal cord* and *brain*; abbr. CNS; opp. *peripheral nervous system*

central retinal artery embolism *central retinal artery occlusion*

central retinal artery occlusion obstruction of retinal artery, sometimes caused by an embolism, which can result in sudden blindness

central retinal veins *veins* of the *retina* that flow into the *superior ophthalmic vein*

central scotoma visual impairment in the center of the visual field, e.g. from *inflammation* of the *optic nerve*

central venous pert. to *central veins*; opp. *peripheral venous*

central venous catheter *catheter* whose tip rests in the *superior vena cava* near the right *atrium* of the heart; used to give drugs and infusions, as well as to measure *central venous pressure*; opp. peripheral venous catheter, abbr. CVC

central venous pressure pressure in the superior vena cava, which can be measured with the patient in supine position using a central venous catheter or pulmonary artery catheter; zero point is determined with a *Burri sliding caliper* at 3/5 of the lateral thoracic diameter, oriented from the base; normal value 28 mmHg or 311 cm H_2O; elevated in right *heart failure*, e.g. due to heart *infarction*, *pulmonary embolism*, *hypervolemia*, *tricuspid insufficiency*, *pericardial tamponade*, and secondarily in left *heart failure*; reduced in *hypovolemia*; abbr. CVP

centralization autoregulation of the body in *shock*; constriction of the peripheral blood vessels results in increased circulation to the most vital internal organs (heart, brain, liver, lungs)

centrifugation separation of materials using a centrifuge

centrifuge device for separating solid components from fluids using centrifugal force, e.g. for examination of *urinary sediment*

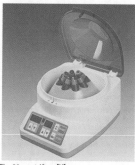

Fig. 88: centrifuge [H]

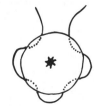

Fig. 89: cerclage

centriole (centrosome) central body in a *cell* with an important role in cell division

centrosome *centriole*

cephal– combining form: head

cephalalgia headache

cephalic vein *vein* located on the thumb side of the forearm, which flows into the *axillary vein*

cephalohematoma *hematoma* between the bone and the periosteum of the skull

cephalosporin *antibiotic* related to *penicillin*

–ceptor combining form: receptor

cerclage circular suture used in *surgery*, e.g. to close a *cervix* that has dilated too far during pregnancy, see Fig. 89

cerebell– combining form: cerebellum

cerebellar pert. to the *cerebellum*

cerebellar cortex outer layer of the cerebellum

cerebellar veins *veins* that transport blood out of the *cerebellum*

cerebellum section of the brain located between the *cerebrum* and *medulla oblongata*; controls balance and coordination

cerebr– combining form: *cerebrum*

cerebral pert. to the *cerebrum*

cerebral compression pressure on the brain; serious head trauma with unconsciousness lasting longer than 24 hours and substantial damage to the brain

cerebral concussion mild *head trauma* with loss of consciousness lasting a maximum of 1 hour, with no lasting damage

cerebral contusion moderately severe head trauma with unconsciousness lasting a maximum of 24 hours

cerebral cortex outer layer of the cerebrum

cerebral palsy congenital nervous system disorder; often results from premature birth; and is characterized by spastic limb movements

cerebral paresis *paresis* caused by brain damage

cerebral perfusion pressure mean pressure in the vessels leading into the brain; especially important in monitoring a head trauma; obtained by subtracting intracranial pressure from mean systemic arterial pressure; abbr. CPP

cerebral sclerosis *arteriosclerosis* of the vessels in the *brain*

cerebral veins *veins* that transport blood out of the cerebrum

cerebrospinal pert. to the *brain* and *spinal cord*

cerebrospinal fluid (liquor cerebrospinalis) fluid formed in the ventricles of the *brain* that circulates in the *subarachnoid* space of the brain and *spinal cord* between the *arachnoid membranes* and *pia mater*; abbr. CSF

cerebrospinal fluid leak discharge of *cerebrospinal fluid*

cerebrovascular pert. to the blood vessels in the *brain*

cerebrum largest section of the brain; the part of the *central nervous system* located within the skull; all voluntary and mental processes take place here, as well as conversion of sensory stimuli into sensations

certificate legal form required after a death or a declaration of metal incompetenca, e.g.

certification legal proof indicating that a person or facility has either met published standards or passed testing

ceruloplasmin *protein* for transport and storage of copper in the body

cerumen (earwax) secretion of the *sebaceous glands* in the *external auditory canal*

ceruminal pert. to *cerumen*

cervi(c)- combining form: neck, nape

cervical pert. to the *cervical spine* or the *cervix uteri*

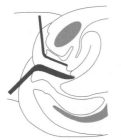

Fig. 90: speculum examination of the cervix

cervical canal canal in *the cervix uteri* or *spinal column*

cervical cap plastic cap that is placed over the *cervical* opening as a barrier method of contraception

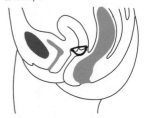

Fig. 91: cervical cap

cervical carcinoma malignant tumor at the neck of the *uterus (cervix uteri)*

cervical dystonia abnormal tonicity and movements affecting the neck

cervical insufficiency inability of the *cervix* to remain closed for the duration of a *pregnancy*, which can lead to a miscarriage

cervical os opening of the birth canal, consisting of the *ostium uteri* (external os toward the *vagina*) and isthmus uteri (internal os toward the uterine cavity)

cervical plexus nerve *plexus* in the neck area (branches of the 1st-4th cervical nerves), which contains the *nervus suprascapularis* et al.

cervical spine (C-spine) uppermost part of the spinal column, consisting of the 7 cervical vertebrae; abbr. CS

cervical syndrome nonspecific collective term for diseases or injuries involving pain or other complaints in the *cervical spine* area

cervical vertebrae see *cervical spine*

cervicitis *inflammation* of the mucosa of the *cervix uteri*

cervix neck

cervix (uteri) neck of the *uterus* extending from the internal os to the external os

cesarean birth delivery of an infant by *cesarean section*

cesarean section C-section
C-grip maneuver for anchoring a mask for *manual* ventilation, e.g. with an *Ambu bag*; the thumb and forefinger form a C shape to hold the mask in place

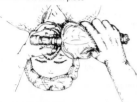

Fig. 92: C-grip (from paramedic's point of view)

Ch abbr. *Charrière*
-chalasia combining form: relaxation
chalazion (meibomian cyst) *chronic noninfectious granulomatous inflammation* of the meibomian gland in the eyelid; pl. *chalazia*
chalcosis bulbi (intraocular chalcosis, copper cataract) eye damage caused by foreign body containing copper
chancre ulcer associated with sexually transmitted diseases; see also *syphilis* (hard chancre) und *chancroid* (soft chancre)
chancroid (ulcus molle, soft chancre) *infectious disease* caused by *Haemophilus ducreyi* that causes *ulceration* at the pathogen's point of entry; transmitted by sexual contact
change of life menopause
Charcot-Marie-Tooth Disease inherited disease producing progressive loss of use and sensation in the limb; nerve impulses are poorly transmitted because the myelin coating on motor and sensory nerves deteriorates, abbr. CMT
chasmus yawning fit
Chassaignac's luxation *Chassaignac's paralysis*
Chassaignac's paralysis (Chassaignac's luxation, Chassaignac's syndrome)

subluxation of the head of the *radius* in children aged 2-6 years due to traction and pronation of the child's extended arm
Chassaignac's syndrome *Chassaignac's paralysis*
CHD abbr. *coronary heart disease*
CHE abbr. *cholinesterase*
cheek buccal cavity
cheilitis *inflammation* of the lips
cheilo- combining form: lip
cheilognathopalatoschisis congenital cleft from the lip back to the soft palate, occurring unilaterally or bilaterally
cheilos (labium) lip
chemical burn *wound* caused by corrosive substances; see *alkali burn, acid burn*
chemoembolization blockage of a vessel using chemical substances in the treatment of malignant neoplastic diseases
chemosis *edema* of the *cornea*
chemotherapeutic agent drug used to fight disease-causing agents or tumor cells
chemotherapy treatment with *chemotherapeutic agents*, e.g. for *infections* or tumors
Cheyne-Stokes respiration pathological breathing pattern marked by gradually increasing depth of respirations with periods of *apnea*; occurs with brain injuries and/or increased *intracranial pressure*

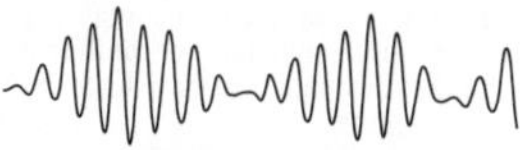

Fig. 93: Cheyne-Stokes respiration

CHF abbr. congestive heart failure
chiasm crossing point, e.g. of *nerves*
chicken pox (varicella) *infectious disease* caused by the *varicella zoster virus*, leading to a vesicular skin rash that can leave scars, mainly on the head and trunk, as well as itching and sometimes fever; in severe cases *meningitis* can result; transmitted by droplet infection or smear infection
childbed fever puerperal fever
Child-Pugh classification system for assessing the degree of severity of *cirrhosis*

chill(s) involuntary shivering motions of the skeletal muscles that increase heat production within the *organism*, e.g. with a rising *fever* or for *compensation* in *hypothermia*

chin mentum

chiragra hand pain

chiropractic form of *chirotherapy* for treating misalignment of the spinal column

chirotherapy (manual therapy) physical manipulation for treatment of functional structural disorders, usually involving the musculoskeletal system

chisel fracture fracture of the radial head

Fig. 94: chisel fracture

Chlamydia *microorganism* that can cause *infectious diseases*, e.g. *ornithosis* (C. psittaci) *trachoma* (C. trachomatis) or *pneumonia* (C. pneumoniae)

chlor(o)- combining form: green

chloride vital *electrolyte* for maintaining water and electrolyte balance, production of stomach acid and acid-base balance; chemical symbol: Cl

choana posterior nasal opening communicating with the posterior nasopharyngeal space; pl. choanae

choanal atresia congenital occlusion of one or both choanae

chol(e)- combining form: bile

cholangi(o)- combining form: bile duct

cholangiocarcinoma rare malignant tumor of the *bile ducts*, usually an *adenocarcinoma*

cholangiography radiography of the *bile ducts* using a *contrast medium*

cholangioma tumor of the *bile ducts*

cholangiopancreatography *endoscopy* of

the *duodenum* and radiography of the pancreatic and bile ducts using a *contrast medium*; abbr. ERCP

cholangitis *inflammation* of the *bile ducts*

chole *bile*

cholecystectomy *surgical* removal of the *gallbladder*

cholecystitis *inflammation* of the *gallbladder*

cholecysto- combining form: gallbladder

cholecystokinin *hormone* produced in the intestinal mucosa that causes *contraction* of the gallbladder, resulting in release of *bile* into the small intestine

cholecystolithiasis presence of *gallstones* in the *gallbladder*

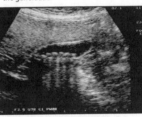

Fig. 95: cholecystolithiasis (ultrasound)

choledocholithiasis presence of *gallstones* in the *common bile duct*

choledochus, ductus *common bile duct*

cholelithiasis presence of *gallstones* in the *bile duct* system

cholera *infectious disease* that causes severe diarrhea; caused by toxins produced by the pathogen Vibrio cholerae, among others; transmitted mainly via contaminated drinking water or food

choleresis formation and secretion of *bile* by the liver

choleretic 1) drug used to stimulate production and secretion of *bile* by the liver cells; 2) pert. to production and secretion of bile

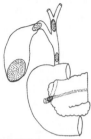

Fig. 96: cholelithiasis

cholestasis (cholestasia) interruption in the flow of *bile*, e.g. due to tumors in the *bile ducts*

cholesteatoma benign tumor of the gallbladder

cholesterol substance found in all of the body's *cells* and blood lipids; important for the metabolism of *vitamins*, *hormones* and *bile acids*; *cholesterol* is ingested with food but can also be produced by the body itself; excess cholesterol in the blood forms deposits on the vascular walls and causes *arteriosclerosis*; classified as *HDL* and *LDL cholesterol*

cholinergic agent (parasympathomimetic*)* drug used to stimulate the *parasympathetic nervous system*

cholinesterase enzyme produced in the liver that breaks down acetylcholine into choline and acetic acid; abbr. CHE

cholinolytic agent *parasympatholytic*

chondr(o)– combining form: cartilage

chondral pert. to cartilage

chondritis inflammation of cartilage

chondroma benign tumor originating in cartilaginous *tissue*

chondropathia patellae *(chondromalacia patellae)* degenerative changes in the cartilage of the patella with *retropatellar* exertion-related pain

chondros cartilage

chondrosarcoma malignant tumor originating in cartilaginous *tissue*

chorea collective term for irregular, sudden, brief attacks of violent movement, usually affecting multiple areas of the body

choriocarcinoma malignant tumor composed of *chorionic* villi remaining in the *uterus* after childbirth

chorioepithelioma *choriocarcinoma*

chorion villous membrane; one of the fetal membranes

chorioretinitis (choroidoretinitis) *inflammation of the choroid and the retina of the eye*

choroid vascular layer of the eye; supplies blood to the *retina*

choroiditis *inflammation of the choroid of the eye*

Christmas factor *antihemophilic globulin B*

chrom– combining form: color

chromatin stainable genetic material in the *cell nucleus*

chromatopsia abnormal perception of color

chromosomal pert. to *chromosomes*

chromosome uncoiled *deoxyribonucleic acid* in the *cell nucleus*; a *cell* contains 23 *chromosome* pairs

chron– combining form: time

chronic long-lasting; opp. *acute*

chronic carrier person who continues to harbor a pathogenic organism after having recovered from the *infectious disease*

chronic leg ulcer *ulcer* on the lower leg caused by a circulatory disorder, e.g. blood congestion due to *varicose veins*

chronic lymphocytic leukemia (chronic lymphatic leukemia) form of *leukemia* characterized by a significant increase in the number of *lymphocytes*; abbr. CLL

chronic myelocytic leukemia (chronic myelogenous leukemia, chronic myeloid leukemia) form of *leukemia* with markedly elevated *leukocyte* count; abbr. CML

chronic myelogenous leukemia *chronic myelocytic leukemia*

chronic myeloid leukemia *chronic myelocytic leukemia*

chronic obstructive lung disease synonym for *chronic obstructive pulmonary disease* abbr. *COPD*

chronic obstructive pulmonary disease COPD

chronotropic affecting the heart rate; positive chronotropic: increasing the heart rate; negative chronotropic: decreasing the heart rate

chrys– combining form: gold

Chvostek's sign sign of hyperexcitability of the *nerves*, e.g. in *tetany*, tapping on the facial nerve causes facial spasms

chyle fluid found in the *lymphatic vessels* of the intestine, which takes on a milky/cloudy color after eating due to increased fat content

chylothorax collection of *chyle* in the *pleural cavity*, e.g. from a stab wound

chylous pert. to *chyle*

chyme partially digested food mass in the stomach

chymotrypsin *enzyme* produced in the *pancreas* that is released into the *duodenum* and breaks down *proteins* for digestion

CI abbr. *cardiac index*

cicatricial contraction contraction of *tissue* due to shrinkage of a scar

cicatrix a scar left by partial healing of the skin

cilia 1) projections of the *ciliated epithelium*; 2) eyelashes; sing. cilium

ciliary body (corpus ciliare) part of the middle layer of the *eye* that produces the *aqueous humor* and contains the *ciliary muscle*

ciliary muscle (musculus ciliaris) ring muscle in the *ciliary body* of the eye that controls the curvature of the *lens*; innervation: *oculomotor nerve*

ciliated epithelium *epithelium* covered with waving *cilia*, e.g. in the respiratory tract

cilium eyelash

Cimino shunt *surgically* created *shunt* between the *radial artery* and *cephalic vein* for *dialysis*

circadian pert. to daily events

circle system *rebreathing system*

circular in the form of a circle

circulation regular circular movement, e.g. of the blood from the heart out to the body parts and back

circulus circle, ring

circum– combining form: around

circumcision surgical removal of the foreskin of the *penis*, e.g. to treat *phimosis*

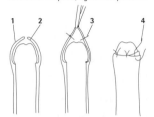

Fig. 97: circumcision
1 Outer layer 2 Inner layer 3 Cut 4 Suture

circumflex artery part of the left *coronary artery* (LCA); supplies the posterior and lateral walls of the left ventricle

circumscribed spreading within a sharply defined boundary; opp. *diffuse*

cirrh– combining form: 1) yellow/orange; 2) hard

cirrhosis irreversible *liver* shrinkage and loss of function, usually following severe liver disease; degree of severity is rated using the *Child-Pugh Classification*

cirrhotic pert. to *cirrhosis*

CIS abbr. *carcinoma in situ*

cis– combining form: on the same side

cistern fluid reservoir

citrated blood blood rendered incoagulable by addition of *sodium citrate*

CK abbr. *creatine kinase*

CK–BB isoform of the *enzyme creatine kinase* that is specific to *brain* and smooth muscle tissue; normally represents only a miniscule portion of total creatine kinase

CK-MB isoform of the *enzyme creatine kinase* that is specific to cardiac muscle tissue; normally represents under 5% of total creatine kinase

CK-MM isoform of the *enzyme creatine kinase* that is specific to *skeletal* muscle tissue; normally represents more than 95% of total creatine kinase

Cl chemical symbol for *chloride*

clap *gonorrhea*

-clasia combining form: break

claudicatio intermittens *intermittent claudication*

claudication cramping pain in the calf of the leg severe enough to cause one to stop walking

claustrophobia anxiety disorder in which the patient fears being in an enclosed space

clavicle collarbone

clavicular pert. to the *clavicle*

clavus corn; callus

claw hand typical hand position in patients with *ulnar nerve* damage

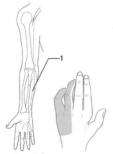

Fig. 98: claw hand
1 Ulnar nerve

clearance elimination from the blood; usually used in connection with *creatinine clearance*

cleft lip (harelip, cheiloschisis) congenital cleft in the upper lip

cleft palate (palatoschisis) congenital fissure in the palate

cleid(o)- combining form: clavicle

climacteric *menopause*

climax sexual orgasm

clinic medical care center

clitoris female sexual organ with *venous* spongy body located in the *genital* area

CLL abbr. *chronic lymphocytic leukemia*

clone genetically identical copy of an organism

clonic pert. to *clonus*; opp. *tonic*

clonus jerking, repetitive muscle *contractions*; opp. *tonus*

closed-angle glaucoma (narrow-angle glaucoma) *glaucoma* due to closure of the iridocorneal angle as a result of protrusion of the base of the iris, or from thickening of the lens associated with *cataracts*

closed pleural drainage *thoracic drain* that is placed in the 5th-7th *ICS* along the anterior *axillary line*

Clostridium genus of *spore*-forming anaerobic gram-negative bacteria

Clostridium botulinum *Clostridium* that causes *botulism*

Clostridium perfringens *Clostridium* that causes *gas gangrene*

Clostridium tetani *Clostridium* that causes *tetanus*

clotting factor *coagulation factor*

clotting time blood clotting test that measures the time interval between blood collection and the formation of *fibrin*; normal time: 5-15 minutes

clubbing (clubbed fingers, hippocratic fingers) enlargement of the terminal phalanx of the fingers due to chronic *oxygen* deficiency; usually occurs in combination with *watchglass* nails

clubfoot *pes adductus*

cluster headache series of intense recurring (usually every 6 weeks) headaches on one side of the head with intense pain localized over one eye

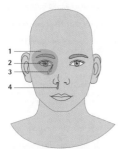

Fig. 99: cluster headache
1 Pain 2 Ptosis, myosis 3 Eye waters
4 Nasal blockage and rhinorrhea

clysis *enema*

CM abbr. *contrast medium*

CML abbr. *chronic myelocytic leukemia*

CMV abbr. *cytomegalovirus*

CNS abbr. *central nervous system*

CO abbr. *cardiac output*

co(m)- combining form: with together

CO$_2$ chemical symbol: *carbon dioxide*

coagul- combining form: clotting

coagulated clotted

coagulation clotting

coagulation factor substances occurring in blood *plasma* (*factors*) that play a critical role in blood coagulation

coagulation necrosis *necrosis* marked by coagulation of *proteins*, e.g. in connection with an *acid burn*

coagulation time *clotting time*

coagulopathy clotting disorder, e.g. in *hemophilia*

coagulum blood clot

cobalamin *cyanocobalamin*

coccus spherical or ovoid *bacterium*, e.g. *Staphylococcus, Streptococcus*; pl. cocci

coccyx (tailbone) lowest part of the *spinal column*, after the *sacrum*

cochle- combining form: snail

cochlea snail-shaped tube in the inner *ear*, vital to hearing

cochlear implant electronic *prosthesis* used to enable hearing where *cochlear* function is absent but the auditory pathway and auditory nerve are still intact

coenzyme substance that supports the action of an *enzyme*

cognitive pert. to thought

cogwheel rigidity symptom of Parkinson's disease where limb shows lead-pipe stiffness followed by a tremor

coherent orderly, logical; opp. *incoherent*

Cohn fraction I *fibrinogen* isolated from blood, given to patients lacking the substance to treat hemorrhages

coincidence simultaneous occurrence

coitarche age at first sexual intercourse

coitus sexual intercourse

coitus interruptus sexual intercourse with intentional ejaculation outside the *vagina* to prevent conception

col(o)- combining form: large intestine

COLD abbr. *chronic obstructive lung disease*

cold agglutinin *antibody* that causes clumping of *erythrocytes* at low temperatures

cold antibody collective term for *cold hemolysin* and *cold agglutinin*

cold hemolysin *antibody* that *destroys erythrocytes* at low temperatures

colibacillus *bacterium* occurring in the human *intestinal flora*, e.g. *Escherichia coli*; some colibacilli produce *vitamin K*

colic cramping pains caused by the spasmodic contraction of hollow organs, e.g. *biliary, colic* intestinal colic

colica, A. *arteria colica*

colitis *inflammation* of the lining of the *colon*

collagen *protein* that serves as a structural element of vessels, skin, bone, cartilage, tendon and teeth

collagenosis disease affecting the entire body that causes *degeneration* of *connective tissue*, e.g. *systemic lupus erythematosus*

collapse decreased circulation with a drop in *blood pressure*

collar crown dental prosthesis in which the *crown* is anchored in the tooth root with a pin

collarbone *clavicle*

collateral circulation circulatory path created to bypass an obstruction, e.g. an occluded blood vessel

Collin forceps (arterial forceps) a locking forceps with sloping blades for grasping the end of a blood vessel until a ligature is applied

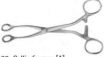

Fig. 100: Collin forceps [A]

colliquative necrosis *necrosis* marked by liquefaction of the affected *tissue*, e.g. in connection with *alkali burn*

colloid gluelike substance with particles dispersed within a liquid

colloid osmotic pressure (*oncotic pressure*) higher concentration of protein in plasma than in interstitial fluid; causes cellular fluids to move

colloidal pert. to *colloid*

collum neck; *cervix* (*uteri*)

collum anatomicum humeri (anatomical neck of the humerus) narrow area of the *humerus* located below the head

collum chirurgicum humeri (surgical neck of the humerus) area of the *humerus* located below the *collum anatomicum humeri*

collum dentis neck of a tooth

collum femoris neck of the *femur*

colon main section of the large intestine; divided into four parts: ascending (colon ascendens), transverse (colon transversum), descending (colon descendens), and sigmoid (colon sigmoideum), the S-shaped final section of the large intestine

colon ascendens ascending *colon*

colon carcinoma malignant tumor of the *colon*

colon conduit *surgically* created diversion of the urine through the *ureters* into a prepared intestinal loop; diversion of the urine outside the body via a *colostomy*

colon descendens descending *colon*

colon sigmoideum sigmoid *colon*

colon transversum transverse *colon*

colonic polyp *polyp* in the *colon*

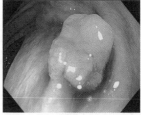

Fig. 101: colonic polyp [I]

colonoscope flexible *endoscope* for performing *colonoscopy*

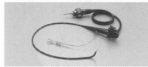

Fig. 102: colonoscope [I]

colonoscopic pert. to *colonoscopy*

colonoscopy insertion of a flexible tube into the rectum to examine the colon *for abnormalities*

colony group of *bacteria* grown in a culture

colorectal pert. to the *colon* and *rectum*

colorectal carcinoma malignant tumor in the *colon* and/or *rectum*

colostomy *surgically* created opening for the colon through the abdominal wall

colostrum pre-milk fluid formed as late as the 4th to 6th day after birth; contains a large amount of *IgA*, among other substances

colp(o)- combining form: vagina

colpitis (vaginitis) *inflammation* of the *vagina*

colpitis senilis inflammation of the *vagina* due to insufficient *estrogenic* stimulation of the *epithelium*, usually occurring in older women

colpocele herniation into the *vagina*

colpocleisis *surgical* closure of the *vagina*

colpos vagina

colposcopy *endoscopy* of the *vagina*

coma altered mental state in which the patient cannot be awakened and shows no reaction to painful stimuli; see also *diabetic coma; hepatic coma*

combination denture denture that combines permanent crowns with a removable *dental prosthesis*

comedo pimple; bump on the skin caused by a blocked sebaceous gland

comminuted fracture *fracture* caused by broad-based application of force creating more than six bone *fragments*; cf. *multifragment fracture*

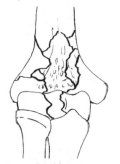

Fig. 103: comminuted fracture

commissure connection

commissurotomy *surgical* dilation of a *stenosed* heart valve

commitment involuntary confinement of a mentally ill person in a hospital

common bile duct main bile duct, which originates at the junction of the *cystic* and the *hepatic* ducts and empties into the *duodenum*

common cold febrile upper respiratory *infection*, usually caused by *viruses*, that resembles a mild case of *influenza*

communis common

compartment space or channel bounded by *fascia*

compartment syndrome impaired circulation caused by an increase in pressure in the muscle fascia compartments, leading to tissue damage (muscle *necrosis*); usually due to bleeding into the muscle below the *fascia* from an injury; see also *fasciotomy*

compatible able to be combined or associated; opp. *incompatible*

compensate to adjust; opp. *decompensate*

compensated adjusted, balanced; opp. *decompensated*

compensation adjustment following a change; opp. *decompensation*

complaint document filed with the court that initiates a lawsuit

complement group of proteins in the blood *serum* that can assist or activate an *antibody*

complement fixation reaction assay used to determine *antigen-antibody reactions* using *complement*; abbr. CFR

complement system special system in an organism's immune defenses that regulates messenger substances in an inflammatory reaction

complexion skin color

compliant adj. of *compliance*; opp. *noncompliant*

complication circumstance that makes a condition worse

component one of the parts constituting a whole

composite mixture, assemblage

compositus composed, put together from parts

compress folded square of gauze to be placed over a wound

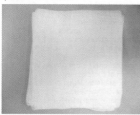

Fig. 104: compress

compression squeezing together

compression bandage pressure bandage used to stop bleeding

compression fracture *fracture* caused by compression of a bone along its long axis

compromise to squeeze shut, close off

compulsion irresistible urge to do something

computed tomography (CT scan) *radiological* examination in which computer-guided sectional images of the body are created; abbr. CT

computerized axial tomography form of radiography that produces cross-sectional images of the body using a computer; abbr. CAT

con- combining form: with; together

concave hollowed out, curved inward; opp. convex

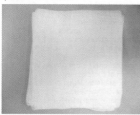

Fig. 105: concave

conception beginning of pregnancy, when the fertilized egg successfully implants in the wall of the *uterus*

concha outer ear; scroll-shaped bone in the nasal cavity

concrement solid mass or formation within a cavity, e.g. stones in the *gallbladder*

condition state of physical health or fitness

conditioning regimen chemotherapy and radiation treatments given over time and prior to stem cell transplantation in order to destroy cancer cells

condom (prophylactic, rubber) rubber sheath to be placed over the *penis* during sexual intercourse to prevent conception and/or protect against sexually transmitted diseases

condom catheter (Texas catheter) *condom*-like *urinal* for males, to which a *urine bag* can be attached for collection of urine

conduit *surgically* created channel-like outlet

condylar plate *osteosynthesis* of a *fracture* at the articular head to neutralize harmful pressure and flexion forces

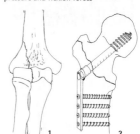

Fig. 106: condylar fracture and repair
1 Condylar fracture 2 Condylar plate

condyle rounded head of a bone that forms a *joint*

condyloma wart growth

condyloma acuminatum textured genital wart caused by *infection* with *papilloma virus*, usually transmitted via sexual intercourse

cone biopsy (conization) removal of a coneshaped tissue sample from the *cervix* for examination

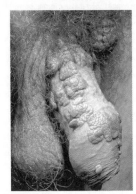

Fig. 107: condyloma acuminatum

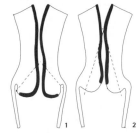

Fig. 108: cone biopsy
1 Cone biopsy in sexually mature female
2 Cone biopsy in menopausal female

cone syndrome radicular compression syndrome due to damage to the *medullary cone* at the level of the 1st to 2nd lumbar vertebrae; usually associated with urinary and bowel *incontinence, saddle block*

anesthesia, and preservation of the *Achilles tendon reflex* (in contrast to *cauda equina syndrome*)

confabulation filling in gaps in memory with fabricated facts and experiences that the person believes to be real

confluent flowing together

congelatio *frostbite*

congenital inborn, present at birth

congenital coxa vara congenital bowed position of both hip joints, which increases as child grows

congenital crus varum congenital unilateral bowing of the lower leg

congenital hip dysplasia disorder of hip joint development resulting in *subluxation* and *dislocation* tendency after birth

congenital megacolon *Hirschsprung's disease*

conglomerate aggregation, cluster

congrade amnesia loss of memory for the time period during an event

coniosis lung disease caused by inhaling dust

coniotomy *(cricothyrotomy)* surgical opening into cricoid and thyroid cartilages

conization *(cone biopsy)* taking of a small amount of tissue for examination

conjoined twins *twins* whose bodies are joined at some point, e.g. the breastbone

conjunctiv– combining form: conjunctiva

conjunctiva mucous membrane of the eye

conjunctival pert. to the *conjunctiva*

conjunctival veins *veins* that transport blood from the *conjunctiva* of the eye to the *superior ophthalmic vein*

conjunctivales, Vv. *venae conjunctivales*

conjunctivitis inflammation of the *conjunctiva*

Conn's syndrome overactivity of the *adrenal cortex* with excessive release of *aldosterone*

connective tissue *tissue* that connects *organs* with their surroundings; present in organ capsules and nerve sheaths, et al.

consent documentation of permission from the patient before any procedure and/ or operation is performed, e.g. transfusion

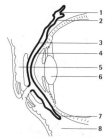

Fig. 109: conjunctiva
1 Upper conjunctival fornix 2 Bulbar conjunctiva 3 Tarsal conjunctiva 4 Cornea 5 Upper lid 6 Lens 7 Lower conjunctival fornix 8 Lower lid

conservative without resorting to *surgery*; opp. *surgical*

consistency texture, solidity

consolidation solidifying; healing esp. of a broken bone

constant continuing, ongoing; opp. *inconstant*

constipated adj. of *constipation*

constipation bowel evacuation disorder with fewer than three stools per week

constitution physical makeup or manifestation

constitutional pert. to the *constitution*

constriction drawing together, tightening

constrictive pericarditis formation of callosities on the *pericardium*, e.g. following *pericarditis*

constructional apraxia see *apraxia*

consult(ation) advice or counsel from one or more additional doctors

consultant physician brought in for a consult

consumption tuberculosis

consumption coagulopathy (disseminated intravascular coagulation) activation of *blood coagulation* within the vessels with increased consumption of *clotting factors* and thrombocytes; abbr. DIC

consumptive pert. to *tuberculosis*

contact infection transmission of an infectious disease through direct contact

contagious catching, transmissible, e.g. *infectious diseases*

contaminate to introduce pathogens or infectious material; opp. *decontaminate*

contaminated pert. to *contamination*; opp. *decontaminated*

contamination introduction of pathogens or infectious material; opp. *decontamination*

continence ability to control bowel or bladder evacuation opp. *incontinence*

continent able to control bowel or bladder evacuation, opp. *incontinent*

continuous regular; opp. *discontinuous*

contra– combining form: against, opposed; opp. *pro-*

contraceptive drug used to prevent conception

contraceptive diaphragm ring with a rubber membrane stretched over it that is inserted into the *vagina* as a barrier method of contraception

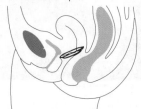

Fig. 110: contraceptive diaphragm

contract to draw or pull together, tighten

contracted kidney *hypoplasia* of the *kidney*

contraction drawing together, tightening; opp. *dilatation*

contracture fibrosis of a joint; limitation in mobility of a joint in a particular direction

contraindicated adj. of *contraindication*; opp. *indicated*

contraindication justification for not performing a medical procedure; opp. *indication*

contralateral on the opposite side of the body

contrary opposed

contrast medium substance used to improve visibility of normally indistinct structures during radiological examination; abbr. *CM*

contrecoup injury to the side of the brain opposite to the site of a trauma, e.g. bleeding in the cerebral cortex on the side of the head opposite to the injury site

controlled release delayed or slow action of a drug

controversial disputed

contusion crushing, bruising

contusion cataract *cataract* resulting from contusion of the eyeball, with a contusion rosette that penetrates into the deeper layers of the lens

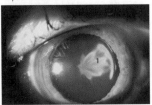

Fig. 111: contusion cataract
1 Contusion rosette

conus cone

conus medullaris lower conical end of the *spinal cord*

convalescence recovery period following an illness

convalescent recovering

converge to move together; opp. *diverge*

convergence turning the bulbar axes inward for near vision

convex curved outward; opp. *concave*

convulsion muscle spasms, e.g. in *epilepsy*

Fig. 112: convex

Coombs' test blood test for detection of *antibodies* to *erythrocytes;* used with *hemolytic anemia,* reactions to a *transfusion,* or as an *antibody* screening test during pregnancy

Cooper scissors surgical scissors with a slight upward curve to the blades

Fig. 113: Cooper scissors [A]

COPD abbr. for *chronic obstructive pulmonary disease;* productive cough and sputum occurring on most days for at least 3 months of each of 2 successive years

coping dealing mentally with a disease and its consequences

copper chemical element; important trace element necessary for formation of red blood cells, et al.; copper is transported and stored in the body by the *protein;* chemical symbol: Cu

copremesis vomiting of fecal material, e.g. due to *ileus*

coprophagy (scatophagy) eating feces, e.g. in dementia

coprostasis fecal impaction, e.g. due to intestinal hypomotility and constipation

cor heart

cor pulmonale enlargement of the right ventricle of the heart due to increased *pulmonary blood pressure*

coracoid process beak-shaped process of the *scapula*

cord blood transplant type of transplant in which stem cells are obtained from the umbilical cord and placenta following birth and subsequently frozen for future use

corium dermis; part of the *cutis*

cornea transparent layer on the front of the eyeball

cornea transparent part of the front of the eyeball

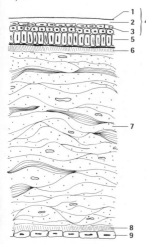

Fig. 114: cornea
1 Lipid layer 2 Fluid layer 3 Mucin layer 4 Film of tears 5 Multilayered epithelium 6 Anterior limiting lamina (Bowman's membrane) 7 Stroma
8 Posterior limiting lamina (Descemet's membrane) 9 Endothelium

corneal reflex (blink reflex) *physiological* polysynaptic *reflex* in which tapping on the *cornea* causes the eyelid to close; mapping: *trigeminal nerve*

corneal ulcer (ulcus corneae) ulcer on the *cornea* of the elye

corona crown, wreath

corona dentis *dental corona*

coronal plane (frontal plane) vertical body plane dividing the body into anterior and posterior portions, e.g. in the context of imaging procedures

coronaris, A. see *coronary artery*

coronary pert. to the *coronary arteries*

coronary angiogram *coronary angiography*

coronary angiography (coronary angiogram) *radiography* of the *coronary arteries* using a contrast medium

coronary arteries *arteries* that supply the heart with oxygen and nutrients

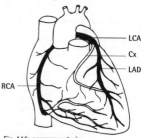

Fig. 115: coronary arteries
LCA Left coronary artery **Cx** Circumflex branch (of LCA) **LAD** Left anterior descending branch (of LCA) **RCA** Right coronary artery

coronary bypass see *bypass*

coronary heart disease clinical manifestation of insufficient blood flow in the *coronary arteries*; abbr. CHD

coronary infarct *myocardial infarction*

coronary sclerosis *arteriosclerosis* of the *coronary arteries*

coronary sinus (sinus coronarius) vein located at the back of the heart; collects blood from the *venae cordis*

coronary spasm spasm of the *coronary arteries*

coronary stenosis narrowing of a *coronary artery*

coronary therapeutic agent drug used to treat *coronary artery* diseases

coronary veins *venae cordis*
corp(o)- combining form: body
corpus body
corpus ciliare *ciliary body*
corpus luteum *yellow body* of the *ovary*
corpus luteum hormone *progesterone*
corpus uteri body of the *uterus*, adjacent to the *cervix*
correlation mutual relationship
cortex outer layer, shell
cortical pert. to a *cortex*
cortical blindness form of blindness caused by disease or injury of the visual cortex in the occipital lobe of the cerebrum
cortical deafness deafness caused by damage to the hearing center of the cerebral cortex
cortical substance of bone bone layer below the periosteum
corticalis cortical substance of bone
cortico- combining form: cortex
corticoid collective term for *hormones* produced in the *adrenal cortex*; types are *mineralocorticoids* and *glucocorticoids*
corticosteroid *hormone* produced in the *adrenal cortex*; main types: *aldosterone* and *cortisol*
corticotropin *adrenocorticotropic hormone*
corticotropin-releasing hormone *hormone* produced by the *hypothalamus* that controls the release of *ACTH* in the *adenohypophysis*; abbr. *CRH*
cortisol *hormone* produced in the *adrenal cortex* (*glucocorticoid*) that influences *carbohydrate* metabolism
cortisone *hormone* with anti-*inflammatory* and detumescent qualities; derived from *cortisol*
Corynebacterium genus of non-*spore*-forming rod-shaped *gram-positive bacteria*
cost- combining form: rib
costa rib
costal nerves nerves of the ribs, innervating the *rectus abdominis muscle* et al.
costal(is) pert. to the ribs
Costen's syndrome *temporomandibular joint syndrome*
costotomy *surgical* division of a *rib*

Coude (catheter) *bladder catheter* with a curved tip for *transurethral* placement, designed for easier insertion into the male *urethra*; see also *Nelaton catheter*

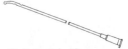

Fig. 116: Coude catheter [C]

counter-incision (counteropening) a second *incision* made on the opposite side in order to improve drainage, e.g. of pus from an *abscess*
counting chamber (hemocytometer) *microscope slide* with an incised grid for counting *cells*, e.g. in blood tests
coupled pulse see *bigemini*
Courvoisier sign painless palpable enlargement of the *gallbladder* in *chronic jaundice*, e.g. due to pancreatic cancer
cover denture special type of dental *prosthesis* for patients with very few remaining teeth; can be used for anchoring
cover test procedure used to test for *strabismus*
cox- combining form: hip
coxa hip

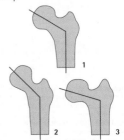

Fig. 117: coxa valga and coxa vara
1 Normal CCD angle 2 Coxa valga 3 Coxa vara

coxa valga deformity resulting from increase in the *caput-collum-diaphysis angle* to greater than 120°; opp. *coxa vara*

coxa vara deformity resulting from decrease in the *caput-collum-diaphysis angle* to less than 120°; opp. *coxa valga*

coxalgia 1) hip pain; 2) nonspecific collective term for painful conditions of the hip joint

coxarthrosis hip joint degeneration due to cartilage wear

coxitis inflammation of the hip joint

CP abbr. *chronic polyarthritis*

CPP abbr. *cerebral perfusion pressure*

crab louse pediculus pubis

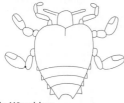

Fig. 118: crab louse

Cramer splint flexible wire ladder splint for immobilization of injured limbs

cramp painful muscle spasm, e.g. in the calf muscle

crani(o)– combining form: skull

cranial 1) pert. to the *skull*; 2) toward the head, upward; opp. *caudal*

cranial base base of the skull, on which the *brain* rests

cranial nerves nonspecific collective term for the 12 paired (except for IV) nerves emerging from the base of the brain:
I. olfactory (*nervus olfactorius*)
II. optic (*nervus opticus*)
III. oculomotor (*nervus oculomotorius*)
IV. trochlear (*nervus trochlearis*)
V. trigeminal (*nervus trigeminus*)
VI. abducens (*nervus abducens*)
VII. facial (*nervus facialis*)
VIII. vestibulocochlear (*nervus vestibulocochlearis*)
IX. glossopharyngeal (*nervus glossopharyngeus*)
X. vagus (*nervus vagus*)
XI. spinal accessory (*nervus accessorius*)
XII. hypoglossal (*nervus hypoglossus*)

cranial sinus vessel located in the *dura mater* that transports blood from the veins in the brain to the *internal jugular vein*

craniotabes softening of the skull, e.g. due to *rickets*

craniotomy *surgical* opening of the skull

cranium skull, bones of the skull

Crea abbr. *creatinine*

C-reactive protein *protein* produced by the liver that activates the body's defense system as a response to *inflammatory* reactions, among other things

creatine kinase *enzyme* involved in metabolic energy production within muscle cells; important clinical laboratory parameter used primarily in testing for *myocardial infarctions* or musculoskeletal diseases, since muscular damage causes the release of the *enzyme* into the blood; abbr. CK; there are three main groups of creatine kinases CK-MB = heart muscle; CK-MM = skeletal muscles; CK-BB = brain and smooth muscles

creatinine clearance measurement of renal excretion of *creatinine* per minute; used for assessing renal function; abbr. C_{Crea}

creatinine end product of muscle metabolism; excreted via the kidneys in urine; important laboratory parameter for assessing renal function; abbr. Crea

credential document showing evidence of qualifications

credentialing process used by healthcare organizations to obtain, verify, assess, and validate previous experience (e.g. licensure, education) or qualifications

Credé's method maneuver for detachment of the *placenta* in cases of *placenta* separation disorders during the *postpartum* period

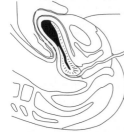

Fig. 119: Credé's method

cremaster muscle abdominal muscle that extends to the *testicles* along with the *spermatic cord*

cremaster reflex *physiological* polysynaptic *reflex* in which stimulation of the inner surface of the *testicle* on that side causes retraction of the thigh; mapping: L2-L3 *dermatome*

crepitation friction between the bone *fragment* ends in a *fracture*

CRH abbr. *corticotropinreleasing hormone*

cricoid cartilage (cartilago cricoidea) lowermost cartilage in the *larynx*, below the *thyroid cartilage*

cricothyrotomy (coniotomy) emergency incision of the *trachea* between the cricoid and thyroid *cartilages*, severing the cricothyroid ligament; employed in acute obstruction of the airway when it is not (or is no longer) possible to perform *intubation*, emergency *bronchoscopy* or *tracheotomy*; see illustration under *tracheotomy*

Crimean Congo hemorrhagic fever *viral hemorrhagic fever*

-crine combining form: secretion

crista iliaca iliac crest

Crohn's disease (enteritis regionalis) *chronic inflammatory* disease of the intestine, usually affecting the lower portions of the *ileum*

cross-examination to question a witness already examined by the opposing side in a trial

cross-infection mutual contagion between two persons with different *infectious diseases*

cross-matching blood test to determine *blood group* and *Rh* factor prior to *transfusion*

cross fracture transverse *fracture* line in a broken bone

crossbite malocclusion of the teeth such that the upper teeth point slightly inward and the lower teeth slightly outward

crosseye *strabismus*

croup life-threatening inflammation of the larynx with danger of asphyxiation, e.g. in *diphtheria*

crowding discrepancy between the size of the jaw and the *teeth*

crown dental procedure for replacing the natural crown of a *tooth* where the tooth can no longer be saved using simple fillings

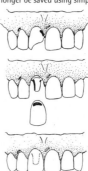

Fig. 120: crown

CRP abbr. *C-reactive protein*

cruciate ligament (ligamentum cruciatum) major ligament in the *knee*

crura pl. of *crus*

crus leg, shin; pl. crura

crush intubation (rapid induction) basal anesthesia method that takes into account an increased risk of *aspiration* (e.g. in *ileus*) during intubation and minimizes the time between reflex loss and *intubation*

crush syndrome *necrosis* and *parenchymal* damage to the liver and kidneys following crushing injury or muscle compression; due to *proteins* released from *hemoglobin* or *myoglobin*, which block the renal *tubules*

crust(a) scab; *secondary efflorescence* caused by dried blood or *secretions*

Crutchfield tongs device used to stabilize *cervical spine fractures*, in which traction is placed on the neck using a device that grips the skull with pins inserted into either side

cry(o)- combining form: cold, frost

cryotherapy treatment with cold

crypt sac in mucosal tissue, e.g. in the *tonsils*

crypt(o)- combining form: hidden

cryptococcosis *mycosis* caused by *Cryptococcus neoformans* that primarily affects immunocompromised persons; may lead to *pneumonia, meningoencephalitis* and *hepatosplenomegaly*

Cryptococcus neoformans type of yeast that causes *cryptococcosis*

cryptorchidism (cryptorchism) malposition or failure of the testicles to descend during embryonic development

CS abbr. *cervical spine*

CSF abbr. *cerebrospinal fluid*

CSF fistula connection between the *CSF space* and the outside, caused by injury to the *meninges*

CSF space see *subarachnoid space*

CT (CT scan) abbr. *computed tomography*

Cu chemical symbol: *copper*

cubit- combining form: elbow

cubitus elbow

cuboid bone one of the *tarsal bones*

cuff inflatable balloon on an *endotracheal tube* for sealing off the *trachea* during ventilation

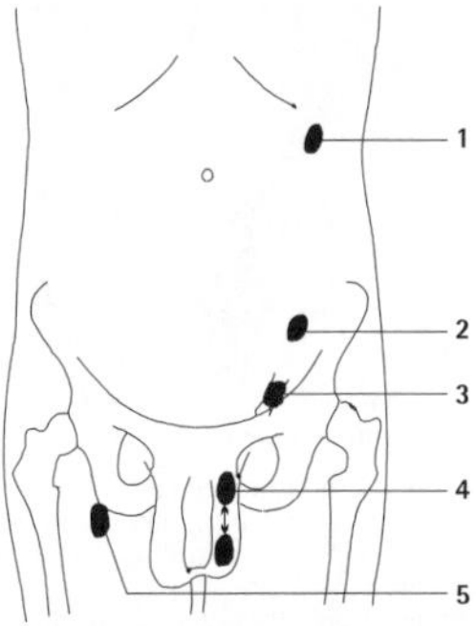

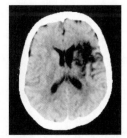

Fig. 121: cryptorchidism (testicular malposition)
1 Position of testis 2 Intraabdominal 3 Inguinal
4 Ectopic femoral 5 Wandering testicle

Fig. 122: computed tomography (head)

cuff pressure monitor device for measuring the cuff pressure of an *endotracheal tube*

cuneiform bone wedge-shaped bone in the ankle joint

CUP abbr. carcinoma of unknown primary [site]; presence of *metastases* of an undetected malignant tumor

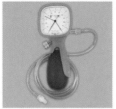

Fig. 123: cuff pressure monitor [N]

cupr- combining form: copper
curable able to be healed; opp. *incurable*
curative healing, bringing about a cure; opp. *palliative*
curettage scraping away, scraping out, scratching down with a *curette*, usually in the context of scraping the inside of the *uterus*

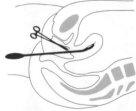

Fig. 124: curettage

curette 1) fenestrated scraping instrument; *surgical* instrument used to scrape off tissue (*curettage*); 2) to scrape out

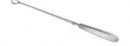

Fig. 125: curette [A]

curvature curved or bent part, e.g. of the stomach
Cushing's disease *Cushing's syndrome*
Cushing's syndrome clinical picture with moon-shaped face, muscle wasting, trunk obesity, osteoporosis, etc.; caused by excess production or increased supply of *glucocorticoid hormones*

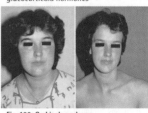

Fig. 126: Cushing's syndrome

-cusis combining form: hearing
cut(an)- combining form: skin
cutaneous pert. to the skin
cutaneous leukocytoclastic angiitis type of *vasculitis* that affects the small *arteries* and *veins* of the skin
cutaneous nerves sensory innervation of the skin; see Fig. 127
cutaneous ureterostomy *surgically* created diversion of the *ureters* through the skin
cutis skin; *epidermis* and *corium*
cuvette small glass vessel for specimens, e.g. for lab work
CVC abbr. *central venous catheter*
CVP abbr. *central venous pressure*
CVVH abbr. continuous venovenous hemofiltration
cyan(o)- combining form: blue
cyanocobalamin (vitamin B_{12}) a water-soluble *vitamin* with an important role in metabolic processes and *erythropoiesis*; vitamin B_{12} deficiency can lead to *pernicious anemia* et al.
cyanosis bluish discoloration of skin and/or lips caused by decreased amount of oxygen in the blood

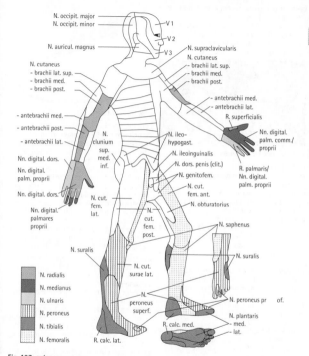

Fig. 127: cutaneous nerves

N. occipit. major
N. occipit. minor
N. auricul. magnus
V 1
V 2
V 3
N. supraclavicularis
N. cutaneus
- brachii lat. sup.
- brachii med.
- brachii post.
N. cutaneus
- brachii lat. sup.
- brachii med.
- brachii post.
- antebrachii med.
- antebrachii lat.
R. superficialis
- antebrachii med.
- antebrachii post.
- antebrachii lat.
Nn. digital. palm. comm./ proprii
N. clunium sup. med. inf.
N. ileo-hypogast.
N. ileoinguinalis
N. dors. penis (clit.)
N. genitofem.
R. palmaris/ Nn. digital. palm. proprii
Nn. digital. dors.
Nn. digital. palm. proprii
N. cut. fem. ant.
N. obturatorius
Nn. digital. dors.
Nn. digital. palmares proprii
N. cut. fem. lat.
N. cut. fem. post.
N. saphenus
N. suralis
N. cut. surae lat.
N. suralis
N. radialis
N. medianus
N. ulnaris
N. peroneus
N. tibialis
N. femoralis
N. peroneus superf.
N. peroneus pr of.
N. plantaris
- med.
- lat.
R. calc. lat.
R. calc. med.

cyanotic pert. to *cyanosis*

cycle regular recurrence, e.g. *menstruation*

cyclic pert. to a *cycle; circular*

cyclitis *inflammation* of the *ciliary body* of the eye

cycloplegia paralysis of the *ciliary muscle* in the eye, with *accommodation* disorders and *mydriasis*

cyclotron particle accelerator

C

cylinder pathological component of *urine sediment* in kidney disease

cyst hollow fluid-filled saclike structure of varying size; true cysts (lined with *epithelium*) are distinguished from pseudocysts (surrounded with *connective tissue*)

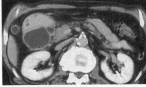

Fig. 128: pancreas, pseudocyst

cyst(o)– combining form: bladder or cyst

cystadenoma *adenoma* with cyst-like components

cystectomy removal of a *cyst* or of the *bladder*

cystic duct occlusion blockage of the *cystic duct*, e.g. by a *gallstone*

cystic fibrosis (mucoviscidosis) congenital metabolic disorder that leads to thickening of the mucus in the respiratory tract, among other things

cystic vein *vein* in the *gallbladder* that joins the *portal vein*

cysticercosis disease caused by infestation with *larvae* of the pork tapeworm

cysticotomy (choledochotomy) *surgical incision* of the *cystic duct*

cystitis *inflammation* of the *bladder*

cystocele *prolapse* of the *bladder*

cystogram cystography

cystography (cystogram) *radiography* of the *bladder* using a *contrast medium*

cystopyelitis *inflammation* of the *bladder* and *renal pelvis*

cystopyelonephritis *inflammation* of the *bladder* and *renal pelvis* and *kidneys*

cystoscope flexible *endoscope* for performing *cystoscopy*

cystoscopy *endoscopy* of the *bladder* using a *cystoscope*

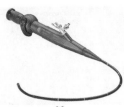

Fig. 129: cystoscope [F]

cyto– combining form: cell

cytochrome P450 enzymes group of enzymes in all cells of the body, esp. the liver and intestine; they may be responsible for the metabolism of approximately 75% of all drugs; many drugs affect or are affected by the cytochrome P450 enzymes, e.g. grapefruit juice inhibits the affects of many neurologic drugs

cytodiagnostics *microscopic* examination of *cells*, usually o7btained from a *smear*, e.g. a *Pap smear*

cytokeratin 19 fragments important *tumor marker* primarily for non-small cell *bronchial* or *bladder* cancer; abbr. CYFRA 211

cytokine messenger substance formed by the *cells* that influences the functions of other cells, e.g. interleukin, interferon

cytological pert. to *cytology*

cytology study of the structure and function of body *cells*

cytomegalovirus *DNA virus* that causes *cytomegalovirus infection*, as well as other infections, e.g. *hepatitis* or *retinitis*, and a clinical picture resembling *mononucleosis*; abbr. CMV

cytomegalovirus infection (CMV infection) *infectious disease* caused by the *cytomegalovirus* that leads to severe *liver* and *brain* damage in the *fetus*, although the mother may not show any signs of disease; transmitted via the *placenta*, *transfusion*, *smear infection* and *droplet infection*

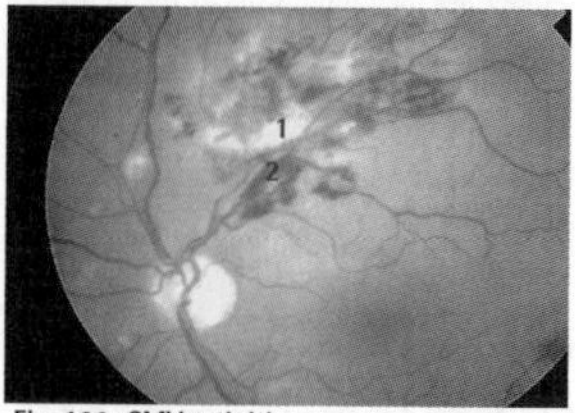

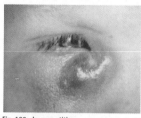

Fig. 130: CMV retinitis

-cytopenia combining form: deficiency of *cells*; opp. *cytosis*

cytoplasm contents of a *cell* apart from the *nucleus*; contains numerous *organelles* and fluid

cytoprotective protective of the *cells*; drug used to protect *cells*, e.g. during treatment of malignant neoplastic disease with *cytostatics*

-cytosis combining form: multiplication of *cells*; opp. *cytopenia*

cytostatic 1) drug used to inhibit growth of *cells*, e.g. for treatment of malignant neoplastic diseases; 2) inhibiting the growth of *cells*

cytotoxic damaging to *cells*

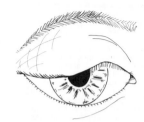

Fig. 131: acute dacryoadenitis

Fig. 132: dacryocystitis

D

Dacron prosthesis vascular *prosthesis* made of synthetic material, usually used in the *aortoiliac* area

dacry(o)- combining form: tears

dacry(o)adenitis *inflammation* of a lacrimal gland with redness and swelling of the gland next to the upper lid, which gives the lid an indented shape

dacryocystitis *bacterial* infection of the lacrimal sac

dacryostenosis *stenosis* of the tear ducts

dactyl- combining form: finger

dakryon (lacrima) *tear*

dashboard injury *trauma* resulting from a knee colliding with the dashboard during a car accident

DAT abbr. dementia, *Alzheimer* type

database collection of related data, usually stored in a computer

dB abbr. *decibel*

DBS abbr. deep brain stimulation

D/C discharge

D/D abbr. *differential diagnosis*

D-dimers by products of the degradation of *fibrinogen* and *fibrin* that appear in the blood in connection with *thromboses* or *emboli* and can be measured for *diagnostic* purposes

DDS abbr. *dialysis disequilibrium syndrome*

de- combining form: from, away, down

deadspace ventilation *insufficient* respiration or ventilation in which no gas exchange can take place in the alveoli due to low respiratory volume

deaf–mutism congenital or acquired deafness leading to loss of the ability to speak

débridement severing of adhesions or removal of superficial *necroses* in the context of *surgical wound* cleaning

decapitation removal of the head

decerebrate posturing observed in brain stem compression; the arms are extended and internally rotated and the legs are extended with the feet pointing down (plantar flexion)

decerebration removal or disabling of the brain

decibel unit of measurement for sound (loudness); abbr. dB

decidua mucous membrane that lines the *uterus* during pregancany; one of the *fetal membranes*

decompensate undergo *decompensation*; opp. *compensate*

decompensated not adjusted; opp. *compensated*

decompensation inability to adjust or balance out; opp. *compensation*

decompression reduction of pressure

decontaminated cleansed; opp. *contaminated*

decontamination cleansing; opp. *contamination*

decubital pert. to a *decubitus*

decubitus (decubitus ulcer) pressure sore; damage to the skin from the effects of continued local pressure, e.g. when a bedridden person does not change position often enough; classified into four levels according to *NPUAP*, which replaced the Seiler scale in 1989:
stage 1: decubitus with sharply circumscribed skin redness and intact skin; darker-skinned people may exhibit skin discoloration; other signs may include edema, thickening or local hyperthermia of the skin;
stage 2: decubitus with partial loss of the

epidermis, including parts of the dermis; the surface damage is usually in the form of vesicles,
stage 3: decubitus with damage to all three skin layers (epidermis, dermis and subcutis) down to the fasciae, which are not affected, see Fig. 134-137

deep breathing and coughing intervention used to improve respiratory function, esp. after surgery

deep femoral vein deep vein in the thigh consisting of branches of the *femoral vein*

deep flexor muscle of the fingers muscle that flexes the distal phalanges of the fingers; *innervation: anterior interosseous* and *ulnar nerve* disease

deep peroneal nerve *nerve* that innervates the *long extensor muscle of the great toe, anterior tibial muscle* and *long extensor muscle of the toes*

defecation evacuation of the bowels

defibrillation treatment of *ventricular fibrillation*, usually with electroshocks from a *defibrillator*, but also mechanically or with drugs

defibrillator device for inducing *defibrillation* or *cardioversion* with electroshocks; abbr. defib

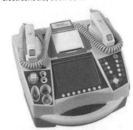

Fig. 133: defibrillator [M]

deficit deficiency, loss, failure to function; see also *prolonged reversible ischemic neurological deficit* (PRIND)

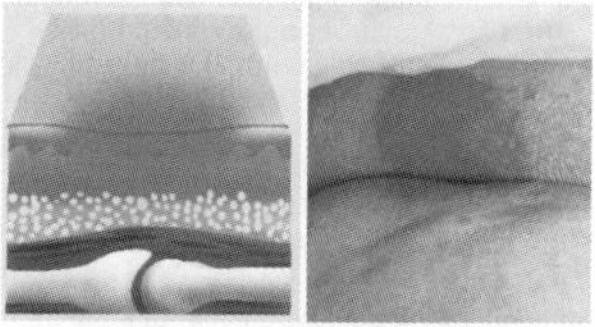

Fig. 134: stage 1 decubitus [E]

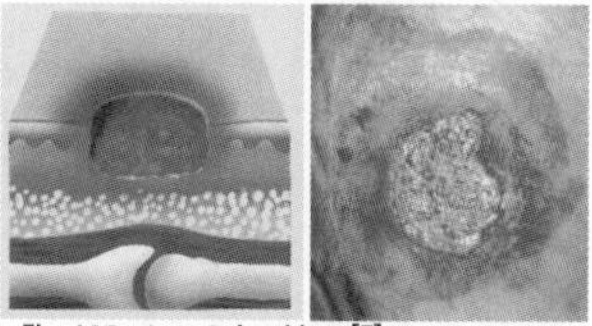

Fig. 135: stage 2 decubitus [E]

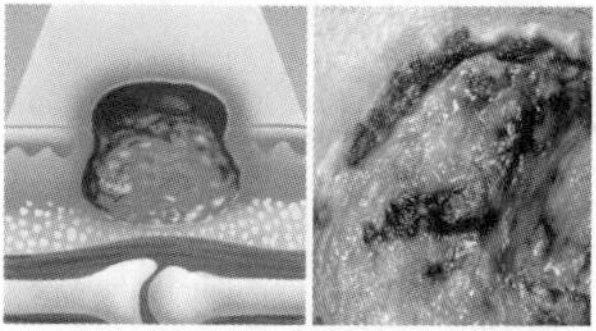

Fig. 136: stage 3 decubitus [E]

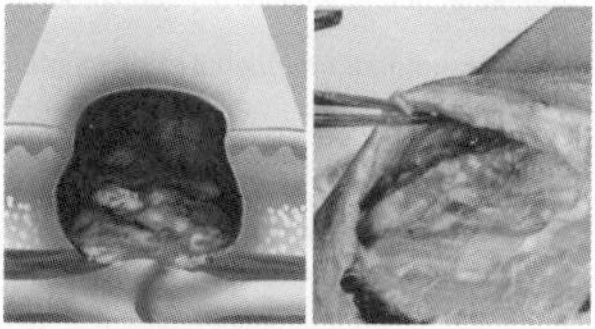

Fig. 137: stage 4 decubitus [E]

defloration rupture of the *hymen* during first sexual intercourse

deformation change in shape

degeneration deterioration, atrophy, degradation, devolution

dehiscence separation of any part or all of a suture line or wound during the healing process

dehydration excessive loss of body water, e.g. due to increased use of diuretic agents; opp. *hyperhydration*

dehydration, hypertonic *hypertonic dehydration*

dehydration, hypotonic *hypotonic dehydration*

dehydration, isotonic *isotonic dehydration*

déjà vu illusion of memory in which one believes one has already experienced or seen something, e.g. when fatigued or in *psychosis*

delayed ejaculation late or absent ejaculation

delayed puberty delayed sexual maturation, e.g. due to *estrogen* deficiency; opp. *precocious puberty*

deleterious harmful, damaging

deletion loss, destruction

delirium form of *psychosis* with decreased level of consciousness, confusion, restlessness and *hallucinations*, e.g. due to *head injury*, alcohol or drug withdrawal

delirium tremens acute psychotic state of severe psychomotor agitation due to withdrawal from alcohol or other addictive drug

delta wave extra wave preceding the *QRS complex* in an *ECG*; seen in *Wolff-Parkinson-White syndrome*

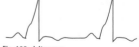

Fig. 138: delta wave

deltoid muscle (musculus deltoideus) muscle on the outer surface of the shoulder joint, which raises the upper arm to the horizontal; *innervation: axillary nerve*

delusion disorder of thought processes marked by loss of contact with reality and *subjective* delusional conviction

demarcation boundary between healthy and diseased *tissue*, e.g. in *frostbite* or *inflammation*

demented cognitively impaired

dementia acquired cognitive impairment due to disease or injury to the brain

demi- combining form: half

demineralization loss of minerals, e.g. decalcification of bones

denaturation change in the structure of *proteins* through chemical or physical processes, e.g. heating

dendrite branching process of a *neuron*

dengue fever (breakbone fever) *hemorrhagic fever* caused by an *arbovirus*, usually transmitted by *Aedes aegypti* mosquitoes

dens tooth; pl. dentes

dens axis (odontoid process) "tooth" on the second vertebra

dens caninus (canine tooth) cuspid tooth with a single root whose function is transfixing food; there is one in each quadrant (see dental chart)

dens incisivus incisor tooth with a single root whose function is biting off pieces of food; there are two in each quadrant

dens molaris molar tooth with in the buccal area for grinding food; there are three in each quadrant, one of which is a wisdom tooth, each with two or three roots

dens premolaris anterior grinding tooth in the buccal area; located in front of the *molars*

dens serotinus wisdom tooth with one to three roots; one of the *molars*

density *tissue* density, as related to imaging procedures such as x-rays

dent- combining form: tooth

dental pert. to the teeth

dental calculus deposits of salts on and between the *teeth*; usually occurs in the lower jaw

dental chart internationally recognized two-digit scheme for numbering the *teeth*, in which the first digit indicates the quadrant

in the jaw (upper right = 1; upper left = 2; lower left = 3; lower right = 4) and the second indicates the tooth; Roman numerals are used for the *primary dentition*

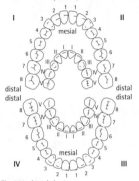

Fig. 139: dental chart
I Right maxillary quadrant **II** Left maxillary quadrant **III** Left mandibular quadrant **IV** Right mandibular quadrant

dental corona portion of the *tooth* visible within the mouth, showing either a cutting or grinding surface according to the type of tooth

dental fluorosis disorder of *dental enamel* formation due to long-term overexposure to *fluoride*

dental granuloma *granuloma* of the dental root

dental implant tooth replacement that is anchored in the jawbone

dental neck (collum dentis) neck of a tooth; the zone between the *crown* and *root*

dental periosteum *periosteum* of the dental root, which anchors and cushions the *tooth* in the dental *alveolus*

dental root (radix dentis) portion of the tooth that is concealed inside the jawbone and thus must be examined by x-ray

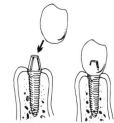

Fig. 140: dental implant

dentes pl. of *dens*
dentin part of the tooth enclosing the *pulp*, covered by the *enamel* towards the *crown* and by the *cementum* toward the root; it develops from the *ectoderm*
dentitio difficilis difficult eruption of the teeth, usually affecting the *wisdom teeth*
dentition 1) permanent dentition of adults (32 teeth); 2) teething; process by which the teeth break through the gums

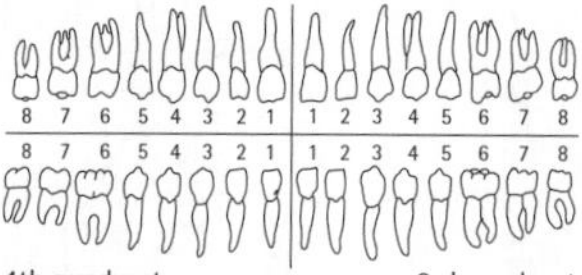

Right   Left
1st quadrant   2nd quadrant

8 7 6 5 4 3 2 1 | 1 2 3 4 5 6 7 8
8 7 6 5 4 3 2 1 | 1 2 3 4 5 6 7 8

4th quadrant   3rd quadrant
Fig. 141: permanent dentition

deoxyribonucleic acid molecule present in the *cell nucleus* that contains complete genetic information; abbr. DNA
depersonalization syndrome *neurotic* disorder of self-concept, marked by the feeling of being detached from one's own personality and body
depigmentation loss of the natural skin coloration due to disease

depilation hair removal
depression pathological state of dejection characterized by a feeling of (emotional) numbness, reduced sense of self-worth or others' worth, psychomotor and thought inhibition, etc.
depressive adj. of *depression*
derivative substance derived from a chemical source substance; usually associated with drugs
derm(at)– combining form: skin
derma skin
dermatics drugs to treat diseases of the skin
dermatitis *inflammation* of the skin
dermatitis solaris *sunburn*
dermatologic(al) pert. to *dermatology*
dermatologist specialist in *dermatology*
dermatology study of skin diseases
dermatome 1) device for creating a *mesh graft* (Fig. 142); 2) sensory landmarks on the skin to localize nerve root and spinal cord lesions, see Fig. 143

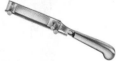

Fig. 142: dermatome [A]

dermatomyositis *poliomyositis* with skin involvement; abbr. DM
dermatophytes collective term for fungi that cause superficial *mycoses*, e.g. *tinea*
dermatoscope small illuminated *microscope* for examination of skin changes, that can be placed directly on the patient's skin, see Fig. 144
dermoid 1) resembling skin; 2) *cystic* germ cell tumor that can contain hair, skin or teeth
Desault's apparatus bandage for immobilization of the shoulder and elbow joints after *reduction* of a *dislocated* shoulder
Descemet's membrane posterior basal membrane of the *cornea*

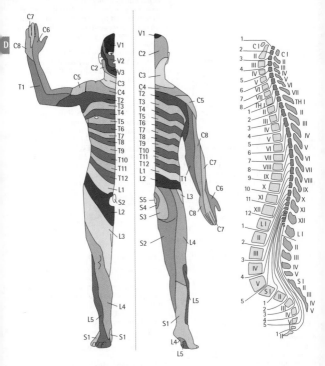

Fig. 143: sensory dermatomes

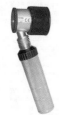

Fig. 144: dermatoscope [H]

descendens moving downward; opp. *ascendens*

descensus (descent) falling, dropping down

descensus uteri prolapse of the *uterus*, e.g. due to weak pelvic floor muscles

Deschamps needle *surgical* instrument with a loop at the tip that can be used to *ligate* blood vessels, etc.

Fig. 145: Deschamps needle [A]

desensitization process by which the body's *immune system* is trained to overcome an *allergy* through administration of small amounts of the *allergen*; opp. *sensitization*

desensitize to treat by *desensitization*

-desis combining form: stiffening; attachment; binding

desm- combining form: band, ligament

desmoid slow-growing *connective tissue* tumor

desquamation flaking of the uppermost layer of the skin

detergent substance that reduces the surface tension of water, e.g. laundry soap

determination establishing the qualities or identity of an object or event

detritus *cell* or *tissue* debris

detrusor vesicae muscle (musculus detrusor vesicae) muscle in the wall of the *bladder* that enables emptying of the bladder

detumescence shrinkage of a swelling or of engorged tissue

deviation turning away from the regular standard or course

dext(r)- combining form: right (side); opp. *sinist(r)-***dexter** on the right side; opp. *sinister*

dextrose *glucose*

di(plo)- combining form: two, double

dia- combining form: through; between; completely

diabetes insipidus reduced ability of the kidneys to concentrate urine due to reduced renal availability or production of *ADH*

diabetes mellitus (diabetes) hereditary or acquired chronic metabolic disorder caused by *insulin* deficiency; abbr. DM

diabetic coma coma caused by *hypo-* or *hyperglycemia* associated with uncontrolled *diabetes mellitus*

diagnosis identification of a health condition; pl. diagnoses

diagnostic pert. to *diagnosis*

diagnostics 1) entirety of all measures taken to diagnose an illness; 2) drugs or medical devices used to make a *diagnosis*

dialysate fluid used in *dialysis*; flows along a *semipermeable* membrane in order to remove urophanic substances from the body

dialysis (hemodialysis) blood filtration for renal insufficiency et al. using a shunt or a dialysis catheter; removal from the blood of substances to be excreted in the urine on the reverse flow principle through a semipermeable membrane; in addition, fluid may also be withdrawn from the body if there is a physical pressure gradient (ultrafiltration); abbr. HD; *peritoneal* **dialysis:** catheter is inserted into peritoneal cavity and a dialysate solution is allowed to flow into and then out of the peritoneal cavity space; the exchange cycle and type of solution vary from patient to patient; can also be performed in the home

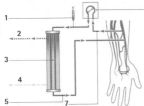

Fig. 146: dialysis [D]
1 Anticoagulant 2 Dialysis fluid 3 Dialyzer
4 Fresh dialysis fluid 5 Blood to patient
6 Blood pump 7 Blood from patient

dialysis disequilibrium (disequilibrium syndrome) cerebral symptoms resulting from dialysis performed too quickly, with delayed *brain edema*; abbr. DDS

dialysis encephalopathy *progressive fatal demential syndrome* that can occur after *dialysis* lasting over a year

diameter distance from one side of an object to the other, measured through its center

diaphanoscopy examination of a body part using transillumination, e.g. of the maxillary sinus

diaphragm 1) septum between individual *organs* or body parts; 2) dome-shaped muscle separating the thorax and abdomen; 3) a barrier method of contraception (contraceptive diaphragm)

diaphragmatic pert. to the *diaphragm*

diaphyseal pert. to the *diaphysis*

diaphyseal fracture isolated fracture of the shaft of a bone; opp. *intraarticular fracture*

diaphysis shaft or middle portion of a long bone; cf. *epiphysis* and *metaphysis*

diaplacental via the *placenta*

diarrhea liquid or unformed feces

diastasis separation of body parts, e.g. the abdominal muscles

diastasis recti separation of the straight anterior abdominal muscles, e.g. during pregnancy or due to *connective tissue* weakness

diastema space or fissure, e.g. between teeth

diastole cardiac muscle relaxation phase; opp. *systole*

diastolic pert. to the *diastole*; opp. *systolic*

diathesis predisposition or tendency to disease

DIC abbr. disseminated intravascular coagulation; see *consumption coagulopathy*

didym– combining form: testicles

didymitis *orchitis*

didymus *testicle*; pl. didymi

diencephalon interbrain; section of the brain located between the *cerebrum* and the *brain stem* with important *hormonal* and *autonomic* functions

diet eating plan tailored to the body's nutritional needs

Diff abbr. *differential blood count*

differential blood count blood smear to determine the number, type and composition of *leukocytes* (*granulocytes lymphocytes monocytes*); abbr. Diff

differential diagnosis distinguishing one disease from another similar one; abbr. D/D

diffuse 1) to penetrate or pass through; 2) without clear boundaries; opp. *circumscribed*

diffusion intermixture of materials in order to achieve equal concentration

digestion process by which enzymes break down a substance, e.g. food in the digestive tract

digestive system alimentary tract from the mouth to the *anus*

digit finger or toe

digital examination examination by palpating with a finger, e.g. *prostate* exam

digital subtraction angiography *angiography* in which a *native image* is derived from x-rays created using *contrast medium*, such that an isolated image of the vessels results; abbr. DSA

digitus pedis (daktylos) toe; pl. digiti pedis; abbr. D

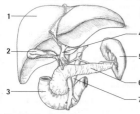

Fig. 147: digestive system
1 Liver (hepar, jecur) 2 Gallbladder (vesica fellea)
3 Duodenum 4 Portal vein 5 Spleen 6 Pancreas
7 Aorta

dilatate to enlarge an existing hollow
structure
dilatation enlargement, typically of an
existing hollow structure; opp. *contraction,
constriction*
dilation stage (first stage of labor) phase of
childbirth from the first *contractions* to
complete dilation of the *cervix*

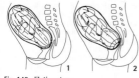

Fig. 148: dilation stage
1 Non-dilated cervix 2 Dilated cervix

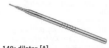

Fig. 149: dilator [A]

dilator 1) muscle that expands an organ, e.g.
the pupil; 2) instrument for enlarging a
cavity

dilution thinning, weakening; attenuation
Dinamap automatic *sphygmomanometer*
that measures *systolic* and *diastolic* blood
pressure, *mean arterial pressure* and *pulse
rate* over a given time interval

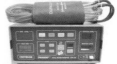

Fig. 150: Dinamap

diopter measure of refractive power of the
lens of the eye; abbr. *dpt*
diphtheria *infectious disease* caused by the
toxins produced by the pathogen
Corynebacterium diphtheriae, which can
lead to *croup*; transmitted mainly via
droplet or *smear infection*
diplopia double vision
dips– combining form: drink(ing)
dis– combining form: apart, between
discharge planning multidisciplinary
activities aimed at providing continuity of
patient care after hospital discharge;
process begins on admission
discontinuous interrupted; opp. *continuous*
discordance conflict, lack of agreement
discordant in conflict
discus disk
discus intervertebralis *intervertebral disk*
disinfect to destroy pathogenic organisms
disinfectant substance used to destroy
pathogenic microorganisms
disinfection *hygienic* measures taken to
destroy pathogenic microorganisms
disk prolapse (*disk protrusion, herniated
disk, nucleus pulposus prolapse*) rupture of
the *anulus fibrosus* with prolapse of the
inner tissues of the disk, usually due to
degene-ration in the *cervical* or *lumbar
spine*; abbr. DP
disk protrusion 1) *disk prolapse;*
2) protrusion of the anulus fibrosus
dislocated displaced, out of position

dislocatio ad latus *lateral dislocation*
dislocatio ad longitudinem *longitudinal dislocation*
dislocatio ad peripheram *peripheral dislocation*
dislocation displacement, malposition
dislocation fracture *fracture* in which the adjacent bone or bone fragments are dislocated

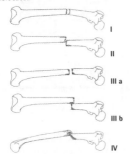

Fig. 151: dislocation fracture
I Angular dislocation II Lateral dislocation
IIIa Longitudinal dislocation with distraction
IIIb Longitudinal dislocation with contraction
IV Peripheral dislocation

disposable catheter *catheter* that is used only once to collect urine from the bladder, e.g. to obtain a specimen; opp. *indwelling catheter*
disobliteration reopening of an *occluded* or *stenosed* vessel
disorientation confusion as to time place and/or identity
disposed liable, having a tendency
disposition 1) tendency to develop disease; 2) behavior, mood
dissection cutting apart, separation of tissues or parts
disseminated intravascular coagulation *consumption coagulopathy*; abbr. DIC

disseminated widespread, scattered
dissemination spreading, scattering distribution
dissociated separated, split
dissociation separation, parting; opp. *association*
distal distant (from the trunk); opp. *proximal*
distension dislocation *dislocation* due to expansion of the joint capsule, usually caused by joint effusion
distillation condensation of a liquid that has been heated and converted to steam
distortion 1) artifacts seen in x-ray films; 2) negative misinterpretation of the truth
distraction pulling apart bone *fragments* in a *fracture*, e.g. using a traction bandage
diuresis excretion of urine
diuretic 1) drug used to promote excretion of urine; 2) pert. to *diuresis*
diver's paralysis *(caisson disease)* decompression syndrome from nitrogen bubbles in a diver's tissues
diverge to move apart; opp. converge
divergence deviation of the eyes from their normal parallel position, e.g. in *strabismus*
diverticulitis *inflammation* of the wall of a *diverticulum*
diverticulosis presence of multiple *diverticula*, usually in the large intestine
diverticulum protrusion of the wall of a hollow organ, e.g. the intestine or esophagus; pl. diverticuli
DM abbr. *diabetes mellitus*
DNA abbr. *deoxyribonucleic acid*
DNA virus virus that uses *DNA* as its genetic material
DOA abbr. dead on arrival
dolicho– combining form: narrow
doll's eyes see *oculocephalic reflex*
dolor pain
dolor– combining form: pain
dominant predominating, prevailing, e.g. in relation to an inherited trait; opp. *recessive*
Donati suture special *surgical* suturing technique for closing a wound
donor one who donates blood, tissue or an organ for transplantation

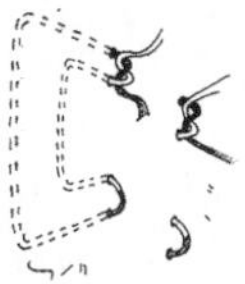

Fig. 152: Donati suture

dopamine circulatory acting *hormone*; important *neurotransmitter* in the *autonomic nervous system*; one of the *catecholamines*

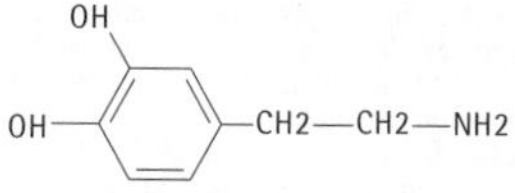

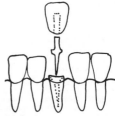

Fig. 153: dopamine

doping use of *anabolic* agents or other substances to improve physical performance

Doppler sonogram *Doppler sonography*

Doppler sonography (Doppler) special examination with *ultrasound*, e.g. to measure flow velocities in the blood

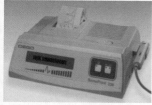

Fig. 154: Doppler sonography [J]

dorsal toward the back, backwards; opp. *ventral*

dorsal muscles collective term for the back muscles

dorsal root ganglion (spinal ganglion, intervertebral ganglion) *ganglion* located in the intervertebral spaces of the spine at the dorsal root of a *spinal nerve*

dorsales linguae, Vv. *venae dorsales linguae*

dorsalis pedis, A. *arteria dorsalis pedis*

dorsi, Mm. *musculi dorsi*

dorsum back of the body

dosage *dose(s)* of a drug or radiation administered within a given time period

dose amount of medication or radiation administered at one time

dosimeter device for measuring radiation output, e.g. x-rays

Douglas' cul-de-sac (pouch of Douglas, Douglas' pouch) space between the *rectum* and *uterus*

Douglas pain specific type of pain during rectal examination; occurs with *retrocecal appendicitis*

dowel crown pin placed into a root canal for the purpose of providing retention for a crown

Fig. 155: dowel crown

Down syndrome (trisomy 21) mental retardation and physical disorders caused by the presence of an extra *chromosome*

dpt abbr. *diopter*; *diphtheria/pertussis/tetanus*

drain 1) to draw fluids out of the body (see also *drainage*; 2) a rubber tube inserted into the body for this purpose

drainage *drain*

drawer test test to assess the stability of the cruciate ligaments in the knee joint

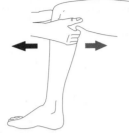

Fig. 156: drawer test

dressing forceps *surgical* instrument used for holding swabs, passing *sterile* instruments or opening *abscesses*, among other tasks

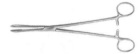

Fig. 157: dressing forceps [A]

Dressler's syndrome *immunological* complication of *myocardial infarction* with formation of *antibodies* against the cardiac muscle *cells* occurring 10-20 days after the *infarction*

DRG abbr. diagnosis related group; code used to insurance companies for reimbursement

drom- combining form: running

dromotropic affecting cardiac conduction velocity; positive dromotropic: increased conduction velocity; negative dromotropic: decreased conduction velocity; cf. *inotropic, bathmotropic, chronotropic*

droplet infection transmission of pathogens through coughing, sneezing or speaking

dropped hand (wrist drop, carpoptosis) typical hand position in *radial nerve* damage

dropped foot inability to dorsiflex the foot because of peroneal nerve damage

drug substance that affects the body's functions, used for medicinal or recreational purposes

dry pleurisy "dry" form of *pleurisy*, e.g. in *pneumonia*; opp. *exudative pleurisy*

DSA abbr. *digital subtraction angiography*

DTR abbr. deep tendon reflex

duct- 1) combining form: duct, canal; 2) vessel, canal

ductus arteriosus *Botalli's duct*

ductus Botalli *Botalli's duct*

ductus choledochus *common bile duct*

ductus cysticus (cystic duct) duct leading out of the *gallbladder*, emptying into the *common bile duct*

ductus deferens *spermatic duct*

ductus hepaticus *hepatic duct*

ductus nasolacrimalis *nasolacrimal duct*

ductus pancreaticus *pancreatic duct*

ductus thoracicus thoracic duct

dumping syndrome digestive and circulatory disorders due to excessively rapid emptying of a *surgically* reduced stomach

duoden- combining form: duodenum

duodenal pert. to the *duodenum*

duodenal atresia congenital, usually complete obstruction of one or more sections of the small intestine, with or without interruption in its continuity

duodenal ulcer (ulcus duodeni) *ulcer* in the *duodenum*, usually leading to *hunger pains* in the epigastrium

duodenum section of the *small intestine* between the pylorus and the *jejunum*

Duplay's disease (periarthritis humeroscapularis, frozen shoulder) collective term for painful restriction of shoulder movement, usually in *abduction*

duplex 1) double; 2) *duplex sonography*

duplex sonogram *duplex sonography*

duplex sonography (*duplex sonogram*) combined *ultrasound* examination consisting of *Doppler sonography* plus a *B scan*, which supplements the Doppler results with a color image of flow patterns within the body, e.g. blood flow in the heart where valve damage is suspected

duplication presence of two organs rather than one; see also *renal duplication, ureter fissus, ureter duplex*

dura mater hard outer membrane of the *brain* and *spinal cord*

dural pert. to the *dura mater*

dural veins *venae meningeae*

DVT (deep vein thrombosis) venous blood clot with an affinity for the lower leg and thigh

dynamometer device for measuring the contractile strength of muscles that functions on the principle of mechanical deformation

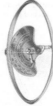

Fig. 158: dynamometer [H]

–dynia combining form: pain

dysacusis (dysacousis, dysacousia) hearing impairment

dysarthria speech disorder with poor articulation

dysautonomia functional disorders of the mind and internal organs (e.g. *cardiovascular* or *gastrointestinal* complaints) with no *organic* cause, due to over- or underactivity of the *autonomic nervous system*

dysbacteria atypical populations of *bacteria* in the *intestinal flora*

dysbasia difficulty in walking

dysentery *infectious disease* caused by *bacteria* (e.g. *Shigellas*) or *amebas,* leading to *inflammation* of the intestinal mucosa with severe diarrhea; mainly transmitted

from human to human by *smear infection* or in contaminated food and water

dysesthesia abnormal sensations triggered by touch

dysfunction impaired action or function

dysgenesis abnormal development of an *organ* or part

dysgnathia abnormal position of the teeth due to jaw abnormalities; opp. *eugnathia*; see also *prognathism, progenia*

dysgraphia inability to write normally

dyskinesia painful muscle cramps, e.g. in the facial muscles as a side effect of *psychotropic drugs*

dyslalia stammering; speech impairment with substitution or inability to pronounce certain sounds or combinations

dyslexia isolated reading and writing disorder with normal overall *intelligence*

dysmelia *congenital* deformity or absence of limbs

dysmenorrhea painful cramps shortly before and during *menstruation,* usually in girls and young women

dysnomia inability to find words or name objects

dyspareunia difficulties during sexual intercourse, e.g. due to pain

dyspepsia digestive disorder, usually functional, marked by gas and bloating

dysphagia painful swallowing disorder

dysphonia difficulty in speaking, including the production of sounds

dysplasia malformation

dysplastic pert. to *dysplasia*

dyspnea difficulty in breathing

dyspneic pert. to *dyspnea*

dysprosody disorder of speech rhythms

dystelectasis diminished ventilation in a part of the lung

dystonia involuntary phasic or *tonic* muscle *contractions* that lead to abnormal movements or malpositions, e.g. in *neurological* diseases

dystopic kidney kidney located in an atypical place (e.g. in the minor pelvis) and usually abnormally small

dystrophy defective nutrition
dysuria difficult, often painful urination
dysuric pert. to *dysuria*

E

e(x)– combining form: out of
E. coli abbr. *Escherichia coli*
ear paired organ of auditory perception, consisting of the external, middle and inner ear

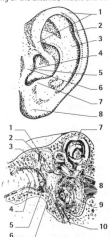

Fig. 159: ear
I **External ear** 1 Helix 2 Scapha 3 Ant(i)helix
4 External auditory meatus 5 Cavum conchae
6 Tragus 7 Antitragus 8 Earlobe
II **Middle and inner ear** 1 Stirrup (stapes)
2 Anvil (incus) 3 Hammer (malleus) 4 External
auditory meatus 5 Eardrum 6 Tympanic cavity
7 Vestibular organ 8 Vestibulocochlear nerve
9 Cochlea 10 Auditory tube

ear forceps *forceps* with curved arms

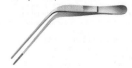

Fig. 160: ear forceps [A]

ear infection *otitis media*
ear speculum interchangeable tip for an
otoscope for insertion into the external
auditory canal
eardrum membrane between the external
auditory canal and the middle ear cavity,
which transmits sound waves directly onto
the ossicles

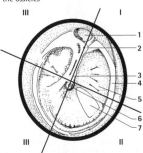

Fig. 161: eardrum
I Anterior superior quadrant II Anterior inferior
quadrant III Posterior inferior quadrant IV Posterior
superior quadrant 1 Pars flaccida 2 Short process of
malleus 3 Handle of malleus 4 Limbus 5 Pars tensa
6 Umbo 7 Cone of light

earwax *cerumen*
Ebola fever *hemorrhagic fever* caused by
the *Ebola virus* and transmissible from
human to human
Ebola virus *virus* that causes *Ebola fever*

EBV abbr. *Epstein-Barr virus*

EC abbr. *erythrocyte concentrate*

ec(to)- combining form: outer, outside

ECC abbr. *extracorporeal circulation (heartlung machine)*

ecchymosis small hemorrhage, e.g. from *hemorrhagic diathesis*

ECF abbr. *extracellular fluid*

ECG electrodes *electrodes* for taking readings in *electrocardiography*; see *Einthoven* and *Wilson* entries for positioning

ECG lead lead used in *electrocardiography*; see also *chest lead, Wilson lead, limb lead, Einthoven lead, Goldberger lead*

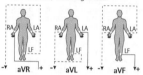

Fig. 162: unipolar leads according to Goldberger

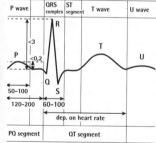

Intervals in milliseconds, amplitudes in mV
Fig. 163: ECG normal values

ECG strip printed copy of heart monitoring readings

echinococcosis *infectious disease* that causes cysts in the liver, spleen and lungs; transmitted by ingestion of the eggs of the dog or fox tapeworm

Echinococcus genus of tapeworm that causes *echinococcosis*, or more specifically its larval stage

ECHO virus (enteric cytopathogenic human orphan virus) any of a group of intestinal *viruses* that can cause diarrhea, summer flu or *meningitis*

echocardiogram ultrasound test that outlines movements of the heart's structures; a transducer is used to obtain the image

echocardiogram *echocardiography*

echocardiograph to perform *echocardiography*

echocardiography echocardiogram

echogram *ultrasound* imaging of heart structures; noninvasive

echography *ultrasound*

echolalia repetition of sentences or fragments spoken by others

echopraxia (echomimia) imitation of another person's motions

eclampsia disorder of pregnancy characterized by *pre-eclampsia* and *tonic-clonic* seizures

-ectasis (-ectasia) combining form: enlargement

ecthyma *pyogenic* skin *infection* caused by *bacteria*, extending deep into the *epidermis*

ectoderm outer *blastodermic* layer of the human embryo, from which the *central* and *peripheral nervous system, epidermis, pituitary gland*, sweat and mammary glands develop

-ectomy combining form: removal

ectopia displacement of *tissues* or *organs*

ectopic outside; located or developing in an unusual place

ectopic ureter opening of a *ureter* in an abnormal location

ectromelia disorder of skeletal development marked by *hypo-* or *aplasia* of individual or multiple bones

ectropion eversion, e.g. of the lower eyelids due to age or *inflammation*; opp. *entropion*

ectropionization eversion of the eyelid over a cotton swab in order to remove a foreign body or examine the *conjunctiva*

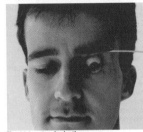

Fig. 164: ectropionization

eczema itchy, red, scaly and thickened skin eruption

edema pathological swelling of *tissue* due to accumulation of fluid

edematous pert. to *edema*

EEG abbr. *electroencephalogram*

EF abbr. *ejection fraction*

efferent descending or leading out, e.g. *nerves* leading from the brain to the spinal cord; opp. *afferent*

efflorescence skin eruption caused by disease; types are *primary* and *secondary efflorescences*

effusion accumulation of fluid in a body cavity; see also *exudate*, *transudate*

EEG abbr. (electroencephalogram) test to measure electrical activity generated by the cerebral cortex

EGD abbr. *esophagogastroduodenoscopy*

Einthoven leads *(standard leads)* limb leads used for *electrocardiography*; ECG leads I, II and III branch off from these; see also *Goldberger* and *Wilson* leads

Einthoven's triangle theoretical model for determining *electrical position* of the heart in an *ECG*

ejaculate seminal fluid released at *ejaculation*

ejaculatio praecox *premature ejaculation*

ejaculatio retarda *delayed ejaculation*

ejaculation expulsion of *semen*

ejection click early systolic ejection sound in the heart

ejection fraction amount of blood expelled from the heart with each heartbeat; abbr. EF

elbow cubitus

elective optional, by choice; opp. *obligatory*

electric response audiometry *audiometry* using computer-aided measurement of fluctuations in *auditory evoked potentials* in the *EEG*; abbr. ERA

electrocardiogram *(electrocardiography)* graph of heart activity patterns for analysis of the electrical impulses and excitation processes in the heart; a normal ECG reading consists of *P wave*, *QRS complex*, *T wave* and *U wave*; see also *Einthoven* and *Goldberger limb leads* and *Wilson precordial leads*; for placement of leads, see entries for *Einthoven* and *Wilson*; abbr. ECG, EKG

electrocardiography *electrocardiogram*

electrocauter (cauter) device for performing *electrocoagulation*

electrocautery wound cauterization during surgery with an *electrocauter*

electrocoagulation use of electrical current to cauterize tissues during *surgery* with an *electrocauter*

electrode electrical lead that conducts current, e.g. in an *ECG*; collective term for *cathodes* and *anodes*

Electrode placement for limb leads:
red = right arm; yellow = left arm; black = right foot; green = left foot

Electrode placement for precordial leads: see *Wilson (leads)*

electroencephalogram (electroencephalography) graph of brain activity patterns for analysis of the electrical impulses and excitation processes in the brain; abbr. EEG

electroencephalography *electroencephalogram*

electrolyte particle that can be decomposed by eletricity

electromyogram *electromyography*

electromyography (electromyogram) examination that records the electrical impulses in a muscle using a needle *electrode*, e.g. as a test for muscle *atrophy*; abbr. EMG

electron negatively charged subatomic particle; opp. *proton*

electroneurogram *electroneurography*

electroneurography (electroneurogram) examination that records the *motor* and *sensory* nerve conduction velocity e.g. in *polyneuropathy*; abbr. ENG

electrophoresis analysis of blood proteins (*albumins* and *globulins*) by separation using electricity

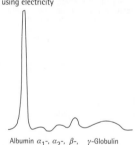

Albumin α_1-, α_2-, β-, γ-Globulin

Fig. 165: normal electrophoresis

elephantiasis massive swelling of the limbs due to lymph congestion

elevation 1) raising of a physical object, e.g. a limb; 2) increase in a measured value, e.g. blood pressure

elimininate to excrete or remove

elimination excretion or removal of waste

ELISA abbr. enzyme-linked immunosorbent assay

em- combining form: in, into

embolectomy *surgical* removal of an *embolus*

embolism obstruction of a blood vessel by an *embolus*

embolus detached blood clot or debris that causes an *embolism*

embrace reflex *Moro reflex*

embryo unborn child, from egg fertilization stage until the end of the first trimester of pregnancy; see also *fetus*

embryoblast component of the blastocyst at ca. 45 days after fertilization

embryonic pert. to the *embryo*

embryonic period interval between fertilization and the end of the 3rd month of pregnancy; see also *fetal period*

embryopathy disease of the embryo during pregnancy

emergency cesarean *cesarean section* performed when there is acute danger to the mother or child

emergent requiring immediate admission

emesis vomiting

emesis gravidarum *hormone*-related *physiological* vomiting during pregnancy, usually occurring between the 4th and 16th weeks of gestation; see also *hyperemesis gravidarum*

emetic 1) drug used to induce *vomiting*; 2) pert. to or causing vomiting

EMG abbr. *electomyography*

–emia combining form: blood

emmetropia normal vision

emotion feeling, mental state

emotional incontinence lack of *affective* control

emotional lability (labile affect, affective instability) increased susceptibility to *affects* with rapid mood changes

empathy awareness and comprehension of others' feelings

emphysema excessive accumulation of gas in the *tissues* or the lungs (pulmonary emphysema)

emphysematous pert. to *emphysema*

empirical based on experience

empyema collection of pus in a body cavity

EMR abbr. electronic medical record

emulsifier substance that enables the creation of an *emulsion* by reducing surface tension

emulsion mixture of two substance that are not mutually soluble

en- combining form: in into

enamel (dental enamel, enamelum, *substantia adamantina*) hardest substance in the human body, which surrounds the *dentin* in the *crown* of the tooth; originates in the *ectoderm*; cannot regenerate

enamel hypoplasia congenital or acquired disorder of dental *enamel* formation due to abnormalities in formation of the *organic* matrix and *mineralization* of the hard structures

enanthem(a) eruption on a mucous membrane; opp. *exanthem(a)*

encephal- combining form: brain

encephalitis inflammation of the brain

encephalocele protrusion of brain tissue through a fissure in the skull

encephalomalacia softening of brain tissues due to *necrosis*, e.g. from circulatory disorder

encephalomyelitis inflammation of the *brain* and *spinal cord*

encephalon brain

encephalopathy (Binswanger's dementia) noninflammatory disease of the brain

encopresis voluntary or involuntary evacuation of the bowels, into clothing or in inappropriate locations, occurring after age 4

end(o)angiitis (endangiitis, endarteritis, endophlebitis) *inflammation* of the inner wall of a blood vessel

endangiitis obliterans *thromboangiitis obliterans*

endarterectomy *thromboendarterectomy*

endbrain *telencephalon*

endemic pert. to a disease that spreads to a limited extent within a population

endo- combining form: inside, interior

endobronchial in the *bronchi*; abbr. EB

endocardial pert. to the *endocardium*

endocarditis inflammation of the *endocardium*, typically also involving the valves; usually caused by *bacteria* or fungi

endocardium inner lining of the heart

endocrine substance (e.g. *hormone*) secreted into the bloodstream; opp. *exocrine*

endocrinologic(al) pert. to *endocrinology*

endocrinology study of *hormones* and endocrine gland function

endoderm inner *blastoderm layer* of the human embryo, from which the *epithelium* of the *gastrointestinal tract, respiratory tract* and *bladder* develop, as well as the *parenchyma* of the *tonsils, thymus,* thyroid gland, *liver* and *pancreas*

endodontics (endodontia) branch of dentistry dealing with the *dental pulp*

endogenous developing or originating within the *organism*; opp. *exogenous*

endometrial carcinoma malignant tumor in the body of the *uterus*

endometrial cycle *menstrual cycle*

endometriosis presence of *endometrium*like *tissue* outside of the uterine cavity

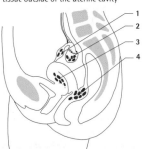

Fig. 166: endometriosis
1 Tubal 2 Ovarian 3 Uterine 4 Retrocervical

endometritis inflammation of the *endometrium*, e.g. from an *IUD*

endometrium mucous membrane lining the *uterus*; consists of columnar *epithelium* and glands

endoplasmic reticulum cell organelle that is involved in *synthesis* and *transport* of *proteins*

endoprosthesis artificial replacement for an internal body part, e.g. a *joint*; see also *total endoprosthesis*

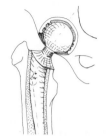

Fig. 167: total endoprosthesis

endorphin substance produced in the *brain* that has an *analgesic* effect and lowers the pain threshold

endoscope to examine by *endoscopy*; instrument used to perform *endoscopy*

endoscopic pert. to *endoscopy*

endoscopic retrograde endoscopy examination (visualization) of internal *organs* and body cavities with a rigid or flexible *endoscope* equipped with a light source and optical system; minor *surgery* can also be performed with smaller instruments introduced via the endoscope

endosonography *ultrasound* examination of the gastrointestinal tract and adjacent structures using a special *endoscope* with an ultrasound transducer at its tip that enables examination from the inside

endostoma tumor that develops inside a bone

endothelial pert. to the *endothelium*

endothelium inner membrane of the heart and of the blood and *lymph vessels*

endotoxin toxin released within the body, e.g. produced by *bacteria* or from the destruction of *cells*

endotracheal anesthesia *anesthesia* requiring *intubation* of the patient, who must be ventilated

endotracheal tube elastic *tube*, usually equipped with a distal inflatable balloon (*cuff*) that enables sealing of the *trachea*; see also *intubation*

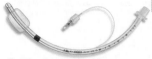

Fig. 168: endotracheal tube [K]

enema 1) (clysis) *irrigation* of the bowel with small amounts of fluid, e.g. for *obstipation*; 2) *irrigation* of the *rectum* and *colon*

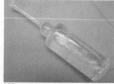

Fig. 169: enema

ENG abbr. *electroneurography;* engraftment (the process whereby stem cells move into the marrow of the patient and produce RBC's of all types)

enophthalmos backward displacement of the eyeball within the *orbit*, e.g. due to *exsiccation*; opp. *exophthalmos*

ENT abbr. otolaryngology (ear, nose and throat medicine)

enter(o)– combining form: intestines, viscera

enteral pert. to the intestines; via the intestines

enteric coated tablet tablet with a protective coating

enteric cytopathogenic human orphan see ECHO virus

enteric fever *enteritis* caused by *Salmonellas*, transmitted via contaminated food; typhoid fever

enteritis *inflammation* of the small intestine

enteritis regionalis *Crohn's disease*

enteroclysis enema given to cleanse the transverse and descending parts of the colon

Enterococcus genus of *bacteria* belonging to the *Streptococcus* family; part of the *intestinal flora*

enterocolitis *inflammation* of the small and large intestine

enterolith intestinal calculus

enteron *intestine*

enterostomy creation of an opening between the gastrointestinal tract and the body surface, e.g. for nutrition or as an artificial anus (e.g. *colostomy*)

enterotomy *surgical* opening of the intestinal lumen

entropion inversion, e.g. of the lower eyelids due to age or *inflammation*; opp. *ectropion*

enucleatio bulbi *surgical* removal of the eyeball

enucleation *surgical* removal of an encapsulated portion of *tissue*, e.g. of the eyeball (cf. *enucleatio bulbi*)

enuresis involuntary urination occurring more than sporadically after the age of 4

enzymatic pert. to *enzymes*

enzyme substance that produces or accelerates chemical/biological reactions without any change in itself

EOM abbr. extraocular movement

eosin- combining form: red

eosinophilic 1) staining readily with the red acidic dye eosin; 2) consisting of structures or *cells* with this property

ependyma single-layered cellular membrane lining the ventricles of the brain and the spinal canal

ependymoma brain tumor originating in the *ependyma*

ephelis freckle; pl. ephelides

epi- combining form: on, upon, above

epicanthus vertical fold of skin at the inner corner of the eye

epicardial pert. to the *epicardium*

epicardium outer membrane of the *heart*

epicondyle prominence at the articular end of a bone

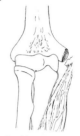

Fig. 170: epicondyle

epicondylitis inflammation of the *epicondyle* of the *humerus* and associated tissues

epicrisis critical analysis or discussion of a case of disease after its termination

epicutaneous pert. to the *epidermis*

epidemic widespread occurrence of an *infectious* disease within a population at the same time; see also *pandemic*

epidemic typhus (typhus exanthemicus) febrile *infectious disease* caused by the pathogen *Rickettsia prowazekii*; transmitted in louse droppings, via skin wounds or inhalation

epidemiological pert. to *epidemiology*

epidemiology study of the frequency and distribution of diseases in the population

epidermal pert. to the *epidermis*

epidermis outermost layer of the skin; part of the *cutis*; pl. epidermides

epidermoid cyst *atheroma*

epidermolysis loosening of patches of *epidermis*, e.g. due to an *allergy*

epidermophytosis *mycosis* of the *epidermis*

epididym- combining form: epididymis

epididymis small organ resting against the *testis* and connecting to the *vas deferens*

epididymitis *inflammation* of the *epididymis*

epidural anesthesia (peridural anesthesia) *block anesthesia* for local numbing of the lower part of the body, in which a *local anesthetic* is applied in the *epidural space*

epidural bleed bleed in the *epidural space* due to rupture of the medial meningeal *artery*, leading to an *epidural hematoma*; usually occurs in connection with a *head injury* with immediate loss of consciousness, awakening (lucid interval) and return of unconsciousness; cf. *subdural bleed*

epidural hematoma *hematoma* in the *epidural space*

epidural space space between the skull bones and the *dura mater*

epigastrica, A. *arteria epigastrica*

epigastrium area of the upper abdomen below the *sternum* and between the costal arches

epiglott- combining form: epiglottis

epiglottis cartilaginous structure that closes off the *trachea* while swallowing

epiglottitis *acute inflammation* of the *epiglottis* with life-threatening respiratory distress; usually occurs in children

epilation *depilation*

epilepsy *seizure disorder*

epileptic seizure sudden rhythmic and synchronic electrical discharge of limited duration in the *neuronal cell* bundles, which can involve the entire brain under certain circumstances

epinephrine (adrenaline) circulatory acting *hormone* produced primarily by the *adrenal medulla*; important *neurotransmitter* of the *autonomic nervous system*; one of the *catecholamines*

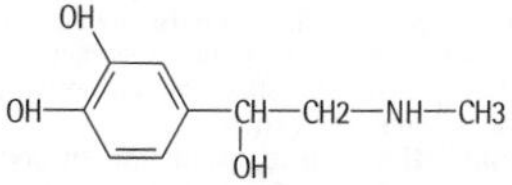

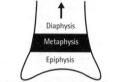

Fig. 171: epinephrine (adrenaline)

epipharynx nasopharynx

epiphora (dacryorrhea) watering eyes, e.g. due to *dacryocystitis*

epiphyseal pert. to the *epiphysis*

epiphyseal cartilage (epiphyseal plate) layer of cartilage between the *diaphysis* and *epiphysis* in long bones (growth layer for longitudinal growth)

epiphyseal growth plate injury type of injury in growing children, involving still-open growth plates; see *Aitken* classifications

epiphyseolysis separation of an *epiphysis*

epiphysis 1) *pineal gland* at the base of the brain; 2) ossification center of a bone; cf. *metaphysis* and *diaphysis*

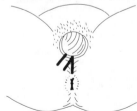

Fig. 172: epiphysis, metaphysis, and diaphysis

episclera outer surface of the *sclera*, resembling *connective tissue*

episcleral veins *veins* that run along the surface of the *sclera* and flow into the *superior ophthalmic vein*

episcleritis *inflammation* of the *episclera*

Fig. 173: episiotomy

episiotomy procedure performed during childbirth to relieve pressure on the *perineum* and to protect the deep pelvic floor musculature if there is the threat of *laceration*, or to avoid fluctuations in the infant's *intracranial* pressure

epispadia, congenital abnormal opening on the underside of the male urethra

epistaxis nosebleed

epithelial pert. to the *epithelium*

epithelialization growth of new *tissue* over a *wound* during the healing process

epithelioma tumor originating in *epithelial tissue*

epithelium surface tissue having no blood vessels; uppermost cell layer of the skin or a mucous membrane

epithesis custom-built *prosthesis* for the facial area

EPO abbr. *erythropoietin*

Epstein-Barr virus *DNA virus* that causes *mononucleosis infectiosa* et al.; abbr. EBV

epulis localized gingival tumor; swelling of the gums during pregnancy

equi- combining form: equal

equilibration restoration of *physiological autonomic* equilibrium; measurement of fluid intake and output to assess fluid balance in the body

equivalent equal in value, amount or effect; substitute, replacement

ER abbr. emergency room

ERA abbr. *electric response audiometry*

ERCP abbr. *endoscopic retrograde cholangiopancreatography*

erect stiffened

erection stiffening of the *penis*, *clitoris* or nipples under sexual stimulation

erethism state of irritability associated with mercury poisoning

ergo- combining form: work

ergomania compulsion to be busy

ergometer device for measurement of work performed; used to assess reactions to exertion, e.g. in a *stress test*

ergotherapy therapy aimed at functional improvement of particular sequences of movements occurring in daily life using appropriate ergonomic practices

erogenous causing sexual arousal

erosion eating away of tissue, destruction by inflammatory processes, e.g. of *organs* or blood vessels

eruption breaking out; usually associated with a skin disease

ERV abbr. *expiratory reserve volume*

erysipelas *infectious disease* caused by toxin-forming beta-hemolyzing group A *streptococci*; leads to widespread *inflammation* of the *subcutis*; in severe cases it can spread along the *lymphatics*; *infection* usually occurs when the pathogen enters the body via small skin lesions

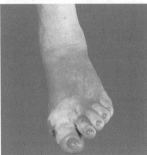

Fig. 174: erysipelas

erysipeloid *infectious disease* caused by *Erysipelothrix rhusiopathiae*, leading to a reddish-purple, painful swelling in the hands; in severe cases it can spread along the *lymphatics*; *infection* usually occurs among workers who handle raw meat, poultry or fish, via small skin lesions where the pathogen can enter

Erysipelothrix rhusiopathiae rod-shaped *gram-positive bacterium* that causes *erysipeloid*

erythema chronicum migrans specific skin changes following a tick bite; an early sign of *Borrelia* infection, e.g. *Lyme* disease

erythema nodosum red rash occurring specifically on the shins, with formation of painful red nodes; often associated with *streptococcus* infections

erythr(o)– combining form: red

erythrasma skin condition caused by *bacteria*, marked by red-brown patches in the skin folds, esp. the groin, inner thighs or armpits

erythroblast immature stage of an *erythrocyte*, found in the bone marrow

erythroblastosis disease marked by increased presence of *erythroblasts* in the blood; occurs in *Rh*-positive children of *Rh*-negative mothers

erythroblastosis fetalis (hemolytic disease of the newborn) *hemolytic anemia* triggered by the mother forming *antibodies* against the fetus' *blood group*

erythrocyte red blood cell produced in the bone marrow, which gets its red color from *hemoglobin*; main function: transport of *oxygen* and *carbon dioxide* in the blood

erythrocyte concentrate *stored blood* for *transfusion*, consisting of the *erythrocytes centrifuged* from blood after separation of the *buffy coat*; abbr. EC

erythrocyte sedimentation rate see also blood sedimentation rate; Westergren's blood test uses blood to which *sodium citrate* is added as an anticoagulant; blood sedimentation testing enables detection of changes in blood protein composition, and thus is useful for monitoring *infections* and neoplastic diseases; abbr. ESR, BSR

erythrocytic pert. to the *erythrocytes*

erythrocyturia presence of *erythrocytes* in the urine

erythroderm(i)a disease affecting the entire skin, marked by severe redness and scaling

erythropoietic pert. to *erythropoiesis*

erythropoietin important *hormone* produced in the kidneys and liver, which stimulates the production of *erythrocytes* in the bone marrow

erythropoiesis formation of *erythrocytes*

ES abbr. *extrasystole*

eschar dead matter sloughed from the skin following a burn or other wound

escharotomy surgical removal or *incision* of sloughed skin tissue from a wound or burn, e.g. with circumferential burns to prevent *compartment syndrome*

Escherichia coli rod-shaped *gram-negative bacterium*, part of the *intestinal flora*; abbr. E. coli

Esmarch–Heiberg maneuver emergency maneuver for maintaining an airway in an unconscious patient by pulling the lower jaw forward, which keeps the tongue from dropping back

eso– combining form: into, inward

esophageae, Vv. *venae esophageae*

esophageal pert. to the *esophagus*

esophageal atresia congenital obstruction of the *esophagus*, usually with a *fistula* into the *trachea*

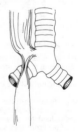

Fig. 175: esophageal atresia with tracheal fistula

esophageal carcinoma malignant tumor of the *esophagus*

esophageal diverticulum protrusion of the entire thickness of the wall of the *esophagus* (true diverticulum) or of the *mucosa* and *submucosa* (pseudodiverticulum)

esophageal varix *varix* in the *esophagus* due to *portal hypertension*; usually occurs in severe *liver* disease; abbr. EV

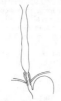

Fig. 176: esophageal carcinoma

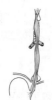

Fig. 177: esophageal diverticulum

esophageal veins *veins* that transport blood from the *esophagus* to the *brachiocephalic* or *azygos vein*

esophagism(us) spasm of the esophageal muscles

esophagitis inflammation of the *esophageal* mucosa, usually near the stomach

esophagogastroduodenoscopy combined *endoscopy* of the *esophagus, stomach* and *duodenum*; abbr. EGD

esophagus muscular tube 23–26 cm in length that carries food into the *stomach*; has three physiologic areas of narrowing: 1) at the cricoid cartilage; 2) at the bifurcation; 3) at the cardia

ESR abbr. *erythrocyte sedimentation rate*

essential necessary to life; pert. to the essence of a thing

essential tremor involuntary trembling associated with purposeful movement; this is not related to Parkinson's Disease

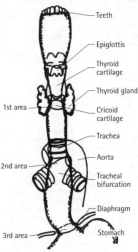

Fig. 178: esophageal areas of physiologic narrowing

–esthesia combining form: perception, sensation

estradiol strong *estrogen* made in the *ovaries*

estriol *estrogens* made from *estradiol*

estrogens collective name for *hormones* made in the *ovaries* and *placenta*; main function: development of female sexual characteristics and regulation of the *menstrual cycle*

estrone (estrogenic hormone) the second most important *estrogen* after *estradiol*

ethical being in accordance with the rules or standards for right conduct or practice, esp. the standards of a profession

ethmoid (os ethmoidale) bone in the *cranial base*, located between the eye sockets and containing the ethmoid sinuses (ethm. *cells*), which connect to the *paranasal sinuses*

ethmoiditis *inflammation of the ethmoid sinuses*

etio– combining form: cause

etiologic(al) pert. to *etiology*

etiology the cause of a disease

EU abbr. *excretory urography*

eu– combining form: good, normal

EUG abbr. *extrauterine gestation; see extrauterine pregnancy*

eugnathia (neutral bite) upper and lower *teeth* meet in a shearing bite with the crowns of the upper teeth slightly in front and those of the lower teeth slightly behind; opp. *dysgnathia*

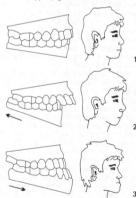

Fig. 179: eugnathia
1 Balanced bite 2 Overbite 3 Underbite

eumenorrhea normal *menstruation*

eunuch male castrated pre-*puberty*

EUP abbr. *extrauerine pregnany*

euphoria feeling of elation

eupnea normal regular breathing at rest with 14 to 20 breaths per minute in adults

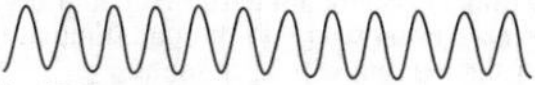

Fig. 180: eupnea

eustachian tube (auditory tube, otopharyngeal tube) tube extending from the middle ear to the nasopharynx

euthanasia mercy killing; assisted suicide

euthyroid pert. to normal *thyroid gland* function

EV abbr. *esophageal varix*

eversion turning outward; combination movement of the foot consisting of forefoot abduction, dorsal extension and pronation; opp. inversion

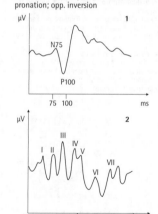

Fig. 181: evoked potentials
1 Visually evoked potentials (VEP)
2 Acoustically evoked potentials (AEP)

evoked potential (evoked response) *EEG* record of *CNS* response to various forms of stimulation, e.g. visual evoked potential (VEP) through stimulation of the vision with a checkerboard pattern, or auditory evoked potential (AEP) through stimulation of the hearing with click sounds

Ewing's sarcoma (Ewing's tumor) fast-growing malignant tumor originating in the *bone marrow*

ex- combining form: out of

exo- combining form: outward, outside

exa- combining form: quintillion (10^{18}); symbol: E

exacerbation flareups, episodes of worsening symptoms, e.g. in multiple sclerosis

exanthem(a) skin eruption; opp. *enanthem(a)*

exarticulation *amputation* of a limb at the joint

exchange transfusion (replacement trans-fusion) *transfusion* in which the patient's entire blood supply is replaced with *stored blood*

excisate excised *tissue*

excise to perform an *excision*

excision cutting out diseased tissue without regard for *organ* boundaries

excitation stimulation

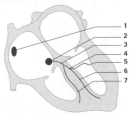

Fig. 182: excitation and conduction system
1 Sinoatrial node 2 AV node 3 Bundle of His
4 Left bundle branch 5 Left posterior branch
6 Left anterior branch 7 Right bundle branch

excitation and conduction system system that regularly generates electrical impulses in the *heart* and thus leads to regular

contraction of the cardiac muscle; components are the *sinoatrial node*, *atrioventricular node*, *bundle of His*, *Tawara branches* and *Purkinje fibers*

excitation state excessive muscle stimulation during the process of general anesthesia

excoriation *secondary efflorescence* caused by superficial defect extending to the *dermis*, e.g. due to abrasion

excrement excreted waste (urine and feces)

excretory pert. to excretion

excretory urography (descending urography, intravenous urography) *radiography* of the urinary tract using *contrast medium*; abbr. EU

exercise ECG *ECG* recorded before, during and after standardized physical exertion, e.g. using an *ergometer*, until a specified heart rate of (220 – age) x 0.85 is reached

exeresis *surgical* removal of vessels or *nerves* by pulling them out

exfoliation shedding, e.g. of cells

exhaustion extreme fatigue

exhibitionism pathological need to attract attention, e.g. by exposing oneself in public

exitus (letalis) death

exocrine substance secreted out of the body via the skin or a mucous membrane; opp. *endocrine*

exogenous developed or originating outside the organism; opp. *endogenous*

exophthalmos (exophthalmus) protrusion of the eyeballs beyond the *orbits*; e.g. unila-terally due to hemorrhage or inflammation behind the eyeball, or bilaterally in *Graves' disease*; opp. *enophthalmos*

exostosis benign bony growth; pl. exostoses

exotoxin toxin produced by living *bacteria*

expectorant drug used to promote expulsion of mucus from the *bronchi*

expectorate to cough up

expectoration coughing up of mucus or phlegm

expiration exhalation; opp. *inspiration*

expiratory reserve volume amount of air that can still be exhaled following a normal exhalation; abbr. ERV

expire to exhale; opp. *inspire*

explant to remove foreign bodies or *organs* surgically; opp. *implant*

exploration examination, investigation of a body part

exposure subjection to external forces, e.g. radiation, weather, light

exposure therapy behavioral therapy using overstimulation, e.g. for obsessive-compulsive disorder

expulsion period birth phase from the full dilation of the *cervix* to the delivery of the infant

exsiccosis dehydration due to negative fluid balance

exstrophy of the bladder deformity in which the lower portion of the anterior abdominal wall and the anterior vesical wall are absent; results in adhesion of the posterior vesical wall and parts of the base of the bladder to the *abdominal* wall

extension 1) stretching out; opp. *flexion*; 2) mechanical stretching of a limb following a *fracture*

extensor muscle that extends a body part; opp. *flexor*

extensor carpi radialis, M. *musculus extensor carpi radialis*

extensor carpi ulnaris, M. *musculus extensor carpi ulnaris*

extensor digitorum brevis, M. *musculus extensor digitorum brevis*

extensor digitorum communis, M. *musculus extensor digitorum communis*

extensor digitorum longus, M. *musculus extensor digitorum longus*

extensor hallucis longus, M. *musculus extensor hallucis longus*

extensor muscle of the fingers forearm muscle that extends the fingers; *innervation: posterior interosseus nerve*

extensor muscle of the thumb forearm muscle that extends the thumb; *innervation: radial nerve*

extensor pollicis, M. *musculus extensor pollicis*

external on the outside; opp. *internal*

external fixation *osteosynthesis* of a *fracture* using indirect external immobilization of the fracture; usually employed for open fractures

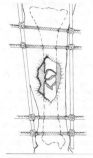

Fig. 183: external fixation

external jugular vein *vein* that collects blood from the occipital neck and shoulder area and joins the *subclavian* or *internal jugular vein*

external rotation rotation away from the midline of the body; opp. *internal rotation*

extirpation complete *surgical* removal of *tumors* or *organs*

extra– combining form: outside; opp. *intra*

extraarticular outside of the joint; opp. *intraartikulär*

extracellular outside a *cell* or cells; opp. *intracellular*

extracellular fluid liquid found outside of *cells*, e.g. in the *interstitial space* or the vessels; comprises approx. 1/3 of total body water; opp. *intracellular fluid*; abbr. ECF

extracorporeal outside of the body; opp. *intracorporeal*

extracorporeal circulation *heart-lung machine*

extract to pull out

extraction pulling or drawing out e.g. of a foreign body or *tooth*

extramedullary outside of the *bone marrow* or *spinal cord*; opp. *intramedullary*

extramural outside the wall of a hollow organ; opp. *intramural*

extraperitoneal outside of the *peritoneum*; opp. *intraperitoneal*

extrasystole heart action occurring outside of the normal heart rhythm, detectable with *electrocardiography*; types are *supraventricular extrasystole* and *ventricular extrasystole*; abbr. ES

extrasystolic pert. to *extrasystole*

extrauterine outside the *uterus*; opp. *intrauterine*

extrauterine pregnancy (graviditas extra-uterina) a rare complication of pregnancy in which the embryo develops outside of the *uterus*; 95% of these occur in the fallopian tube (*tubal pregnancy*), less frequently in the abdominal cavity (*abdominal pregnancy*), ovary or cervix; abbr. EUP

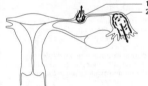

Fig. 184: extrauterine pregnancy
1 Tubal rupture 2 Tubal abortion

extremity limb

extrinsic from the outside; opp. *intrinsic*

extroverted turned outward; opp. *introverted*

extubation removal of an *endotracheal tube*; opp. *intubation*

exudate *inflammatory protein*-rich *effusion* released into body cavities; opp. *transudate*

exudation release of fluid

exudative pert. to *exudate*; opp. *transudative*

exudative pleurisy "wet" form of *pleurisy* e.g. in *tuberculosis*; opp. *dry pleurisy*

exulceration ulcerous degeneration

eye (oculus, ophthalmos) paired sense organs of visual perception

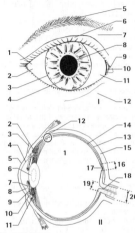

Fig. 185: right eye
I **Anterior view** 1 Lateral angle of eye 2 Conjunctiva (covers sclera) 3 Limbus 4 Cornea 5 Eyebrow 6 Eyelashes 7 Upper eyelid 8 Pupil 9 Lacrimal caruncle 10 Plica semilunaris
II **Horizontal section** 1 Vitreous body 2 Ciliary muscle 3 Conjunctiva 4 Iridocorneal angle 5 Cornea 6 Lens 7 Iris 8 Anterior chamber 9 Posterior chamber 10 Schlemm's canal 11 Zonule fibers 12 Ora serrata 13 Retina 14 Choroid 15 Sclera (white of the eye) 16 Macula lutea 17 Fovea centralis 18 Lamina cribrosa 19 Papilla 20 Optic nerve

eye socket orbit

eyeball ocular bulb, bulbus oculi

eyecup receptacle used for bathing the eye

eyelash cilium

eyelid palpebra

F

fainting *syncope*
FBS abbr. *fasting blood sugar*
face *facies*

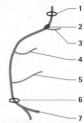

Fig. 187: course of facial nerve
1 Internal auditory meatus 2 Geniculate ganglion 3 Greater petrosal nerve 4 Stapedial nerve 5 Chorda tympani 6 Stylomastoid foramen 7 Parotid plexus

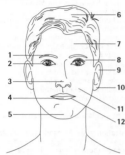

Fig. 186: face (facies)
1 Eyebrow (supercilium) 2 Eye (oculus, ophthalmos) 3 Nose (nasus, rhis) 4 Lip (labium, cheilos) 5 Chin (mentum) 6 Hair (capillus, pili, thrix) 7 Forehead (frons) 8 Eyelashes (cilia) 9 Ear (auris, ous) 10 Earlobe (lobulus auriculae) 11 Cheek (bucca) 12 Mouth (os, stoma)

facet syndrome pain syndrome originating in the articular facets of the smaller vertebral joints
faci– combining form: face
facial nerve *7th cranial nerve*; contains sensory, motor and parasympathetic fibers; primarily controls the tongue's ability to taste and facial expressions (see *facial nerve paresis*)
facial nerve paralysis *paralysis* of the facial muscles caused by damage to the *facial nerve*, e.g. from a *stroke*
facialis, A. *arteria facialis*
facialis, N. *nervus facialis*
facialis, V. *vena facialis*
facies face

Factor I *fibrinogen*; important *coagulation* factor; plasma protein
Factor II *prothrombin*; important *coagulation* factor; plasma protein; FactorIIA is called thrombin
Factor III *tissue factor*; important *coagulation* factor; plasma protein
Factor IV *calcium ion*; important *coagulation* factor
Factor V *proaccelerin*; important *coagulation* factor
Factor VII *proconvertin*; important *coagulation* factor
Factor VIII *antihemophilic globulin A*; important *coagulation* factor; deficient in hemophilia
Factor IX (Christmas factor, plasma thromboplastin component) *antihemophilic globulin B*; important *coagulation* factor
Factor X *Stuart factor*; important *coagulation* factor; needs vitamin K to be synthesized
Factor XI *plasma thromboplastin antecedent*; important *coagulation* factor; deficiency causes hemophilia C
Factor XII *Hageman factor*; important *coagulation* factor

Factor XIII *fibrin-stabilizing factor*; important *coagulation* factor; also called fibrin

factitious disorder *Munchausen syndrome*

facultative possible, optional, by choice; opp. *obligate*

FAG abbr. *fluorescence angiography*

fallopian tube (uterine tube, oviduct, salpinx) paired tube, ca. 12 mm in length, that connects the *ovary* with the *uterus*

fango special type of mud used to treat *rheumatic* complaints

farsightedness *hyperopia*

fascia fibrous membrane that covers muscles and nerves; pl. fasciae

fasciitis *inflammation* of the *fascia*

fasciotomy *surgical* separation of the muscle *fascia* to relieve pressure, e.g. in *compartment syndrome*

fasting blood sugar blood sugar measured in the morning before the first meal; abbr. FBS

fat 1) important dietary substance with 9.3 kcal per gram; 2) adipose tissue of the body

fat embolism *embolism* caused by particles of fat, usually detached due to a *fracture*

fatigue tiredness, general exhaustion

fatty liver (steatosis hepatis) *triglycerides* in less than 50 % of the liver cells; cf. *steatocirrhosis*

favus *mycosis* affecting the scalp

Fe chemical symbol: *iron*

febri– combining form: fever

febrile pert. to *fever*; opp. *afebrile*

febris fever

febris recurrens *relapsing fever*

fecal pert. to *feces*

feces excrement, stool

fecund fertile

fecundity fertility

feedback response, influence of output over input

fel *bile*

fellatio *oral* sex performed on a male

femina woman

feminine characteristic of a female; opp. *masculine*

femoral pert. to the *femur*

femoral hernia (hernia femoralis) *hernia* into the femoral canal

femoral neck fracture *fracture* of the *femur* between the shaft and the head usually in elderly persons from falling on a hip

femoral nerve nerve in the thigh arising from the *lumbar plexus*; innervates the *iliopsoas, femoral, quadriceps* and *sartorius* muscles

femoral pulse *femoral artery* pulse palpable in the groin

femoral vein *vein* that transports blood from the lower extremities to the *inferior vena cava*

femoralis, A. *arteria femoralis*

femoralis, N. *nervus femoralis*

femoralis, V. *vena femoralis*

femoropatellar pain (syndrome) *chondropathia patellae*

femur thighbone; pl. femora

fenestra window or similar aperture, as in a bandage or cast

fenestration surgical creation of a *fenestra*

fentanyl transdermal opioid drug that is placed on the skin in patch form to manage chronic, severe pain

ferr– combining form: iron

ferment to decompose through enzymatic action

fermentation *anaerobic* breakdown of carbohydrates

ferning test used to detect estrogen in mucus from uterine cervix; presence of hormone provides information about ovulation

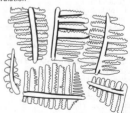

Fig. 188: ferning

ferrum iron
fertile capable of reproduction
fertility ability to reproduce
fertilization penetration of the ovum by a spermatozoon, beginning the process of zygote development

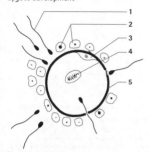

Fig. 189: fertilization
1 Sperm 2 Corona radiata cells 3 Polar body
4 Female pronucleus 5 Zona pellucida

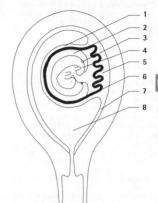

Fig. 190: fetal membranes
1 Decidua capsularis 2 Chorionic sac 3 Amnion
4 Amniotic cavity 5 Decidua basalis 6 Chorion
7 Decidua parietalis 8 Uterine cavity

fet– combining form: fetus
fetal membranes collective term for the membranes that surround the unborn baby consisting of the *amnion*, *chorion* and *deciduas*
fetal period period from the 4th month of pregnancy to birth; see also *embryonic period*
fetal pert. to the *fetus*
fetid foul-smelling
fetishism sexual arousal from viewing specific inanimate objects
fetopathy disease or damage to the *fetus* during pregnancy
fetor hepaticus musty breath due to severe liver disease
fetor oris (halitosis) foul breath
fetor uremicus urinelike mouth and body odor due to severe kidney disease
fetus unborn child from the 4th month of pregnancy to birth; see also *embryo*

FEV$_1$ abbr. forced expiratory volume in one second
fever elevation of body temperature above 38°C; see also *subfebrile*
FFP abbr. *fresh frozen plasma*
fibr(o)– combining form: fiber
fibrin filamentous blood *protein* generated during coagulation by the action of *thrombin* on *fibrinogen* (Factor I); it arrests bleeding by creating a network of individual fibers
fibrin stabilizing factor important blood *coagulation factor* (Factor XIII); abbr. FSF
fibrinogen degradation products breakdown products resulting from degradation of *fibrin* and *fibrinogen* that occur in the body when blood clots dissolve, e.g. *D-dimers*

fibrinogen important *coagulation factor* (*Factor I*) produced in the *liver* and bone marrow; precursor of fibrin

fibrinolysin *plasmin*

fibrinolysis breakdown of a *fibrin* clot

fibrinolytic 1) drug used to cause *fibrinolysis*; 2) pert. to fibrolysis

fibroadenoma tumor consisting of connective and glandular *tissue*

fibroblast precursor of *connective tissue* cells

fibroblast interferon *interferon* produced by the *fibroblasts* (*beta interferon*)

fibrolipoma benign tumor consisting of connective and adipose *tissue*

fibroma benign *connective tissue* tumor

fibromatosis proliferation of *connective tissue*

fibromyalgia syndrome (fibrositis) non-rheumatoid disorder with locomotor system pain; abbr. FMS

fibrosarcoma malignant *connective tissue* tumor

fibrosis pathological proliferation of *connective tissue* in an *organ*

fibrositis *fibromyalgia*

fibrotic pert. to *fibrosis*

fibrous pert. to connective tissue

fibul combining form: fibula, calf

fibula the small bone of the lower leg

fibular veins *venae peronaeae*

fibulares, Vv. *venae peronaeae*

field block infiltration anesthesia

fil(ament)– combining form: thread

filia *metastasis*

filtrate filtered fluid

fimbria fringelike end of an *organ*, e.g. the *fallopian tube*; pl. fimbriae

final (terminal) pert. to an end(ing)

fine–needle catheter jejunostomy placement of a very thin nutrient tube in the jejunum

finger bone *ossa digitorum manus*

finger *digitus* (manus)

finger–to–nose test test in which the patient, with eyes closed and arm extended, attempts to touch the nose with the index finger; in diseases of the

cerebellum there will be *intention tremor* and *ataxia*; abbr. FNT

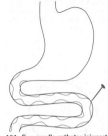

Fig. 191: fine-needle catheter jejunostomy

fingertip valve valve inserted between suction tubes for suction of body secretions that allows temporary interruption of the suction process, e.g. to change a suction catheter

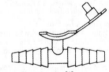

Fig. 192: fingertip valve [C]

fissure 1) groove, furrow, cleft; 2) painful crack in the skin or a mucous membrane; see also *hairline fracture*

fistula unnatural (artificially created or disease-related) connection between hollow organs ,or between a hollow organ and the body surface

fixation fastening, holding in place

flaccid lacking muscle tone

flail chest condition where structural support of the chest is impaired; often results from blunt-force trauma

flapping tremor *asterixis*

flat back spine lacking the normal S-curve
flatfoot *pes planus*
flatulence *(meterorism)* abdominal gas and bloating
flatus intestinal gas
flav- combining form: yellow
flex- combining form: bending
flexion bending; opp. *extension*
flexor muscle of the thumb muscle that flexes the metacarpophalangeal joints and distal phalanges of the thumb; *innervation ulnar* and *median nerve*
flexor carpi radialis, M. *musculus flexor carpi radialis*
flexor carpi ulnaris, M. *musculus flexor carpi ulnaris*
flexor digitorum profundus, M. *musculus flexor digitorum profundus*
flexor digitorum superficialis, M. *musculus flexor digitorum superficialis*
flexor muscle that pulls a limb toward the body; opp. *extensor*
flexor pollicis, M. *musculus flexor pollicis*
flexure bend in an organ, e.g. the *colon*
flight of ideas disorder of thought processes marked by shifting subjects and losing one's train of thought, e.g. in *mania*
floaters small particles floating in the *vitreous* of the *eye*, which the patient sees as they drift across the visual field
florid redness of a wound or the complexion
flowmeter device for measuring the flow of gases and thus, e.g. to monitor the dose of oxygen flowing from an *oxygen tank* or a wall access
fluctuation rapid change or wavelike movement
fluo- combining form flow
fluorescence angiogram *fluorescence angiography*
fluorescence angiography (fluorescence angiogram) visualization of the blood vessels in the *retina* and *choroid* through i.v. *injection* of dye; abbr. FAG
fluoride salt of hydrofluoric acid
fluorine chemical element; present in tooth enamel and bones, et al.; chemical symbol: F

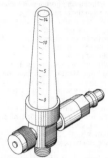

Fig. 193: flowmeter [N]

flush temporary reddening of the skin, e.g. due to *allergies*, *carcinoid* or hot flashes in *menopause*
FMS abbr. *fibromyalgia* syndrome
FNT abbr. *finger-to-nose test*
focal pert. to a *focus*
focal epilepsy (jacksonian epilepsy) *epilepsy* caused by damage to the cerebral cortex, marked by *partial* seizures with no loss of consciousness
focal seizure (partial seizures) seizure in which initial discharge comes from a unilateral area of the brain (temporal, frontal etc.); uncontrollable tremor begins in hand or foot
focal therapy conflict-centered *psychotherapy*
focus center, starting point
Fogarty catheter *balloon catheter* for performing *thrombectomy*
folate folic acid; water-soluble *vitamin* with an important role in formation of blood and *DNA*; folic acid deficiency can lead to *megaloblastic anemia* or (during pregnancy) to birth defects et al.
folic acid *folate*
follicle small sac

follicle-stimulating hormone *hormone* produced in the *adenohypophysis*; function: stimulates maturation of ovarian follicles in women, as well as spermatogenesis and seminiferous tubule development in men; abbr. FSH

folliculin *estrone*

folliculitis inflammation of (hair) follicles

Folstein Mini-Mental State Examination a copyrighted form to help screen patients for dementia; a score below 26 (out of 30) is considered abnormal

Fontaine classification system for rating the degree of severity of *peripheral arterial occlusive disease*

fontanel(le) (soft spot) gap between the unfused cranial bones of a newborn

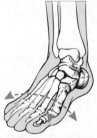

Fig. 195: foot (normal foot with transverse and longitudinal arches)

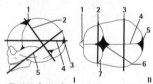

Fig. 194: fontanels
I Fontanels, lateral view 1 Anterior fontanel 2 Suboccipitobregmatic diameter 3 Posterior fontanel 4 Frontoocipital diameter 5 Occipitomental diameter
II Fontanels, superior view 1 Nose 2 Bitemporal diameter 3 Biparietal diameter 4 Sagittal suture 5 Posterior fontanel 6 Anterior fontanel 7 Coronal suture

foot pes

foramen opening, hole, aperture

foramen ovale opening between the right and left atria of the heart; closes shortly after birth

forceps pincerlike *surgical instrument* with long arms used for various holding tasks; basic types are *surgical forceps* with serrated gripping ends and *anatomical forceps* with blunt or ridged gripping ends, e.g. obstetrical forceps

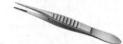

Fig. 196: forceps [A]

forceps delivery (forceps extraction) use of *forceps* to end a difficult delivery; preconditions are complete dilation of the *cervix*, fetal head at the level of the pelvic floor, empty bladder and completed rupture of *fetal membranes*

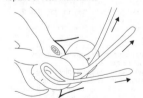

Fig. 197: forceps delivery

forceps extraction *forceps delivery*

forearm antebrachium
Foregger blade straight *laryngoscope blade* for *intubation*, usually used with small children; see also *McIntosh blade*

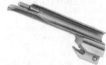

Fig. 198: Foregger blade [A]

forensic medicine medical knowledge used in the service of law enforcement
Forestier's disease disease leading to stiffening of the spine
-form combining form: -like, -shaped
fornix arched structure, e.g. fornix of the stomach
forte strong
fossa depression, furrow
Fournier's gangrene (Fournier's disease) *necrotizing skin inflammation* in the *scrotal* area, usually resulting from a *perianal* infection
fovea centralis retinae point of sharpest vision within the eye
fovea small pit
Fr abbr. *French*
fraction separable part; ratio of one component to a whole
fractionate to separate into component parts
fracture 1) breakage of a bone following direct or indirect application of force; main types are open fracture (involving a wound open to the exterior) and closed fracture (completely internal); cf. *infraction, hairline fracture*; 2) to break
fractured broken
fragile easily broken or fractured
fragility proneness to *fractures*
fragment 1) (broken) piece; 2) to break into pieces
Francisella tularensis nonmotile rod-shaped *gram-negative bacterium* that causes *tularemia*

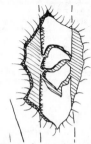

Fig. 199: open (compound) fracture

Frank Starling law rule in cardiopulmonary circulation: as *diastolic* stretch of heart muscle fibers increases, so does the *cardiac output*
FRC abbr. *functional residual capacity*
free radicals highly reactive molecules that damage *cells*
fremitus audible or palpable vibration e.g. tactile fremitus, where the vibrations of the chest during speech can be felt by laying a hand on the chest
French (Charrière) unit of measurement for the diameter of a *catheter*; 1 French = 1/3 mm; abbr. *Fr*
frenulum small band or fold
frenulum of the tongue (frenulum linguae) *frenulum* connecting the underside of the tongue to the floor of the mouth
frenulum of the lip mucous membrane fold connecting the lip to the alveolar mucosa; upper lip: frenulum labii superioris; lower lip: frenulum labii inferioris
frenulum preputii frenulum connecting the *foreskin* to the *glans penis*
frequency number of occurrences within a given time period
fresh frozen plasma *plasma* for *transfusion* *centrifuged* from blood immediately after donation; contains a high percentage of

coagulation factors, esp. *Factor V* and
Factor VIII; abbr. FFP

Friedreich's ataxia hereditary *progressive
ataxia,* usually with onset prior to age 25

frig(id)- combining form: cold

frigid pert. to *frigidity*

frigidity (sexual arousal disorder) lack of
sexual response

Fritsch retractor *surgical* instrument used
to retract *wounds* or the abdominal wall

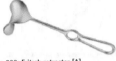

Fig. 200: Fritsch retractor [A]

Froment's sign sign of damage to the *ulnar
nerve* with *paresis* of the *musculus adductor pollicis;* when the patient grasps a sheet
of paper between the thumb and forefinger,
the distal phalanx of the thumb flexes to
compensate for inadequate *adduction*

frons forehead

frontal pert. to the forehead or the *frontal
bone*

frontal bone bone of the forehead/brow

frontal plane *coronal plane*

frontal sinus see *paranasal sinuses*

frontal sinusitis *inflammation* of the
frontal sinuses

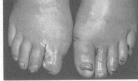

Fig. 201: frostbite

frostbite freezing injury classified according
to degree of tissue damage: 1st degree

frostbite (congelatio erythematosa):

frostbite with slight pain and redness when
the area is rewarmed; 2nd/3rd degree
frostbite (congelatio bullosa): frostbite
with blistering and pain in the frozen area;
4th degree frostbite (congelatio
necroticans): frostbite with deep tissue
necrosis and gangrene in the frozen area

frotteurism sexual gratification from
rubbing the genitals against another
person in a crowd

fructose (levulose) fruit sugar

frustration feeling of being thwarted or
disappointed

FSH abbr. *follicle-stimulating hormone*

fulminant (fulminating) with a rapid and
intense onset

funct- combining form: performance,
capability

functio laesa loss of function; see also *signs
of inflammation*

functional 1) pert. to a function; 2) without
a recognizable *organic* cause

functional residual capacity amount of air
that remains in the lungs after a normal
expiration; abbr. FRC

fundal varix *varix* in the upper curvature of
the stomach caused by portal flow disturbances, e.g. associated with *liver* disease

fundoplication *surgical* formation of a
sleeve of gastric *fundus* surrounding the
distal esophagus for prevention of *reflux
esophagitis* in cases of cardial
insufficiency, *hiatal hernia* or *achalasia*

fundoscopy visualization of the *fundus* of
an *organ,* esp. of the *fundus oculi*
(ophthalmoscopy)

fundus base, body or largest part of an organ

fundus hypertonicus pathological changes
in the *fundus oculi* due to *arterial
hypertension*

fundus oculi posterior inner part of the eye;
visualized through the pupil with an
ophthalmoscope to diagnose pathological
changes, e.g. *papilledema* or *fundus
hypertonicus*

fundus uteri (fundus of the uterus) upper
end of the *uterus*

fung- combining form: fungus

fungemia presence of fungi in the blood

fungicidal fungus-killing

fungistatic 1) inhibiting the growth of fungus; 2) drug to inhibit growth of fungus

funicular myelosis progressive disease of the *spinal cord* that can lead to *paresthesias* and *paralysis*

funiculitis *inflammation* of the *spermatic cord*

funiculus spermaticus *spermatic cord*

funiculus umbilicalis *umbilical cord*

funnel chest (pectus excavatum) deformity of the chest with indentation of the lower sternal area, usually congenital

furuncle purulent inflammation of the hair follicle; see also *carbuncle*

fusc- combining form: dark brown

fused vertebrae fusion of vertebral bones

fusion uniting, blending, fusing together

G

G 1) symbol: billion (10^9), prefix: giga; 2) abbr. *gauge*

g symbol: gram

GABA abbr. *gamma-aminobutyric acid*

Gaenslen's sign sign in *rheumatoid arthritis*: compression of the metacarpophalangeal joints results in painful pressure on the hand

gag reflex *physiologic* polysynaptic *reflex* in which touching the back of the throat results in elevation of the palate and *contraction* of the pharynx

gala (*lac*) milk

galact- combining form: milk

galactagogue drug used to promote milk secretion

galactogram *galactography*

galactography (galactogram) form of *mammography* in which the milk ducts of the mammary glands are visualized using a *contrast medium*

galactorrhea secretion of milk after nursing has ended

galactose a *carbohydrate*; building block of *lactose*

galactose intolerance *galactosemia*

galactosemia (galactose intolerance) serious disease occurring in infants, marked by inability to tolerate *galactose* due to *enzyme* deficiency; the galactose then accumulates in the blood and is excreted in the urine

galactostasis retention of milk in the mammary glands and their ducts, usually due to flow obstruction or incomplete emptying; can lead to *mastitis puerperalis*

galea helmet-like structure

Galeazzi's fracture *diaphyseal fracture* of the radius with dislocation of the *distal ulna*

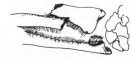

Fig. 202: Galeazzi's fracture

gallbladder (vesica fellea) hollow organ located below the *liver* that stores *bile*

gallbladder carcinoma rare malignant tumor of the *gallbladder*, usually an *adenocarcinoma*

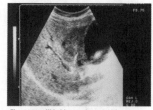

Fig. 203: gallbladder carcinoma with infiltration of the right lobe of the liver (ultrasound)

gallbladder empyema collection of pus in the *gallbladder*

gamet- combining form: reproductive cells

gametes male or female reproductive cells (sperm or ova)

gamma globulin (immune globulin) high-molecular-weight blood *protein* with *antibody* properties

gamma interferon *immune interferon*

gamma–aminobutyric acid important *neurotransmitter* in the brain; abbr. *GABA*

gamma–glutamyl transferase *enzyme* present in all body cells; plays a role in *amino acid* transport; sensitive laboratory parameter for detection and progression control of *liver* and *bile duct* disorders; abbr. GGT

gammacism form of *dyslalia* in which the G sound is pronounced as D

gangli(o)– combining form: ganglion

gangliocyte *neuron*

ganglion nerve tissue mass

ganglionectomy *surgical* removal of a *ganglion*

gangrene *necrotic tissue* destruction with autolysis and blackening of tissues

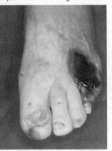

Fig. 204: dry gangrene due to AOD

Garcin's syndrome *cranial nerve* deficit on one side caused by changes in one half of the *cranial base*, e.g. due to *meningitis* or trauma

gas gangrene *infectious disease* caused by *Clostridium perfringens* toxins, which under anaerobic conditions leads to a life-threatening gas-forming *wound infection* with *necrosis*; transmission is mainly via contamination of *open wounds*

gastr(o)– combining form: stomach

gastralgia stomach pain

gastrectasia (gastrectasis) dilation of the *stomach*

gastrectomize to perform a *gastrectomy*

gastrectomy *surgical* removal of the *stomach*, e.g. due to tumors; can lead to *vitamin B₁₂* deficiency

gastric pert. to the *stomach*

gastrica, A. *arteria gastrica*

gastric bypass surgical intervention for obesity

gastric carcinoma malignant tumor of the *stomach*

gastric perforation hole in the stomach wall, e.g. caused by a *gastric ulcer* or foreign body

gastric ulcer stomach ulcer; *ulcer* in the *gastric mucosa*

gastric volvulus lengthwise or crosswise twisting of the stomach

gastrocnemius muscle calf muscle that flexes the foot at the ankle; *innervation tibial nerve*

gastrin *hormone* produced in the *stomach* that stimulates the production of gastric juice

gastrinoma (Zollinger-Ellison syndrome) *gastrin*-producing tumor, usually localized in the *pancreas* or *duodenum*

gastritis *inflammation* of the *stomach* lining

gastrocnemius, M. *musculus gastrocnemicus*

gastroenteritis *inflammation* of the mucosa of the *stomach* and small intestine, usually with vomiting and diarrhea, caused by *infection* with *rotavirus* or other pathogens, among other things

gastroenterological pert. to *gastroenterology*

gastroenterologist specialist in *gastroenterology*

gastroenterology study of diseases of the gastrointestinal tract

gastrointestinal pert. to the digestive tract; abbr. GI

gastrointestinal tract digestive tract; abbr. GIT

gastrojejunostomy *Billroth operation*

gastroscope flexible *endoscope* for performing *gastroscopy*

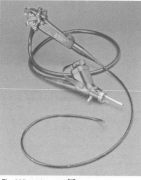

Fig. 205: gastroscope [F]

gastroscopic pert. to *gastroscopy*

gastroscopy *endoscopy* of the *stomach*, usually as part of an *esophagogastroduodenoscopy*

gastrostomy *surgical* opening of the *stomach*

gauge unit of measurement for the external diameter of a *catheter* or *needle*; abbr. G

gauze pad *compress*

GBS abbr. *Guillain-Barré syndrome*

GCS abbr. *Glasgow Coma Scale*

gelasmus laughing fit

gemelli *twins*

geminus *twin*; pl. gemini

gen(o)- combining form: origin

gene portion of a *chromosome* consisting of *DNA*

gene technology (genetic engineering) procedures for altering the genetic material of a life form

gene therapy treatment of disease by injection of intact *genes* to repair hereditary factors

general anesthesia reversible general numbing of the body with artificial unconsciousness and analgesia induced for performing *surgery*; opp. *regional anesthesia*

generalized not confined to one area; opp. *local*

generalized seizure (grand mal) no focal component is present. This seizure is a major motor seizure involving all extremities and having tonic and clonic movements; urinary incontinence is common

generic drug sold under a generic name based on its main active substance

generic name (nonproprietary name) internationally recognized WHO designation for chemical substances such as drugs

-genesis combining form: generation, origin

genetic pert. to the *genes*

genetics study of heredity

-genic combining form: generating, producing

genit(o)- combining form: reproduction sex

genital herpes (herpes genitalis) *infectious disease* caused by the *herpes simplex 2 virus* which leads to vesicle formation on the genitals; transmitted mainly via sexual contact or by reactivation of *viruses* lying dormant in the *cells* after recovery from an infection

genital wart *condyloma acuminatum*

genitalia sexual organs

genitals *genitalia*

genome complete set of all the *genes* in a *chromosome*

genotype all of the genetic information in an *organism*; cf. *phenotype*

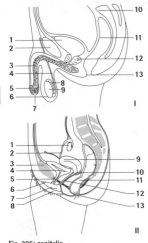

Fig. 206: genitalia
I Male genital organs 1 Bladder (vesica urinaria)
2 Pubic bone (os pubis) 3 Penis 4 Spermatic duct
(vas deferens) 5 Glans (head of penis) 6 Scrotum
7 Urethra 8 Epididymis 9 Testis (didymus, orchis)
10 Sacrum 11 Rectum 12 Prostate 13 Anus
II Female genital organs 1 Ovary 2 Fallopian tube
(uterine tube, salpinx) 3 Pubic bone (os pubis)
4 Bladder (vesica urinaria) 5 Urethra 6 Clitoris
7 Labia minora 8 Labia majora 9 Uterus (metra,
hystera) 10 Cervix 11 Rectum (proctos) 12 Anus
13 Vagina (kolpos)

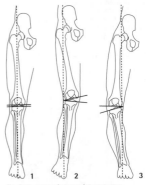

Fig. 207: genu valgum and genu varum
1 Normal position 2 Genu valgum 3 Genu varum

genu knee
genu valgum (knock-knee) *physiological*
knock-kneed leg position in children
between age 2 and 5; normal position after
age 6
genu varum (bowleg) *physiological* bowed
leg position in children before age 2
geriatric pert. to old age

geriatrics *gerontology*
germ layer collective term for the *ectoderm
mesoderm* and *endoderm*
German measles *rubella*
germinal tumor tumor originating in the
reproductive cells
gero- combining form: age, elder
geron elderly person
gerontologist specialist in diseases
of old age; geriatrician
gerontology (geriatrics) the study of
diseases of old age
gest- combining form: pregnant
gestagen female progestational *hormone,*
e.g. *progesterone*
gestation pregnancy
gestational diabetes manifestation of
impaired *glucose* tolerance or *diabetes
mellitus* during pregnancy
gestosis *pre-elampsia*
-geusia combining form: taste
GFR abbr. *glomerular filtration rate*
GGT abbr. *gamma-glutamyl transferase*
GH abbr. *growth hormone (somatotropin)*

GHRH abbr. *growth hormone-releasing hormone*

GI abbr. *gastrointestinal*

Giardia genus of flagellate protozoa that can cause *giardiasis*

giardiasis *inflammation* of the intestine and *bile ducts* caused by *Giardia lamblia*

gibbus hump; extreme *kyphosis*

Giemsa stain contrast staining for better visualization of *cells* and their components

giga– combining form: billion (10^9); symbol G

gigantism abnormally large size

Gilbert's disease hereditary disease marked by impaired *bilirubin* conjugation and reduced uptake of bilirubin into the liver cells, resulting in *intermittent jaundice*

gingiv– combining form: gums

gingiva (gums) oral mucosa surrounding the necks of the teeth and covering the *alveolar* processes and *cementum* attached to the *periosteum* of the jaw; isolates the alveoli from the oral cavity

gingivitis *inflammation* of the *gingiva*

groin *inguen*

GIT abbr. *gastrointestinal tract*

glabella (intercilium) hairless spot between the eyes

glabella reflex *orbicularis oculi reflex*

glanders (malleus) *infectious disease* caused by *Actinobacillus mallei*; main forms are melioidosis (malleus humidus), which causes ulcerous changes in the upper respiratory tract and farcy (malleus farciminosus), which causes purulent eruptions on the skin, muscles and internal organs; transmitted mainly by ungulates (horses, donkeys, mules)

glandula gland

glandula lacrimalis *lacrimal gland*

glandula parotis *parotid gland*

glandula pinealis *pineal gland*

glandula pituitaria *pituitary gland*

glandula prostatica *prostate*

glandula salivariae (salivary gland) collective term for the *parotid* and *sublingual glands*

glandula sublingualis *sublingual gland*

glandula suprarenalis *adrenal gland*

glandula thyreoidea *thyroid gland*

glandulae sebaceae *sebaceous glands*

glandulae sudoriferae *sweat glands*

glans penis (head of the penis) bulbous area of the corpus spongiosum at the end of the *penis*

Glasgow Coma Scale scoring system for levels of altered mental status, e.g. associated with a *head injury*; abbr. GCS

glauco– combining form: blue/green/gray

glaucoma damage to the optic nerve caused by an increase in intraocular pressure to above 20 mmHg (normal: 10-20 mmHg) due to impaired aqueous humor drainage

GLDH abbr. *glutamic dehydrogenase*

neuroglia; supporting substance of the *central nervous system*; present in the spaces between *nerve* cells, their branches and blood vessels

gliadin *allergenic* component of *gluten*; can lead to *celiac disease*

glioblastoma malignant brain tumor originating in the *glia*

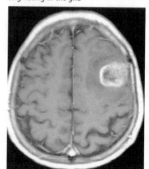

Fig. 208: glioblastoma (MRI)

glioma brain tumor originating in the *glia*

glioma retinae *retinoblastoma*

Glisson's sling apparatus for *extension* of the spinal column

global insufficiency right- and left-sided *heart failure*; see also *respiratory insufficiency*; opp. *partial insufficiency*

globulin plasma *protein* with important transport and defense functions

globus syndrome sensation of having a lump in the throat

glomerular filtration rate amount of *primary urine* that the *glomeruli* filter out of the blood per minute, measured in milliliters; abbr. GFR

glomerular pert. to the *glomeruli*

glomeruli plural of *glomerulus*

glomerulonephritis *inflammation* of the *kidney*, affecting primarily the *glomeruli*; abbr. GN

glomerulus small bundle of *capillaries* in the *renal cortex*; function: filtration of *primary urine*; pl. glomeruli

gloss(o)- combining form: tongue

glossa tongue

glossitis *inflammation* of the of the tongue's mucous membranes

glossopharyngeal nerve 9th contains nerve; contains sensory, motor and parasympathetic fibers; mainly provides *motor* innervation of the *pharynx* (with the *vagus nerve*) and *sensory* innervation of the *pharynx*, *larynx* and posterior auditory canal

glottis sound-producing apparatus of the larynx

gluc- combining form: sugar; glucose

glucagon pancreatic *hormone*; manufactured in the islet cells (A cells); function is to raise *blood sugar*

glucagonoma *glucagon*-producing tumor of the *pancreas*, typically malignant

glucocorticoid collective term for a type of *hormone* produced in the *adrenal cortex* with an important role in *carbohydrate* metabolism, e.g. *cortisol*

glucose (dextrose) monosaccharide found in fruits and other sources; central substance in sugar metabolism; a building block for starches

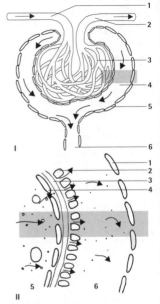

Fig. 209: glomerulus
I **Glomerulus** 1 Afferent arteriole 2 Efferent arteriole 3 Capillary loops 4 Bowman's space 5 Bowman's capsule 6 Proximal tubule
II **Glomerular membrane** 1 Bowman's capsule epithelium 2 Epithelial cells 3 Basement membrane 4 Capillary endothelium 5 Plasma 6 Filtrate

glucose meter (glucometer) device for measuring blood sugar using a drop of blood placed on a treated strip

glucosuria excretion of *glucose* in the urine

glutamic dehydrogenase *enzyme* found primarily in the *mitochondria* of *liver cells* that is released into the blood as a result of *cell* damage and therefore can be used as a laboratory parameter to assess the extent of the damage; abbr. GLDH

Fig. 210: glucose meter [H]

glutamic-oxaloacetic transaminase (aspartate transaminase, AST) *enzyme* found primarily in the *liver, heart* and skeletal muscles that is released into the blood as a result of *cell* damage and therefore can be used as a laboratory parameter to assess disorders of the *heart* and *liver*; abbr. SGOT

glutamic-pyruvic transaminase (alanine transaminase, ALT) *enzyme* found primarily in the *liver* that is released into the blood as a result of *cell* damage and therefore can be used as a laboratory parameter to assess disorders of the *liver*; abbr. SGPT

gluteal pert. to the buttocks

gluten *protein* found in grains

gluteus buttocks muscle

gluteus maximus *(musculus gluteus maximus)* largest buttocks muscle, which straightens the pelvis and extends the thigh; innervation: *inferior gluteal nerve*

gluteus medius, M. *musculus gluteus medius*

gluteus medius (middle gluteal muscle) medium-sized buttocks muscle that abducts the leg at the hip and turns the pelvis to the side; innervation: *superior gluteal nerve*

gluteus minimus smallest buttocks muscle, which abducts the leg at the hip and turns the pelvis to the side; innervation: *superior gluteal nerve*

gluteus minimus, M. *musculus gluteus minimus*

gluteus..., N. *nervus gluteus...*

glyc(o)– combining form: sugar; glucose

glycogen *glucose* molecule compound; function: storing energy in the *cells*

glycogenolysis breakdown of *glycogen*

glycogenosis metabolic disorder marked by pathological accumulation of *glycogen* in the muscles and other *organs*, caused by *enzyme* defects in *glycolysis* or *glycogenolysis*

glycolysis breakdown of *glucose* in the body's *cells*

glycoside *cardiac glycoside*

glycosuria (glucosuria) excretion of *glucose* in the urine

GN abbr. *glomerulonephritis*

gnatho– combining form jaw

-gnos, gnos– combining form: knowledge

goiter (struma) visible or palpable enlargement of the *thyroid gland*

Goldberger lead *unipolar limb leads* used for electrocardiography, connecting with the *Einthoven* ECG leads; the *aVR*, *aVL* and *aVF* leads branch off from these; see also *Einthoven limb leads* and *Wilson precordial leads*

Goldblatt's mechanism mechanism whereby *stenosis* of the renal arteries causes an increase in *blood pressure* from activation of the *renin-angiotensin-aldosterone* system; the lack of circulation to the kidneys activates the system, leading to elevation of blood pressure

GON abbr. greater occipital nerve

gon(o)– combining form: reproductive organs

gonadal dysgenesis absence of gametes due to dysfunctional *gonads*

gonadotropin *hormone* produced by the *adenohypophysis* that acts on the *gonads*

gonadotropin-releasing hormone a *hormone* produced by the *hypothalamus* that controls the release of *follicle-stimulating hormone* and *luteinizing hormone* in the *adenohypophysis*; abbr. GnRH

gonads reproductive organs (*ovaries* and *testes*)

gonarthrosis degeneration of the knee *joint* due to *cartilage* wear

goniometer instrument used for measuring diameters and angles, e.g. *joint* angles

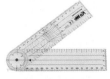

Fig. 211: goniometer

gonoblenorrhea (gonococcal conjunctivitis) purulent *inflammation* of the *conjunctiva* caused by *gonococci*, usually occurring in newborns

gonococcal urethritis infection of the urethra caused by gonococci

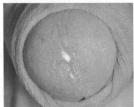

Fig. 212: gonococcal urethritis

gonococci genus of nonmotile *gram-negative bacteria* that cause *gonorrhea*, e.g. *Neisseria gonorrhoeae*

gonorrhea (clap) *infectious disease* caused by *Neisseria gonorrhoeae*, affecting mainly the mucous membranes of the *urethra*, *cervix uteri*, *cornea* and *pharynx*, as well as

the *rectum*; transmitted mainly via sexual intercourse

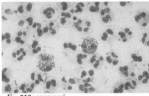

Fig. 213: gonococci

gony knee

Gordon reflex similar to *Babinski's reflex* but triggered by pressure on the calf

GOT abbr. *glutamic-oxaloacetic transaminase*

gout (gouty arthritis) relapsing-remitting disease in which increased *uric acid* in the blood leads to deposition of uric acid salts (urates) in peripheral joints, resulting in recurrent inflammation; affects primarily the metatarsophalangeal joint (*podagra*)

gouty arthritis gout

GPT abbr. *glutamic-pyruvic transaminase*

Graafian follicle vesicular follicle in the *ovary* that holds the ovum before it is released at *ovulation*

gracilis, M. (musculus gracilis) *gracilis muscle*

gracilis muscle slender hip muscle that draws the thigh toward the body and extends the knee joint; *innervation: obturator nerve*

–grade combining form: steps, progression

gradient degree of change

grading of muscle strength 0 = no contraction; 1 = muscle contraction; 2 = movement with gravity eliminated; 3 = movement against gravity; 4 = movement against moderate resistance; 5 = full strength

grading *histological* categorization of *tumors* to rate their malignancy

graft–versus–host disease *rejection reaction* in which the *cells* in a *graft* react against the recipient's *tissues*

-gram combining form: written, record

Gram stain (Gram's method) staining of *bacteria* for better identification under the microscope; see also *gram-positive, gram-negative*

gram-negative *bacteria* that do not take on a blue color in *Gram's method* of staining, e.g. *gonococci, meningococci, Salmonella, Shigella, Pseudomonas, Enterobacter, Brucella, Haemophilus* and *Yersinia*

gram-positive *bacteria* that take on a blue color in *Gram's method* of staining, e.g. *staphylococci, streptococci, pneumococci, Listeria, Corynebacteria, Bacillus anthracis*

grand mal (seizure) most severe form of *epileptic seizure*, in which both halves of the brain are affected; opp. *petit mal (seizure)*

granular conjunctivitis *trachoma*

granulate drug in powder form

granulation formation of scar *tissue*

granulation tissue *tissue* from which scar tissue is created through deposition of *collagen* fibers

granulocyte plasma cell belonging to the *leukocyte* group; function in immune defense: can absorb other *cells* and activate defensive substances to fight tumor cells or other *infected* white blood cells and foreign substances; differentiated in the laboratory into *neutrophils eosinophils* and *basophils* according to dye affinity

granuloma tumor consisting of *granulation tissue*, e.g. on a *dental root*

granulomatosis presence of multiple *granulomas*

-graph combining form: recorder, writer

-graphy combining form: recording, writing

Graves' disease *hyperthyroidism*

gravid- combining form: pregnancy

gravid pregnant

gravidity pregnancy

Gray unit of measurement for energy dose e.g. in radiation therapy; symbol Gy

great saphenous vein *vein* that takes blood from the inner edge of the foot to the *femoral vein* along the inner side of the leg

great toe hallux

greater pectoral muscle (pectoralis major) large muscle of the chest that adducts the upper arm, etc.; *innervation: ventral* branches of the *thoracic nerve*

greater trochanter (trochanter major) bony process below the head of the *femur*

greenstick fracture *fracture* occurring in children and adolescents in which the *periosteum* remains intact on at least one side of the bone

grippe *influenza*

gtt(s). abbr. *drop(s)*

guaiac test for presence of blood in the stool

Guedel tube (oropharyngeal tube) short rubber tube that is introduced into the oropharyngeal area; used for patients with impaired consciousness to prevent them swallowing the tongue and thus obstructing the airway; see also *Wendl tube*

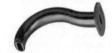

Fig. 214: Guedel tube [K]

Guillain–Barré syndrome (acute inflammatory polyradiculopathy, acute inflammatory polyneuropathy) ascending *inflammation* and paralysis of the *spinal nerves*, usually occurring after febrile *infections* of the respiratory or gastrointestinal tract; abbr. GBS

gums *gingiva*

gunshot wound penetrating injury from a bullet; variable damage depending on location of injury, deflection by bones, amount of soft tissue injury; abbr. GSW

gust(a)- combining form: taste

gut *intestines; large intestine; small intestine*

Gy symbol *gray*

gyn(eco)- combining form: female, woman

gyne woman

gynecologic(al) pert. to *gynecology*

gynecologist specialist in *gynecology*

gynecology study of diseases of the female reproductive system

gynecomastia abnormal increase in the size of the male breast due to *hypertrophy* of glandular or fatty tissue, e.g. in *Klinefelter's syndrome*

gyrus convolution on the surface of the *brain*; pl. gy

H

H chemical symbol *hydrogen*

h symbol: hour; hundred (10^2); combining form: *hecto-*

H_2CO_3 chemical symbol: *carbonic acid*

H_2O chemical symbol: water

H_2O_2 chemical symbol: hydrogen peroxide

habitual repeated by habit, recurring

habituation becoming accustomed, e.g. to a drug

habitus outward appearance of the body

Haemophilus rod-shaped *gram-negative bacterium* that is able to grow in anaerobic conditions, but always requires blood or *hemoglobin* to do so; can cause a wide variety of *infectious diseases*, including *chancroid* (H. ducreyi) *conjunctivitis* (H. aegyptius) *laryngitis*, *meningitis*, *endocarditis*, or *pneumonia* (H. influenzae)

Hageman factor important blood *coagulation* factor (*Factor XII*)

haima blood

hairline fracture fine fracture with no separation of the bone fragments; few *symptoms*, usually detectable only by *x-ray*; cf. *infraction*, *fracture*

halitosis foul breath

hallucination false perception for which there is no basis in reality and which the patient does not recognize as imaginary; see also *pseudohallucination*

hallucinosis condition marked by frequent recurring *hallucinations*

hallux great toe, big toe

hallux rigidus *arthrosis* of the basal joint of the great toe

hallux valgus displacement of the great toe in the direction of the little toe

hallux varus displacement of the great toe toward the midline of the body

hamate bone one of the *carpal bones*

hamatum, os (os hamatum) *hamate bone*

hand manus

Hansen's disease *leprosy*

Hantavirus genus of *viruses* that cause *hemorrhagic fevers* and hantavirus pulmonary syndrome

haplo- combining form: one, single

hapt- combining form: touch

haptoglobin *protein* that transports *hemoglobin* from hemolyzed *erythrocytes* in the bloodstream into the reticuloendo-thelial system in order to prevent the body from losing *iron*, among other functions

hard chancre typical *syphilitic ulcer*

harelip *cleft lip*

Häring tube wire-reinforced crush-proof *tube* for maintaining a passageway for food in patients with esophageal carcinoma

HAV abbr. *hepatitis A virus*

Hb abbr. *hemoglobin*

HbA$_{1c}$ glycosylated *hemoglobin* that yields information about the metabolic state of *diabetes mellitus* patients over the preceding 48 weeks; based on the average survival time of *erythrocytes*

HbE abbr. *hemoglobin* content of individual *erythrocytes*

HBV abbr. *hepatitis B virus*

HCC abbr. *hepatocellular carcinoma*

HCG abbr. *human chorionic gonadotropin*

HCl chemical symbol: hydrochloric *acid*

HCO$_3$ chemical symbol: *standard bicarbonate*

HCT abbr. *hematocrit*

HCV abbr. *hepatitis C virus*

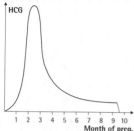

Fig. 215: HCG production during pregnancy

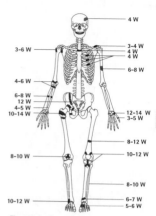

Fig. 216: healing periods

HD abbr. *hemodialysis (dialysis)*

HDF abbr. *hemodiafiltration*

HDL abbr. *high-density lipoprotein;*
lipoprotein with a high molecular weight

HDL cholesterol high-density *lipoprotein*
cholesterol; *cholesterol* that is bound to
protein, which is believed to have vascular-
protective effects; see also *LDL cholesterol*

HDV abbr. *hepatitis D virus*

head injury (head trauma, craniocerebral
trauma) *post-traumatic* combined damage
to the *skull* and *brain*; classified according
to degree of severity: *cerebral concussion,
cerebral contusion, cerebral compression*;
also by damage to the *dura:* injury to dura
= open head injury; no injury to dura =
closed head injury; abbr. HI

healing by first intention (primary healing)
immediate wound healing with closure of
the wound edges and formation of a thin
scar

healing by second intention wound healing
delayed past the *granulation* stage with
epithelialization from the edges of the
wound inward, e.g. following *wound
infection*

healing period time required for stable bone
healing, e.g. following a *fracture*

health condition of physical, mental and
social well-being

hearing test see *Weber test, Rinne test*

heart *organ* situated in the *mediastinal
space*, divided into two atria and two
ventricles; pumps blood through the
circulatory system by means of rhythmic
contractions

heart attack *myocardial infarction*

heart axis electrical axis of the heart during
maximum excitation of the QRS complexes
in an ECG

heart catheterization see *cardiac
catheterization*

heart failure (cardiac insufficiency)
inadequate cardiac performance, such that
the heart can no longer pump the volume
of blood required by the body; can occur as
either left heart failure or right heart
failure; global heart failure affects both the
left and right heart; rated according to
degree of severity in the *NYHA
Classification*; abbr. HF

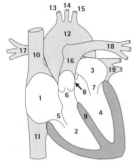

Fig. 217: heart
1 Right atrium 2 Right ventricle 3 Left atrium
4 Left ventricle 5 Triscuspid valve 6 Pulmonary
valve 7 Mitral valve 8 Aortic valve 9 Interventricular septum 10 Superior vena cava 11 Inferior vena
cava 12 Aorta 13 Brachiocephalic (trunk) artery
14 Left common carotid artery 15 Left subclavian
artery 16 Pulmonary trunk 17 Right pulmonary artery 18 Left pulmonary artery 19 Pulmonary vein

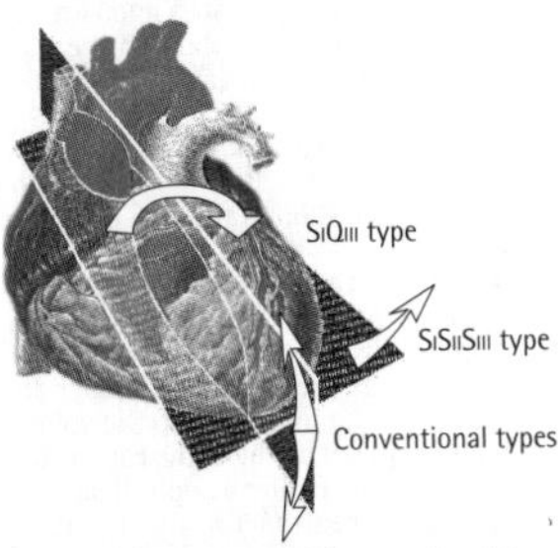

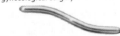

Fig. 218: electrical axes of heart and positions

heart–lung machine (extracorporeal
circulation) device that enables blood to
circulate outside the body, circumventing
the heart and lungs; used for open-heart
surgery; abbr. HLM, ECC

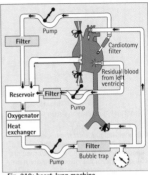

Fig. 219: heart-lung machine

heatstroke buildup of heat in the body due
to inadequate heat regulation, marked by
circulatory problems, headache and
unconsciousness

hebephrenia form of *schizophrenia*
occurring in adolescents or younger adults

hecto- combining form: hundred (10^2);
symbol: h

heel calx

heel pain syndrome nonspecific collective
term for exertion-related pain in the area
from the sole of the foot to the origin of
the *Achilles tendon*

heelbone *calcaneus*

Hegar dilators (Hegar rods) series of metal
rods of varying thickness, used e.g. for
gradual dilation of the *cervical* canal for
gynecological surgery

Fig. 220: Hegar dilator [A]

height of fundus height of the fundus of the *uterus*, determined by palpation, in order to establish week of gestation and/or degree of involution of the uterus following birth

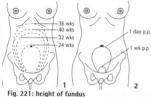

Fig. 221: height of fundus
1 Height of fundus 2 Postpartum height of fundus

Heimlich maneuver emergency maneuver for *aspiration* of foreign bodies with the danger of asphyxiation, in which pressure exerted on the *epigastrium* with both arms creates a sudden increase in *intraabdominal* pressure, which should then result in expulsion of the foreign body, but is more likely to lead to damage to the abdominal organs

helix curled edge of the external ear

HELLP syndrome (**h**emolytic anemia, **e**levated **l**iver enzymes, **l**ow **p**latelets) disease of pregnancy marked by *pre-eclampsia* and clotting disorders, usually with right epigastric pain due to liver capsule distension

helminth– combining form: worms

hema, hemo combining form blood

hemangioma benign tumor consisting of enlarged blood vessels

hemangiosarcoma malignant tumor originating in the blood vessels

hemarthros(is) bloody *effusion* within a *joint*, e.g. due to *trauma*

hematemesis vomiting of blood; color is normally blood-red or dark brown with a coffee-ground look if the blood has previously been in contact with stomach acid

hematin non-protein component of *hemoglobin* in which iron is present as Fe^{3+}

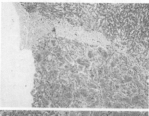
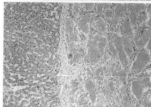

Fig. 222: cavernous hemangioma in liver

hematocele collection of blood in an existing body cavity, e.g. following *surgery*

hematochezia visible blood in the stool

hematocolpos accumulation of blood in the *vagina*, usually *menstrual* blood in cases of *imperforate hymen*

hematocrit percentage of particulate components in whole blood (*erythrocytes*, *leukocytes* and *thrombocytes*); abbr. HCT

hematogenic 1) pert. to blood; 2) originating in the blood; 3) pert. to *hematopoiesis*

hematologic(al) pert. to *hematology*

hematologist specialist in *hematology*

hematology study of blood cells and blood diseases

hematoma bruise

hematometra accumulation of blood in the *uterine* cavity, usually a consequence of backed-up *menstrual* blood from a *hema-tocolpos* in cases of *imperforate hymen*

hematomyelia hemorrhage into the *spinal cord*

hematopneumothorax combination of *pneumothorax* and *hemothorax*

hematopoiesis formation of blood cells

hematopoietic pert. to *hematopoiesis*

hematorrhea copious bleeding

hematothorax (hemothorax) pathological collection of blood in the *pleural cavity*, usually due to injury to the thorax

hematuria excretion of blood in the urine, e.g. due to injuries to the *bladder*

hemeralopia diminished vision in high light

H **hemi-** combining form: half

hemiamaurosis *hemianopsia*

hemiamblyopia *hemianopsia*

hemianop(s)ia (hemiamaurosis, hemiamblyopia) blindness affecting one half of the visual field

hemiazygos, V. *hemiazygos vein*

hemiazygos vein *vein* that runs parallel to the *azygos vein* and then joins it

hemiballism involuntary violent jerking movements of one side of the body; cf. *ballism*

hemicolectomy *surgical* removal of half (or less) of the colon, e.g. due to tumors

hemiglobin *methemoglobin*

hemilateral pert. to one side only

hemiparalysis complete paralysis of one side of the body

hemiparesis incomplete paralysis of one side of the body

hemiparetic pert. to *hemiparesis*

hemiplegia *hemiparalysis*

hemiplegic pert. to *hemiplegia*

hemisphere one of the halves of the *brain*

hemochromatosis 1) bronze diabetes; 2) chronic *iron* storage disease with increased *iron absorption* and *hemosiderosis*

hemoconcentration thickening of the blood due to loss of fluids

hemodiafiltration procedure for removing urophanic substances and liquids from the blood in *renal failure*; combination of *hemofiltration* and *dialysis*; abbr. HDF

hemodialysis procedure for removing impurities and wastes from the blood; the blood is shunted from the body through a machine via an *arteriovenous shunt*

hemodilution blood thinning

hemodynamic pert. to *hemodynamics*

hemodynamics study of blood flow in the vascular system from a physical perspective

hemofiltration procedure for removing high-molecular-weight substances and liquids from the blood in a patient with uremia; types are *arteriovenous hemofiltration* and *venovenous hemofiltration*; abbr. HF

hemoglobin red blood pigment found in the *erythrocytes*; function: transport of *oxygen* and *carbon dioxide*; abbr. Hb

hemoglobinuria excretion of dissolved *hemoglobin* in the urine, e.g. due to *hemolysis*

hemolysis destruction of *erythrocytes*

hemolytic pert. to hemolysis

hemolytic anemia *anemia* caused by destruction of *erythrocytes*

hemolytic–uremic syndrome *hemolytic anemia* with *thrombopenia*, hemorrhagic *diathesis* and *renal failure*, usually occurring in infants and young children; abbr. HUS

hemopathy nonspecific collective term for blood disease

hemoperfusion detoxification procedure in which the patient's blood is run through an *adsorber* (activated charcoal or resin) *extracorporeally*; used to remove *lipophilic protein*-binding *toxins*

hemopericardium collection of blood in the *pericardium*

hemophilia A blood *coagulation* disorder due to deficient *antihemophilic globulin A* (Factor VIII)

hemophilia B blood *coagulation* disorder due to due to deficient *antihemophilic globulin B* (Factor IX)

hemoptysis 1) coughing up larger amounts of bright red, possibly frothy blood; 2) presence of small amounts of blood in expectorated mucus

hemorrhage bleeding
hemorrhagic bloody; pert. to *hemorrhage*
hemorrhagic diathesis tendency to excessive bleeding due to an inherited disease
hemorrhagic fevers a group of viral infections that cause fever, chills, headache, respiratory and GI symptoms, followed by capillary hemorrhages and possibly death if other organs are severely involved; signs and symptoms differ by geographic location
hemorrhoid vascular bundle that is pressed down into the anal canal due to weak connective tissue, *obstipation,* a low-fiber diet or pregnancy
hemosiderin *protein* that stores iron in *organs,* e.g. the *liver, spleen* and *bone marrow*
hemosiderosis increased deposition of *iron* in the *tissues*
hemostasis arrest or cessation of bleeding
hemostat (hemostatic forceps) *surgical* instrument, e.g. according to Adson, used for temporary interruption of blood flow, to clamp off damaged blood vessels, and for general holding tasks

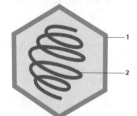

Fig. 223: hemostat [A]

hemostatic 1) drug or device to arrest bleeding; 2) having the ability to arrest bleeding
hemostatic forceps *hemostat*
hemostyptic *hemostatic agent*
Henle's loop U-shaped section of the *renal tubule* where *loop diuretics* take effect

Fig. 224: injection stopper [C]

Hep-Lok plug with a Luer connector for plugging a venous catheter; integrated rubber membrane enables injection through the plug
hepa(to)- combining form: liver
hepar *liver*
hepatic 1) pert. to the *liver;* 2) drug used to treat liver disease
hepatic coma coma with preserved brain stem, caused by an increase in *ammonia* levels due to liver dysfunction
hepatic cyst (liver cyst) single or multiple fluid-filled cavities in the *liver*
hepatic duct (ductus hepaticus) duct leading out of the liver, emptying into the *common bile duct*
hepatic puncture *puncture* of the *liver* to obtain *tissue* samples for testing
hepatic veins collective term for the right, intermediate and left hepatic veins
hepatica, A. *arteria hepatica ...*
hepaticae, Vv. *venae hepaticae*
hepatitis A *infectious disease* affecting the *liver cells,* caused by the *hepatitis A virus;* transmitted mainly via *smear infection,* contaminated shellfish and blood

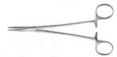

Fig. 225: hepatitis A virus
1 Capsule 2 RNA

hepatitis A virus *virus* that causes *hepatitis A;* abbr. *HAV*
hepatitis B *infectious disease* affecting the *liver cells,* caused by the *hepatitis B virus;* transmitted mainly via blood, unsterilized needles and sexual intercourse

hepatitis B virus *virus* that causes *hepatitis B*; abbr. *HBV*

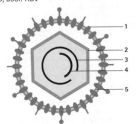

Fig. 226: hepatitis B virus
1 Envelope 2 Capsid (HBc/HBe-Ag) 3 DNA minus strand 4 DNA plus strand 5 HBs antigen

hepatitis C *infectious disease* affecting the *liver cells*, caused by the *hepatitis C virus*; transmission as for *hepatitis B*
hepatitis C virus *virus* that causes *hepatitis C*; abbr. *HCV*
hepatitis D virus *virus* that causes *hepatitis D*; abbr. *HDV*
hepatitis E *infectious disease* affecting the *liver cells*, caused by the *hepatitis E virus*; transmission via *smear infection*
hepatitis E virus *virus* that causes *hepatitis E*; abbr. *HEV*
hepatitis inflammation of the *liver*
hepatocellular carcinoma malignant tumor of the *liver cells* (hepatocytes); abbr. HCC
hepatocyte *liver cell*
hepatogenous originating in the *liver*
hepatolenticular degeneration *Wilson's disease*
hepatolienal pert. to the *liver* and *spleen*
hepatoma *liver* tumor
hepatomegaly pathological enlargement of the *liver*
hepatopathy nonspecific collective term for liver disease
hepatosis nonspecific collective term for noninflammatory liver disease

hepatosplenomegaly pathological enlargement of the *liver* and *spleen*
hept(a)– combining form: seven
hereditary inherited
hereditary spherocytosis *spherocytic anemia*
hermaphrodite (androgyne) individual with physical characteristics of both sexes
hernia (rupture) protrusion of *organ* parts through a gap in muscle or connective tissue, e.g. displacement of a portion of the intestine into a bulge in the peritoneum

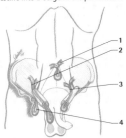

Fig. 227: hernia
1 Umbilical 2 Indirect inguinal hernia 3 Direct inguinal hernia 4 Femoral hernia

herniated disk rupture of the cartilage surrounding an intervertebral disk, causing the nucleus to prolapse into the spinal cord space
herniorrhaphy *surgical* treatment of a *hernia*
herpes (simplex) *infectious disease* caused by the *herpes simplex virus* (HSV) that leads to vesicle formation on the skin and mucosa; HSV 1 *infections* occur mainly in the facial and head area; HSV 2 *infections* mainly on the *genitals*, transmitted mainly via contact or *smear infection*, or by reactivation of *viruses* lying dormant in the cells after recovery from an infection
herpes febrilis *herpes* affecting the lips and nasal mucosa

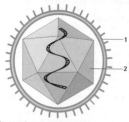

Fig. 228: herpes simplex virus
1 Envelope with spikes 2 Nucleocapsid

herpes labialis cold sore; fever blister; *infectious disease* caused by the *herpes simplex 1 virus*, occurring mainly in connection with a febrile disease and causing vesicle formation on the lips; transmitted mainly via contact or *smear infection* or by reactivation of *viruses* lying dormant in the *cells* after recovery from an infection

herpes simplex virus *DNA virus* that causes *herpes (simplex)*; there are two subgroups, of which type 1 (HSV 1) causes mainly *herpes labialis* and type 2 (HSV 2) *herpes genitalis*; abbr. HSV

herpes zoster *shingles*

hetero– combining form: different

heterochromia difference in *iris* color between the right and left eyes, usually congenital

heterogeneous not uniform; opp. *homogeneous*

heterologous not of the same type; opp. *autologous, homologous*

heterologous graft *xenogeneic graft*

heterosexuality sexual attraction to persons of the opposite sex; opp. *homosexuality*

heterotopic located or appearing in an unusual location; opp. *orthotopic*

heterotransplantation *transplantation* in which the site from which the transplant is taken differs from the site where it is

implanted in the recipient; see also *homotopic graft, isotopic graft*

HEV abbr. *hepatitis E virus*

hex(a)– combining form: six

HF abbr. *hemofiltration; heart failure*

Hg chemical symbol: *mercury*

hGH abbr. *human growth hormone (somatotropin)*

hGH–releasing hormone (somatostatin) *hormone* produced by the *hypothalamus* that controls the release of *somatotropin* in the *adenohypophysis*; abbr. GHRH

hiatal hernia (esophageal hernia) protrusion of part of the stomach into the *mediastinum* through an opening in the *diaphragm*

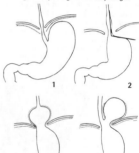

Fig. 229: hiatal hernia
1 Normal 2 Obtuse angle of His C3323 Axial sliding hernia 4 Paraesophageal hernia

hiatus gap; opening

hiccups (hiccoughs) spasmodic closure of the *glottis* caused by rapid *contractions* of the *diaphragm*

Hickman catheter brand name for a surgically inserted triple-lumen catheter inserted for central venous delivery of medications

hidr(o)- combining form sweat

hidros sweat

high-dose chemotherapy administering higher, more effective doses of chemotherapy; the chemo destroys bone marrow, so a stem-cell rescue is required to replenish blood-forming bone marrow cells

high enema (enteroclysis) injection of *contrast medium* for radiography of the entire small intestine

hilum (hilus) entry or exit point in an *organ*, e.g. for nerves or vessels

hip coxa

hip bones *os coxae*, consisting of the *ilium*, *ischium* and *pubic bone*

HIPAA abbr. Health Information Portability and Accountability Act of 1996

hip contracture stiffening of the hip joint in contracted position so that extension is no longer possible

Hirschsprung's disease congenital *megacolon* caused by a narrow segment in the *rectum* or *sigmoid colon*

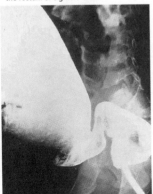

Fig. 230: Hirschsprung's disease

hirsutism male-type hairiness in women due to increased *androgen*dependent terminal hair growth

hirud(in) combining form: leech

histamine *tissue hormone* with multiple functions, e.g. as a messenger substance in *allergic* reactions

histo- combining form: tissue

histologic(al) pert. to *histology*

histology study of the structure of body *tissues*

histopathology study of disease-related tissue changes in the body

Hitselberger's sign *sensory* impairment of the external auditory canal in patients with *acoustic neurinoma*

HIV abbr. human immunodeficiency virus; *virus* that causes the *infectious disease* AIDS

HLM abbr. *heart-lung machine*

HMO abbr. health maintenance organization

Hodgkin's disease malignant disease affecting the *lymph nodes*

holo- combining form: complete, total

holosystolic lasting through the entire *systole* (e.g. heart sounds)

Holter monitor device used to monitor the ECG recordings of the heart for 24 hours or more as the patient carries out his activities of daily living

Homans' sign pain in the calf under passive *dorsal flexion* of the foot; a sign of *phlebothrombosis*

hom(e)o- combining form: same, like

homeopathic pert. to *homeopathy*

homeopathy study of treatment of illness with greatly diluted medicines

homeostasis equilibrium of body's functions

homo human being

homocysteine intermediate product of *protein* metabolism; a high level in the blood is a risk factor for *myocardial infarction*

homogeneic graft *allogeneic graft*

homogeneous uniform; opp. *heterogeneous*

homologous graft *transplantation* of tissue from a donor to a recipient of the same species

homosexuality sexual attraction to persons of the same sex; opp. *heterosexuality*

H

honeymoon cystitis *cystitis* caused by frequent sexual intercourse

hordeolum (stye) acute *inflammation* of the *sebaceous* glands at the edge of the eyelids

horizontal plane (transverse plane) body plane running parallel to the floor, used e.g. in imaging processes

hormonal pert. to *hormones*

hormone chemical messenger substance formed in any of several glands, regulating metabolism and *organ* functions

Horner syndrome neurological symptom identified by a constricted pupil and ptosis of the eyelid, which may be caused by a lesion of the the spinal cord

horseshoe kidney malformation in which the kidneys are joined together, usually at the lower end, by a bridge of *parenchymal* tissue

hospice care facility for terminally ill patients

hospitalism any damages or injuries incurred during a hospital stay

hospitalist physician specializing in inpatient care

Howell-Jolly bodies *cell nucleus* debris in the *erythrocytes*

HPT abbr. *hyperparathyroidism*

HPV abbr. human papillomavirus; HPV causes persisent viral infection that can lead to cancer of the cervix; onset typically in the third to sixth decades of life

HPV vaccination vaccine given for prevention of cervical cancer

HRT abbr. hormone replacement therapy

HSV abbr. *herpes simplex virus*

HTX abbr. *heart transplant*

human pert. to a human being

human chorionic gonadotropin *hormone* normally produced only during pregnancy by the *placenta*; HCG sustains the function of the *corpus luteum* and thus prevents occurrence of *menstruation* during pregnancy; important *tumor marker* for reproductive cell tumors; abbr. HCG

humer– combining form: upper arm

humerus fracture *fracture* of the *humerus* along its shaft, with the risk of vascular or nerve injury, e.g. to the *radial nerve*

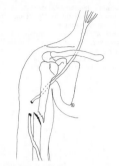

Fig. 231: humerus fracture

humerus upper arm bone

humor fluid

humoral pert. to fluid

humpback (hunchback) abnormal curvature (*kyphosis*) of the *thoracic spine*, e.g. due to *Scheuermann's disease*

hunger pains pain in the epigastrium occurring several hours after the last meal, typical of *duodenal ulcer*

Huntington's chorea (Huntington's disease) hereditary chorea with mental degeneration that results in dementia; age of onset is commonly in the forties

HUS abbr. *hemolytic-uremic syndrome*

hyal– combining form: glassy

hyalin elastic albuminous substance in the cartilage

hyaline transparent

hydrarthrosis *joint effusion*

hydatid tapeworm larva

hydatid torsion acute torsion of the *appendix testis*

hydatiform mole (hydatid mole) malformation of the *placenta* due to cystic degeneration of the *villi* in the *trophoblast* during early pregnancy

hydr– combining form: water

hydramnion (hydramnios) increase in the amount of *amniotic fluid* in the *amnion*; opp. *oligohydramnion*

hydrargyria (mercurialism) *mercury* poisoning

hydrargyrum *mercury*; chemical symbol: Hg

hydrocele accumulation of water or *serous* fluid between layers of *tissue*; usually occurs in the *scrotal* area

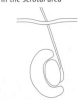

Fig. 232: hydrocele

hydrocephalus (hydrencephalus) enlargement of the ventricles of the brain caused by faulty *CSF* drainage

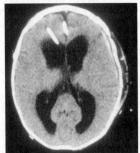

Fig. 233: hydrocephalus in CT

hydrocortisone *glucocorticoid* formed from *cholesterol* in the *adrenal cortex*

hydrogen chemical element present in water and nearly all other organic compounds; chemical symbol: *H*

hydronephrosis (sacculated kidney) stretching of the *renal pelvis* due to impaired outflow through the urinary tract

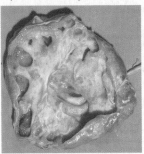

Fig. 234: hydronephrosis

hydrophilous able to be combined with water; opp. *hydrophobic*

hydrophobic 1) unable to be combined with water; opp. *hydrophilous*; 2) intolerant of water; see *rabies*

hydrops (edema) accumulation of fluid in an existing body cavity, e.g. the *gallbladder*

hydros (aqua) water; chemical symbol: H_2O

hydrosalpinx accumulation of fluid in the *fallopian tube*

hydruria increased excretion of water with the urine, e.g. in *diabetes insipidus*

hygiene study of disease prevention and preservation of health

hygienic pert. to *hygiene*

hygro– combining form: moisture

hygroma tumor consisting of water and mucus, usually associated with *chronic inflammation* of a *bursa*

hymen (maidenhead) fold of mucous membrane with a small opening that covers the *vagina*

hymen– combining form: hymen

hyoglossus, M. (musculus hyoglossus) *hyoglossus muscle*

hyoglossus muscle muscle that extends from the *hyoid bone* to the lateral edges of the tongue and moves the tongue upward and back; *innervation hypoglossal nerve*

hyoid bone U-shaped bone beneath the tongue

hyoideum, os (os hyoideum) *hyoid bone*

hypalgesia diminished ability to feel pain; opp. *hyperalgesia*

hypasthesia diminished ability to sense touch

hyper- combining form: over, above, excessive; opp. *hypo-*

hyperacidity excessive production of hydrochloric acid by the *stomach*; opp. *anacidity*

hyperacusis pathologically heightened perception of sound

hyperaldosteronism increased secretion of *aldosterone* by the *adrenal cortex*

hyperalgesia heightened ability to feel pain; opp. *hypalgesia*

hyperalimentation syndrome diminished overall health due to overeating

hyperbilirubinemia increased *bilirubin* in the blood, leading to *jaundice*

hypercalcemia increase in blood *calcium* to levels above 2.6 mmol/l, e.g. due to *osteolysis*; may lead to a *hypercalcemic crisis*; opp. *hypocalcemia*

hypercalcemic crisis disease pattern triggered by excessively high levels of *calcium* in the blood, which may lead to *polyuria, polydipsia,* vomiting, *exsiccosis,* fever, *psychosis* and confusion, and finally to *coma*

hypercapnia (hypercarbia) increased level of *carbon dioxide* in the blood, e.g. due to *hypoventilation*; opp. *hypocapnia*

hypercholesterolemia elevated levels of *cholesterol* in the blood

hyperchromatism 1) increased stain ability; 2) increased amount of *hemoglobin* in the *erythrocytes*

hyperchromic pert. to *hyperchromatism*; opp. *hypochromic*

hyperchylia increased production of gastric juice

hyperdense having increased tissue density usually used in relation to imaging procedures e.g. x-ray; opp. *hypodense*

hyperdynamia excessive muscular activity; opp. *adynamia*

hyperdynamic pert. to *hyperdynamia*; opp. *adynamic*

hyperemesis gravidarum *hormone*-linked severe vomiting during pregnancy, usually between the 4th and 16th weeks; see also *emesis gravidarum*

hyperemia increased quantity of blood in an *organ* or area of the body; opp. *hypoemia*

hyperemic 1) adj. of *hyperemia*; opp. *hypoemic*; 2) drug used to increase blood volume in an *organ* or area of the body

hypergalactia increased milk secretion during the nursing period with the danger of *galactostasis*; opp. *hypogalactia*

hyperglycemia pathological elevation of *blood sugar*; opp. *hypoglycemia*

hyperglycemic pert. to *hyperglycemia*; opp. *hypoglycemic*

hypergonadism overfunctioning of the sex glands

hyperhidrosis increased production of sweat; opp. *anhidrosis, hypohidrosis*

hyperhydration state of excessive water content in the body, e.g. in *renal failure*; opp. *dehydration*

hyperkalemia increase in blood *potassium* to levels above 5.0 mmol/l, e.g. in *renal failure* or due to *hemolysis* in the collected blood sample; may lead to life-threatening cardiac dysrhythmias that could progress to *asystole*; opp. *hypokalemia*

hyperkeratosis thickening of the horny layer of the *epidermis*, e.g. on the feet

hyperkinesia excessive movement, e.g. due to brain damage; opp. *akinesia*

hyperkinetic pert. to *hyperkinesia*; opp. *akinetic*

hyperlipemia increased concentration of fat in the blood

hyperlipoproteinemia increased concentration of one or several *lipoproteins* in the blood

H

hypermagnesemia increase in blood *magnesium* to levels above 1.1 mmol/l, e.g. due to overdosing as a result of parenteral magnesium administration; may lead to impaired consciousness (magnesium narcosis); e.g.; opp. *hypomagnesemia*

hypermenorrhea heavy *menstruation* (> 5 pads/day) lasting the normal length of time; *organic* or *endocrine* causes; opp. *hypomenorrhea*

hypermetropia *hyperopia*

hypermnesia exaggeration of memory, e.g. for individual details; usually occurs in mental retardation; opp. *hypomnesia*

hypernatremia increase in blood *sodium* to levels above 145 mmol/l, e.g. due to *hypertonic dehydration*; may lead to dehydration of *cells* and *tissues*; opp. *hyponatremia*

hypernephroma nonspecific term for tumors originating in the *renal cells*

hyperopia farsightedness caused by inadequate refractive ability due to a shortened eyeball, such that parallel rays are focused behind the retina; opp. *myopia*

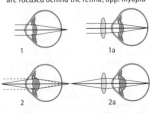

Without correction   With correction
Fig. 235: hyperopia

hyperparathyroidism overactivity of the *parathyroid gland* with increased production of *parathyroid hormone*; abbr. HPT

hyperpathia hypersensitivity to pain

hyperphosphatemia increase in blood *phosphate* to levels above 1.6 mmol/l, e.g.

due to *renal failure*; may lead to calcification; opp. *hypophosphatemia*

hyperpituitarism increased hormone production by the *pituitary gland*, leading in turn to increased hormone production in the affected organs

hyperplasia increase in the size of an *organ* due to excessive proliferation of *cells* in a *tissue*; opp. *hypoplasia*

hyperplastic pert. to *hyperplasia*; opp. *hypoplasia*

hyperproteinemia increased levels of *proteins* in the blood, e.g. due to *inflammation*; opp. *hypoproteinemia*

hyperpyretic pert. to *hyperpyrexia*

hyperpyrexia (hyperthermia) elevation of the body temperature to > 40.5° C

hyperreflexia increased strength of *reflexes*; opp. *hyporeflexia*, *areflexia*

hypersalivation increased production of saliva; opp. *hyposalivation*

hyperspermia *ejaculate volume* > 7 ml; opp. *hypospermia*

hypersplenism increased breakdown of blood cells in an enlarged *spleen*

hypertelorism increased distance between two paired organs, e.g. the eyeballs

hypertension (high blood pressure) pathological elevation of *blood pressure* to values above 160/95 mmHg in adults (WHO definition); borderline hypertension is considered to start at 140/90; opp. *hypotension*

hypertensive pert. to *hypertension*; opp. *hypotensive*

hypertensive crisis life-threatening elevation of *blood pressure* to values > 230/120 with no signs of *acute organ* damage; cf. *hypertensive emergency*

hypertensive emergency critical elevation of *blood pressure* with signs of *acute life-threatening organ* damage, e.g. *angina pectoris*, pulmonary *edema*, intracranial bleeding, etc.; cf. *hypertensive crisis*

hyperthermia (hyperpyrexia) excessive warmth in the body or of a body part; opp. *hypothermia*

hyperthermic pert. to *hyperthermia*; opp. *hypothermic*

hyperthyroid pert. to *hyperthyroidism*; opp. *hypothyroid*

hyperthyroidism overactivity of the thyroid gland, with increased thyroid production and secretion; opp. *hypothyroidism*

hypertonic dehydration disproportional loss of water and *sodium* (higher loss of water), e.g. due to insufficient water intake or excessive sweating; consequence: *ICF* is decreased, *ECF* is decreased

hypertonic hyperhydration disproportional increase of water and *sodium* (sodium excess), e.g. due to excessive administration of sodium-containing *infusion* solution; consequence: *ICF* is decreased, *ECF* is increased

hypertrichosis abnormal increase in body hair; opp. *hypotrichosis*

hypertriglyceridemia increased level of *triglycerides* in the blood

hypertrophic enlarged; opp. *atrophic*

hypertrophy increase in the size of an *organ*; opp. *atrophy*

hyperuricemia increased levels of *uric acid* in the blood; may lead to *gout*

hypervascularization increased formation of blood vessels

hyperventilate to breathe too rapidly; opp. *hypoventilate*

hyperventilation deeper and more rapid breathing, e.g. from excitement, exertion or *hypoxia*; opp. *hypoventilation*

hypervigilance state of increased alertness or awareness, e.g. in drug abuse

hypervitaminosis disease caused by excessive intake of vitamins; opp. *hypovitaminosis*

hypervolemia increase in the volume of fluid circulating in the vessels, e.g. in *renal failure*; opp. *hypovolemia*

hyphema bleeding into the anterior chamber of the *eye*

hypno– combining form: sleep

hypnosis altered, sleeplike state of consciousness induced by suggestion

hypnotic sleep-inducing agent

hypo– combining form: under, below too little; opp. *hyper-*

hypoacidity *anacidity*

hypoalbuminemia decreased *albumin* in the blood

hypocalcemia decrease in blood *calcium* to levels below 2.2 mmol/l, e.g. due to insufficient nutritional supply; may lead to *tetany*; opp. *hypercalcemia*

hypocapnia (hypocarbia) decreased level of *carbon dioxide* in the blood, e.g. due to *hyperventilation*; opp. *hypercapnia*

hypochondria abnormal fear-based concern about one's body, with subjective physical complaints and fear of disease, usually occurring in middle age and beyond

hypochromasia decreased stainability of *chromosomes* and *cell nuclei*

hypochromic having reduced coloration, decreased stainability or decreased amount of *hemoglobin*; opp. *hyperchromic*

hypodense having reduced tissue density; usually used in relation to imaging procedures, e.g. x-ray; opp. *hyperdense*

hypodermic syringe graduated syringe with a needle or Luer connector for drawing blood or injecting drugs

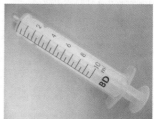

Fig. 236: hypodermic syringe

hypoemia decreased quantity of blood in an organ or area of the body; opp. *hyperemia*

hypoemic pert. to *hypoemia*; opp. *hyperemic*

hypogalactia reduced secretion of milk during the nursing period, e.g. due to infant's sucking weakness; opp. *hypergalactia*

hypogastrium area of the abdomen below the *stomach*

hypoglossal nerve 12*th* cranial nerve; contains motor fibers; mainly controls tongue movement, e.g. *innervation* of the *hypoglossus muscle*

hypoglycemia pathological decrease in blood sugar to values less than 50 mg/dl; opp. *hyperglycemia*

hypoglycemic pert. to *hypoglycemia*; opp. *hyperglycemic*

hypogonadism underactivity of the sex glands

hypohidrosis reduced sweat production; opp. *hyperhidrosis*

hypokalemia decrease in blood *potassium* to levels below 3.5 mmol/l e.g. due to insufficient supply or excessive loss (e.g. due to the use of diuretic agents); may lead to cardiac dysrhythmias; opp. *hyperkalemia*

hypomagnesemia decrease in blood *magnesium* to levels below 0.7 mmol/l e.g. due to insufficient nutritional supply; may lead to cramps in the calf muscles or tremors; opp. *hypermagnesemia*

hypomenorrhea light *menstruation* (< 2 pads/day) lasting the normal length of time; *organic* or *endocrine* causes; opp. *hypermenorrhea*

hypomnesia decreased ability to remember; opp. *hypermnesia*

hyponatremia decrease in blood *sodium* to levels below 135 mmol/l, e.g. in *hypotonic hyperhydration*; may lead to edemas, e.g.; opp. *hypernatremia*

hypoparathyroidism underactivity of the parathyroid gland with reduced production of *parathormone*

hypopharynx lower portion of the *pharynx*

hypophosphatemia decrease in blood *phosphate* to levels below 0.8 mmol/l, e.g. due to insufficient nutritional supply; may lead to *CNS* dysfunction, e.g.; opp. *hyperphosphatemia*

hypophysis *pituitary gland*

hypoplasia underdevelopment of an *organ*; opp. *hyperplasia*

hypoproteinemia decreased levels of *proteins* in the blood, e.g. in *nephrotic syndrome*; opp. *hyperproteinemia*

hypopyon visible accumulation of pus in the anterior chamber of the eye

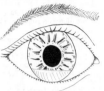

Fig. 237: hypopyon

hyporeflexia weakened *reflexes*; opp. *hyperreflexia*

hyposalivation reduced production of saliva; opp. *hypersalivation*

hypospadias atypical opening of the urethra on the underside of the penis; see also *anaspadias*

hypospermia *ejaculate* volume of < 2 ml; opp. *hyperspermia*

hypotension (low blood pressure) pathological lowering of *systolic* blood pressure to values below 100 mmHg in adults; opp. *hypertension*

hypotensive pert. to *hypotension*; opp. *hypertensive*

hypothalamus organ to which the *hypophysis* is subordinate and with which it is in direct contact; produces *releasing hormones* such as *GnRH, TRH, CRH, GHRH*, and *hormones* such as *oxytocin* and *ADH*

hypothermia cooling of the body or a body part to a temperature below 36°C; opp. *hyperthermia*

hypothermic pert. to *hypothermia*; opp. *hyperthermic*

hypothyroid pert. to *hypothyroidism*; opp. *hyperthyroid*

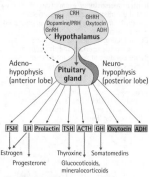

Fig. 238: hypothalamus

hypothyroidism underactivity of the thyroid gland with decreased production and release of thyroid *hormone*; opp. *hyperthyroidism*

hypotonic dehydration disproportional loss of water and sodium (higher loss of sodium), e.g. due to vomiting or diarrhea; consequence: *ICF* is increased, *ECF* is decreased

hypotonic hyperhydration disproportional increase of water and sodium (water excess with *hyponatremia*), e.g. due to *renal failure* or excess supply of free water; consequence, *ICF* is normal, *ECF* is increased

hypotrichia inherited or acquired lack of hair; opp. *hypertrichia*

hypoventilate to breathe too slowly; opp. *hyperventilate*

hypoventilation slower, shallower breathing e.g. due to CNS disease; depressed respiration caused by drugs or metabolic disorder; opp. *hyperventilation*

hypovitaminosis disease caused by inadequate intake of *vitamins*; opp. *hypervitaminosis*

hypovolemia decrease in the volume of fluid circulating in the vessels; opp. *hypervolemia*

hypovolemic shock (oligemic shock) *shock* triggered by *hypovolemia*

hypoxemia decreased *oxygen* content in the blood

hypoxia decreased *oxygen* content in the *tissues*

hypoxic pert. to *hypoxia*

hystera *womb*

hysterectomy *surgical* removal of the *uterus*

hystero– combining form: uterus

hysteroscope rigid *endoscope* used for *hysteroscopy*

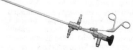

Fig. 239: hysteroscope [F]

hysteroscopy endoscopy of the *uterus*

I

–iasis combining form: disease

iatro– combining form: relationship with medicine and/or physician

iatrogenic adverse effect in a patient caused by a prescribed treatment

IBS *irritable bowel syndrome*

IC abbr. *inspiratory capacity*

ICD abbr. International Statistical Classification of Diseases and Related Health Problems

ICF abbr. *intracellular fluid*

ichthyosis skin disease with extremely dry skin tending to produce thick scales

ICP abbr. *intracranial pressure*

ICS abbr. *intercostal space*

icteric pert. to *icterus*

icterus (jaundice) yellowish discoloration of the skin and mucous membranes due to an elevated level of *bilirubin* in the blood

icterus intermittens juvenilis Gilbert's disease

ictus solis sunstroke

ICU abbr. intensive care unit

ideal weight calculated optimal body weight; formula for females: (height in meters)^2 x 21.5; formula for males: (height in meters)^2 x 23

ideational apraxia see *apraxia*

identical twins see *twins*

ideomotor apraxia (ideokinetic apraxia) see *apraxia*

idio- combining form: individual

idiopathic lacking a recognizable external cause or appearing spontaneously

idiopathic pulmonary fibrosis proliferation of scar tissue in the *lungs*

idiopathic thrombocytopenic purpura (thrombocytopenic purpura, thrombopenic purpura, Schönlein's disease, Werlhof's disease) disease marked by premature destruction of *thrombocytes* from *immunological* causes; *acute* form occurs mainly in children after *viral infections*; *chronic* form involves accelerated breakdown of thrombocytes in the *spleen* and *RES* due to formation of *antibodies* against thrombocytes

IFN abbr. *interferon*

IgA abbr. *immunoglobulin A*

IgD abbr. *immunoglobulin D*

IgE abbr. *immunoglobulin E*

IgG abbr. *immunoglobulin G*

IgM abbr. *immunoglobulin M*

IL abbr. *interleukin*

ILBBB abbr. incomplete *left bundle branch block*

ileitis *inflammation* of the *ileum*

ileitis regionalis Crohn's disease

ileocecal valve (valve of Varolius, valvula coli, Bauhin's valve) fold of mucosa at the transition between the *ileum* and the *cecum*

ileocolostomy *surgical* connection of the *ileum* and *colon*

ileojejunostomy *surgical* connection of the *ileum* and *jejunum*

ileostomy artificial opening for the *ileum* through the abdominal wall

ileotransversostomy *surgical* circumvention of the *transverse colon* by connecting it with the *ileum*, e.g. due to *stenosis* caused by a tumor

ileum section of the small intestine between the *jejunum* and the *appendix*

ileum conduit 1) *surgically* created diversion of the urine through the *ureters* into a prepared *ileal pouch*; 2) diversion of the urine outside the body via an *ileostomy*

ileus disorders of bowel passage due to paralysis or lack of peristalsis (paralytic ileus) or mechanical obstruction (mechanical ileus)

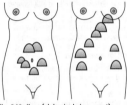

Fig. 240: ileus (abdominal view, erect)

iliac 1) pert. to the *ilium*; 2) pert. to the *iliac artery*

iliac artery arteria iliaca ...

iliac bone (ilium) pelvic bone; one of the *hip bones*

iliac crest puncture technique used to obtain *bone marrow* from the upper pelvic bone

iliopsoas, M. *(musculus iliopsoas) iliopsoas muscles*

iliopsoas muscles collective term for the muscles that flex the hips; *innervation femoral nerve*

ilium *ilium*

illusion perceptual disturbance marked by disordered perception of real objects or situations

IM abbr. *intramuscular*

imbibition soaking up absorption of fluid

immature not fully developed; opp. *mature*

immediate section quick removal of *tissue* from a surgical patient for microscopic examination during the *operation* in order to determine benign or malignant status of a *tumor* and thus to make a decision about the extent of the *surgical* intervention

imminent impending, about to happen; e.g. *imminent abortion*

immobile unmoving, unable to move; opp. *mobile*

immobilization rendering incapable of movement, e.g. a fracture; opp. *mobilization*

immobilization position positioning of a joint for long-term immobilization in order to ensure future functionality

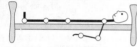

Fig. 241: immobilization position

immune not susceptible

immune complex substance formed during an *antigen-antibody reaction* that neutralizes the bound *antigens*

immune interferon *interferon* produced by the *lymphocytes* (gamma interferon)

immune system *cells, tissues* and *organs* of the body's defense systems, which attack abnormal cells and *antigens*

immunity resistance to a disease-producing agent

immunization (vaccination) stimulation of antibody formation following contact with an *antigen*; see also *active immunization passive immunization simultaneous immunization*

immunization, active formation of antibodies when injected antigen cells come in contact with the plasma reticuloendothelial cells and large lymphocytes

immunoglobulin antibody produced by B *lymphocytes*; abbr. Ig

immunoglobulin A *immunoglobulin* present primarily in saliva, stomach and intestinal secretions, which protects the corresponding body regions from *infections*; abbr. IgA

immunoglobulin D *immunoglobulin* found on the surface membrane of B *lymphocytes* as receptors for *antigens*; abbr. IgD

immunoglobulin E *immunoglobulin* that protects the body from *parasites* and plays an important role in *allergic* reactions; abbr. IgE

immunoglobulin G class of *immunoglobulin* that functions as a "memory cell" to destroy an *antigen* on repeated contact; abbr. IgG

immunoglobulin M *immunoglobulin* that is produced on initial contact with an *antigen*; abbr. IgM

immunostimulant drug used to support the body's immune system

immunosuppressant drug used to suppress the body's immune systems

immunosuppression suppression of the body's immune system

immunosuppressive pert. to *immunosuppression*

impacted cerumen blockage of the *external auditory canal* by a mass of *cerumen*

impacted fracture *compression fracture*

impalement injury special form of *puncture wound*; penetrating injury in the *genital* and *anorectal* area

imperforate hymen (hymenal atresia) absence of the opening in the *hymen*; can lead to *hematocolpos* and *hematometra* among other things; see Fig. 243

impermeable unable to be penetrated; opp. *permeable*

impetiginous pert. to *impetigo*

impetigo contagiosa *infectious disease* caused by pathogens such as *streptococci* or *staphylococci* leading to skin eruptions with yellowish crusting; transmitted via contac

implant 1) implanted object or donor organ; 2) to perform an *implantation*; opp. *explant*

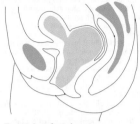

Fig. 242: imperforate hymen

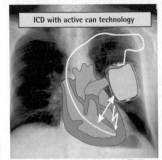

Fig. 244: implantable cardioverter-defibrillator

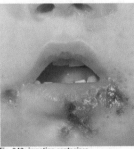

Fig. 243: impetigo contagiosa

implantable cardioverter-defibrillator
(automated implantable cardioverter-
defibrillator) special type of *pacemaker* for
constant monitoring of *cardiac rhythm*; in
the event of *ventricular tachycardia* or
ventricular fibrillation, it generates a small
electrical shock between the metal housing
of the pacemaker and the electrode (active
can technology) for either *cardioversion* or
defibrillation; abbr. ICD; AICD
implantation 1) placement of an *implant* in
the body; 2) penetration of the *trophoblast*
into the *endometrium*

impotence (erectile dysfunction) inability of
a male to achieve erection
impregnation penetration of the *sperm* into
the ovum, rendering the zona pellucida
impenetrable by other sperm
impression 1) perception; 2) depression in a
surface caused by pressure from another
object
impulse stimulus, impetus
in- combining form: inside, into
in vitro outside the body, e.g. in a test tube;
opp. *in vivo*
in vitro fertilization combination of a
sperm cell with a harvested ovum in a test
tube in cases where natural fertilization is
not possible, e.g. due to tubal disorders
in vivo inside the body or on the living
organism, e.g. in connection with scientific
research; opp. *in vitro*
inactive not effective, not acting; opp.
active
inadequate not appropriate, not sufficient;
opp. *adequate*
inanition weakened condition due to
starvation
inappetence lack of appetite or desire; opp.
appetence

inbreeding *incest*

incarceration imprisonment or constriction of a body part, e.g. a *hernia*

incentive spirometer device used to encourage deep breathing and coughing in order to prevent pneumonia

incest (inbreeding) sexual relations between family members or close relatives

incidence statistical term for the number of new cases of a given disease in a given period of time in relation to the total population

incipient beginning

incised wound *wound* with clean edges usually without *dehiscence*

incisors *dentes incisivi*

Fig. 245: incisors

incision 1) a cut; 2) the act of cutting into

incisional hernia *hernia* due to secondary *dehiscence* of a *fascia* in a *laparotomy* scar, most often after medial laparotomy

incisivi, dentes *dentes incisivi*

incisure slit, notch, e.g. in a bone

inclination bending the cervical, thoracic or lumbar spine forward; opp. *reclination*

incoherence disorder of the thought processes marked by absent-mindedness with unconnected illogical thoughts, e.g. in *mania* or *schizophrenia*

incoherent disordered, unrelated; opp. *coherent*

incompatibility inability to be combined or associated; opp. *compatibility*

incompatible unable to be combined or associated; opp. *compatible*

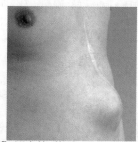

Fig. 246: incisional hernia

incomplete unfinished, not whole; opp. *complete*

inconstant not continuous, fluctuating; opp. *constant*

incontinence inability to control bladder or bowel evacuation; opp. *continence*

incontinent adj. of *incontinence*; opp. *continent*

incorporation 1) taking up a substance into the body; 2) combining into a mass

incrustation formation of a crust

incubation period period from exposure to a pathogen until the outbreak of *infectious disease*

incubator 1) heated cabinet for culturing *microbiological* specimens such as blood or urine *cultures* at body temperature; 2) heated crib for premature or weak infants

incurable unable to be healed; opp. *curable*

incus (anvil) one of the three ossicles in the middle ear, located between the *malleus* and *stapes*

indentation tonometry Schiötz' method for measuring intraocular pressure through indentation of the cornea using a defined weight

indicated medically justified; opp. *contraindicated*

indication justification for performing a medical procedure; opp. *contraindication*

indicator material that makes it possible to measure a chemical reaction

indifferent unspecified; undetermined

induction act of inducing, causing

induration hardening, e.g. due to formation of scar tissue

indwelling catheter *bladder catheter* with a balloon at the end that is left in the bladder for extended periods, e.g. to gauge urine production; opp. *disposable catheter*

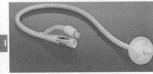

Fig. 247: indwelling catheter [N]

infant child in the period between birth and completion of its first year of life

infantile pert. to a child

infantile glaucoma buphthalmia

infantile paralysis poliomyelitis

infantilism remaining in a childlike state of development

infarcted adj. of infarction

infarction death of tissue in an *organ* due to inadequate blood supply

infaust hopeless, unfavorable

infection contagion caused by pathogenic microorganisms, e.g. *viruses* or *bacteria*

infectious contagious

infectious disease disease caused by infection with a disease-causing agent, e.g. a *virus* or *bacterium*

infectious mononucleosis *mononucleosis*

inferior lower, located beneath; opp. *superior*

inferior mesenteric vein lower *mesenteric vein* that connects with the *splenic vein* behind the *pancreas* or joins directly with the *portal vein*

inferior ophthalmic vein *vein* that joins the *sinus cavernosus* or *superior ophthalmic vein* from the lower orbit

inferior rectus muscle straight ocular muscle that turns the eyeball downward; innervation: *oculomotor nerve*

inferior vena cava *vein* that transports blood from the lower part of the body to the right atrium of the heart; abbr. IVC

infertility inability to achieve pregnancy

infiltrate substance that has penetrated into a *tissue*

infiltration penetration of *tissue* by fluids, tissue fragments or cells from another tissue

infiltration anesthesia (field block) local anesthesia via intra- or subcutaneous *injection* of a local anesthetic into the surgical site in a fan pattern

inflammation the body's reaction to harmful irritants, e.g. to invasion by a *microorganism*; see also *signs of inflammation*

inflow congestion backup of blood ahead of the right heart due to right heart failure; signs include extreme protrusion of the external *jugular vein* and increase in CVP

influenza (grippe) *infectious disease* caused by *influenza viruses*, leading to a severe febrile illness; transmitted via *droplet infection*

influenza virus *RNA virus* that causes *influenza*

infra- combining form: underneath opp. *supra-*

infraction break in a bone without complete separation of the bone structure; cf. *fracture, hairline fracture*

infraspinatus, M. (musculus infraspinatus) *infraspinous muscle*

infraspinous muscle muscle that rolls the upper arm outward; innervation: *suprascapular nerve*

infuse to administer an *infusion*

infusion introduction of larger amounts of fluid into the bloodstream or *tissues*

infusion pump device for administering precise doses of *infusions*, which can be programmed for infusion rates in milliliters per hour, enabling uniform flow through a *venous catheter*

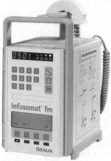

Fig. 248: infusomat [C]

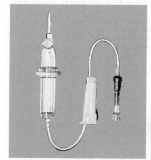

Fig. 250: infusion system [L]

infusion solution drug preparation designed for *infusion*, to be introduced into the body via an infusion system connected to a *venous catheter*

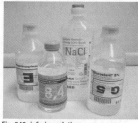

Fig. 249: infusion solutions

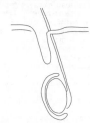

Fig. 251: inguinal hernia

infusion system (infusion device) tube system used to run *infusion solution* through a *venous catheter*

inguinal pert. to the groin

inguinal hernia (hernia inguinalis) *hernia* at the superficial inguinal ring

inhalation inhaling nebulized drugs or vapor

inhale to breathe in nebulized drugs or vapor

inhibit to repress or restrain

inhibited repressed or restrained

inhibitor chemical substance that inhibits a function

initial at first, beginning

initial therapy first treatment of a disease following *diagnosis*

inject to force a drug into the bloodstream or *tissues*

injection forcing a drug into the bloodstream or *tissues* via a syringe

inlay dental filling made of precious metal, plastic or ceramic that is cemented into a *tooth* to close a cavity

inner ear *see ear*

innervation nerve supply

inoperable unable to be treated with *surgery*; opp. *operable*

inorganic not living, mineralic; opp. *organic*

inotropic affecting the force with which the heart muscle contracts; positive inotropic: increasing the force of muscle contraction; negative inotropic: decreasing the force of muscle contraction; cf. *bathmotropic*, *chronotropic*, *dromotropic*

inpatient admitted to a hospital for care; opp. *outpatient*

INR abbr. international normalized ratio; used to report results of blood coagulation (clotting) tests, e.g. prothrombin time

insecticide substance for killing insects

insemination penetration of a *sperm* into the ovum during *fertilization*; artificial fertilization by placement of *semen* on the *cervix*

insertion tendopathy *degenerative* changes of tendon origins and insertions due to *abacterial inflammation* following overuse

insomnia sleeplessness

inspection close visual examination of the body

inspiration drawing in of breath; opp. *expiration*

inspiratory pert. to *inspiration*; opp. *expiratory*

inspiratory capacity maximum amount of air that can be inspired after a normal expiration; abbr. IC; see illustration under *spirometry*

inspiratory reserve volume amount of air that can still be inspired after a normal inspiration; abbr. IRV; see illustration under *spirometry*

inspire to breathe in; opp. *expire*

instill to perform an *instillation*

instillation dripping or other introduction of a solution, e.g. into a cavity

insufficiency inadequate function or performance; opp. *sufficiency*

insufficient adj. of *insufficiency*; opp. *sufficient*

insufflation 1) forcing gases or nebulized drugs into body cavities; 2) blowing air through the fallopian tube to test for patency (*pertubation*)

insulin *hormone* produced in the islet cells (beta cells) of the *pancreas* that causes *blood sugar* to drop

insulinoma (islet cell tumor) *insulin*-producing tumor of the *pancreas*, usually benign

insult injury or trauma, e.g. brain insult from *stroke*

intelligence the entire range of mental abilities

intelligence quotient an individual's measured mental abilities, expressed as a numerical value; abbr. IQ

intention purpose, goal

intention tremor (action tremor) tremor that occurs shortly before the completion of a purposive movement

inter- combining form: between, in between, in the middle

interaction influence that one drug's effects have on another drug

intercostal between the ribs

intercostal neuralgia belt-like pain distributed along the intercostal spaces

intercostal space space between the ribs; abbr. *ICS*

intercurrent intervening

interdisciplinary involving multiple medical specializations

interferon *cytokine* produced by the *leukocytes*, *lymphocytes*, or *fibroblasts* following contact with a *virus*, which inhibits reproduction of the virus

interleukin *cytokine* produced by *leukocytes* that acts as a chemical messenger between *cells* in the body's defense system; abbr. IL

intermediary occurring between two events; located between two objects

intermediary metabolism intermediate stage of metabolism before final waste products are formed

intermediate cuneiform bone second cuneiform bone; one of the *tarsal bones*

intermediate hepatic veins *veins* that transport blood from the caudate lobe of the liver to the *inferior vena cava*

intermittend occurring from time to time; opp. regular

intermittend claudication muscular pain in the legs caused by impaired *arterial* circulation, appearing with exercise and disappearing with rest

internal on the inside; opp. *external*

internal jugular vein *vein* that collects blood from the brain. pharynx and larynx area and joins the *subclavian* to form the *brachiocephalic vein*

internal rotation turning inward; opp. *external rotation*

internist specialist in internal medicine

interossei, Mm. (musculi interossei) *interosseous muscles*

interosseous muscles collective term for the muscles that spread and adduct the fingers; innervation: *ulnar nerve*

interstitial pert. to the *interstitium*

interstitial space the space between *cells, tissues* and *organs*

intertrigo chafing in folds of skin, e.g. in the *genital* area or armpit

interval intervening space or time period

intervene to take action

intervention action or procedure, e.g. an *operation*

intervertebral disk (discus intervertebralis) elastic disk located between *vertebrae*, consisting of the *anulus fibrosus* and *nucleus pulposus*

intervertebral ganglion *dorsal root ganglion*

intestinal pert. to the *intestine*

intestinal flora normal *bacteria* present in the intestine

intestinal grasping forceps *surgical* instrument according to Allis that is used for operating on the intestine, among other things

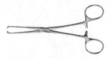

Fig. 252: intestinal grasping forceps [A]

intestinal tube wide-bore tube placed into the intestine for administering fluids or nutrients, or for aspirating substances, to draw off intestinal gas in *meteorism*, or to *irrigate* the *colon*

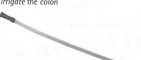

Fig. 253: intestinal tube

intestinal villi projections of the mucous membrane on the inner surface of the intestine that increase its surface area

intestinales, Aa. *arteriae intestinales*

intestine (enteron) bowel

intestinum tenue *small intestine*

intima innermost wall of a vessel

intolerance inability to endure or digest; opp. *tolerance*

intoxication poisoning

intra– combining form: inside of, in, into; opp. *extra–*

intraabdominal in(to) the abdomen

intraarterial in(to) an *artery*

intraarticular in(to) a joint; opp. *extraarticular*

intraarticular fracture *fracture* involving an intraarticular surface; opp. *diaphyseal fracture*

intracellular in(to) the *cells*; opp. *extracellular*

intracellular fluid liquid found within cells; comprises approx. 2/3 of total body water; opp. *extracellular fluid*; abbr. *ICF*

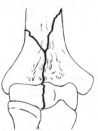

Fig. 254: intraarticular fracture

intracerebral in(to) the *brain*
intracerebral hemorrhage bleeding inside the *brain*, usually caused by *hypertension* or *arteriosclerosis*
intracorporeal in(to) the body; opp. *extracorporeal*
intracranial in(to) the skull
intracranial bleed bleeding inside the skull cavity; see *epidural bleed*, *subdural bleed*, *subarachnoid bleed*, *intracerebral bleed*
intracranial pressure pressure inside the skull (normal: 0–15 mmHg); can be increased in the presence of brain tumors, bleeds or *brain edema*, among other things, leading to headaches, nausea and vomiting, but also to acute life-threatening problems; abbr. ICP

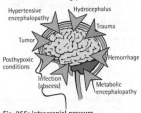

Fig. 255: intracranial pressure

intracutaneous in(to) the skin; abbr. i.c.
intragluteal in(to) the major buttock muscle
intramedullary in(to) the bone marrow or spinal cord; opp. *extramedullary*
intramural in(to) the wall of a hollow organ; opp. *extramural*
intramuscular in(to) the muscle; abbr. IM
intraocular in(to) the eyeball
intraoperative during an *operation*; see also *perioperative*, *postoperative*, *preoperative*
intraperitoneal in(to) the *peritoneum*; opp. *extraperitoneal*
intrapulmonary in(to) the *lungs*
intrathecal in(to) the subdural space
intratracheal in(to) the *trachea*
intrauterine in(to) the *uterus*; opp. *extrauterine*
intrauterine device coil or *pessary* inserted into the *uterus* for contraception; usually has a plastic base and contains copper or *progesterone*; abbr. IUD

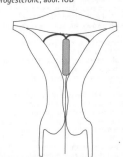

Fig. 256: intrauterine device

intrauterine insemination sperm placed into the uterus
intravaginal in(to) the *vagina*
intravenous into a *vein*; abbr. IV

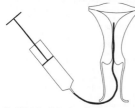

Fig. 257: intrauterine insemination

intraventricular block (bundle branch block) impulse conduction disorder visible in an *ECG*, involving one or more of the *Tawara branches* below the *bundle of His*

intravesical in(to) the *bladder*

intrinsic from within; opp. *extrinsic*

intro– combining form: into

introitus entrance into a hollow *organ*, e.g. the *vagina*

introverted turned inward; *extroverted*

intubation (endotracheal intubation) introduction of an *endotracheal tube* for ventilation via the mouth, usually under visual guidance with the aid of a *laryngoscope* (orotracheal intubation) or via the nose (nasotracheal intubation) past the *epiglottis*, through the rima glottidis, between the *vocal cords* and then into the *trachea*

intussusception (invagination) infolding of hollow organs, e.g. the *intestine*

invagination intussusception

invasion growth of a *tumor* into the surrounding *tissue*

invasive penetrating or invading the body tissues

inversion turning or tilting under; e.g. combination movement of the foot consisting of forefoot *adduction, plantar flexion* and *supination*; opp. *eversion*

involution regression to a previous state; opp. *evolution*

iod– combining form: iodine

iodination absorption of *iodine* into the *thyroid* cells

iodine important trace element, e.g. in production of *thyroid hormones*; chemical symbol: I

iodine deficiency goiter *goiter* caused by *iodine* deficiency

iodization incorporation of *iodine* in a thyroid *hormone*

ion positively or negatively charged electrical particles; see also *cation anion*

ipsilateral on the same side

IQ abbr. *intelligence quotient*

IRBBB abbr. incomplete *right bundle branch block*

irid– combining form: iris

iridocoloboma inherited *iris* defect in the form of a fissure or cleft

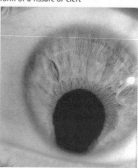

Fig. 258: iridocoloboma

iridodialysis detachment of the edge of the *iris* from the *ciliary body*

iris colored membrane of the eye located between the cornea and the lens

iritis *inflammation* of the *iris*

iron (ferrum) an important component of *hemoglobin* and various *enzymes* that is involved in *oxygen* transport and other metabolic functions; iron is stored as *ferritin* in the liver, spleen and bone marrow; chemical symbol: Fe

iron-deficiency anemia (sideroachrestic anemia) most common form of *anemia*, caused by lack of *iron*, resulting in insufficient ability to produce *hemoglobin*

irradiation exposure to radiation, e.g. to treat tumors

irradiation field area of the body exposed during radiation therapy

irreparable unable to be repaired or restored; opp. *reparable*

irreversible not able to be reversed; opp. *reversible*

irrigation rinsing a hollow organ with a solution, e.g. the intestine for *obstipation* (enema)

irrigator device for performing an *irrigation;* fluid receptacle with tubes for connection to an intestinal tube in order to administer an *enema*

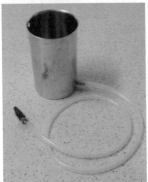

Fig. 259: irrigator

irritable bladder frequent urge to urinate due to *neural* hyperexcitability of the bladder

irritable bowel syndrome (irritable colon) bowel function disorder with alternating *diarrhea* and *constipation;* abbr IBS

irritants chemotherapy drugs that can produce severe reactions to surrounding tissue if infiltration occurs during IV administration, e.g. cisplatin

irritation reaction to a harmful or unpleasant stimulus

IRV abbr. *inspiratory reserve volume*

ischemia inadequate blood supply

ischemic pert. to *ischemia*

ischial bone (ischium) "sit bone"; one of the *hip bones*

ischialgia (sciatica) pain radiating from the sacrum toward the toes, caused by irritation of the *sciatic nerve*

ischii, os *(os ischii)* ischium

ischium bones forming the lower portion of the pelvis

ischuria urinary retention

islet cell carcinoma malignant tumor originating in the islet cells of the *pancreas*

islets of Langerhans (pancreatic islands) *insulin*-producing cells in the pancreas

iso- combining form: like, similar

isocoria equality in pupil size; opp. *anisocoria*

isocoric pert. to *isocoria;* opp. *anisocoric*

isogeneic graft *syngeneic graft*

isolated separated

isolation separation, keeping apart from others, e.g. in *quarantine*

isologous graft *syngeneic graft*

isometric having the same muscle length but increased muscle tension; opp. *isotonic*

isosthenuria excretion of urine with the same osmolality as plasma due to impaired *renal tubule* function

isotonia 1) having constant *osmotic* pressure; 2) change in the length of a muscle under constant muscle tension

isotonic 1) having constant *osmotic* pressure; 2) changing the length of a muscle while maintaining constant muscle tension; opp. *isometric*

isotonic dehydration proportional loss of water and *sodium* with maintenance of blood isotonicity, e.g. in *polyuria*; consequence, *ICF* is normal, *ECF* is decreased

isotonic hyperhydration proportional gain of water and *sodium* outside of the *cell* with maintenance of blood isotonicity, e.g. in *renal failure*; consequence: *ICF* is normal, *ECF* is increased

isotope atom with the same atomic number as the normal element, but with a different number of neutrons, and thus subject to radioactive decay

isotopic graft *transplantation* of the same type of tissue to the same location in the body; see also *orthotopic graft*, *heterotopic graft*

isovolemia normal volume of fluid circulating in the vessels

isthmus constriction or narrow passage

isthmus uteri isthmus of the *uterus*; narrowing of the *uterus* between the *cervix* and uterine body

itch mite *Sarcoptes scabiei*

itching *pruritus*

ITN abbr. *intubation anesthesia*

IUD abbr. *intrauterine device*

IV abbr. *intravenous*

IVC abbr. *inferior vena cava*

IVF abbr. *in vitro fertilization*

ixod– combining form: tick

Ixodes ricinus wood tick

J

J abbr. *joule*

jacket crown *dental crown* made of porcelain or plastic that is placed over the tooth

jacksonian epilepsy (jacksonian march) *focal motor seizure*

Jamshidi needle punch needle for taking *bone marrow biopsies*

jaundice *icterus*

jejunal pert. to the *jejunum*

JCAH Joint Commission on Accreditation of Hospitals (regulatory agency that accredits hospitals)

jejunal ulcer *ulcer* in the *jejunum*

jejunitis *inflammation* of the jejunum

jejunoileostomy *surgical* connection of the *jejunum* and *ileum*

jejunostomy tube (jejunostomy tube) feeding tube placed in the *jejunum* for pump-controlled enteral feeding; used for patients with impaired stomach emptying, increased risk of *aspiration*, or *pyloric stenosis*

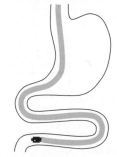

Fig. 261: jejunal feeding tube

jejunum portion of the small intestine between the *duodenum* and the *ileum*

joint (articulatio) articulation point between bones

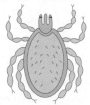

Fig. 260: Ixodes ricinus (wood tick)

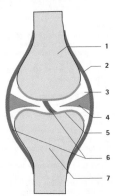

Fig. 262: joint
1 Articular head (convex) 2 Joint capsule with synovial membrane 3 Joint space with synovial fluid 4 Menisci (fibrocartilage) 5 Articular surfaces with hyaline cartilage 6 Ligament 7 Socket (concave)

joint effusion accumulation of fluid (*exudate*) in the joint capsule exceeding the normal *physiological* complement

joint mouse (free body) detached bone fragment floating within a joint, which can cause pain with use

joule unit of heat; 4.2 kilojoules will heat 1 kg of pure water by 1°C; an older unit of measurement is the *calorie*: 1 calorie equals 4.2 joules

jugular pert. to the throat

jugular vein neck vein differentiated into the anterior, internal and external jugular veins

jugularis, vena (vena jugularis) *jugular vein*

jugulum neck, throat

jury a group selected according to law and sworn to inquire into the facts of a case and render a verdict to a court

juvenile immature; youthful

juxta- combining form: near, close to

K

K chemical symbol *potassium*

k symbol: thousand (10^3); prefix: kilo-

kali- combining form: potassium

Kaposi's sarcoma malignant tumor occurring mainly in *HIV*-infected patients, which first affects the skin and mucous membranes and in later stages involves the *lymph nodes* and internal *organs* as well

Kehr's sign pain radiating into the left shoulder due to acute abdomen or *ruptured* spleen

keloid proliferation of scar *tissue*

Kent's bundles muscle fiber bundle occurring in *Wolff-Parkinson-White syndrome*

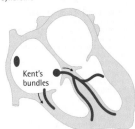

Fig. 263: Kent's bundles in WPW syndrome

keratitis inflammation of the *cornea* of the eye, usually caused by *bacteria*

kerato- combining form: horny

keratoconjunctivitis *inflammation* of the *cornea* and *conjunctiva* of the eye

keratoconus conical protrusion of the center of the *cornea* with reduction of the curvature radius

keratolytic 1) pert. to the softening and shedding of the horny outer layer of the skin; 2) drug used to loosen or soften the horny layer of the skin

keratomalacia softening of the *cornea* due to *vitamin A* deficiency

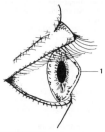

Fig. 264: keratoconus
1 Central thinning of cornea

keratoplasty corneal *transplant*

keratosis severe horny growth on the skin

kernicterus brain damage due to deposition of *bilirubin*, e.g. in *jaundice* of the newborn

Kernig's sign flexion of the knee to relieve the *sciatic nerve*, e.g. in *sciatica*, where *active* extension of the leg is not possible

ketoacidosis *acidosis* caused by excess of *ketone* bodies

ketone chemical compound containing at least one ketone group; ketones, e.g. *acetone*, occur in the body as a result of disorders of *carbohydrate* metabolism

ketonuria excretion of *ketones* in the urine

kg abbr. *kilogram*

kidney paired *organ* situated in the *retroperitoneal space*; function: excretion of metabolic waste products and regulation of water and *electrolyte* balance

kidney basin (emesis basin) kidney-shaped basin used to catch fluids or body secretions

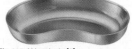

Fig. 265: kidney basin [A]

Kienböck's disease aseptic osteochondrosis of the *lunate bone*, usually occurring in middle-aged men

killer cell *lymphocyte* produced in the *lymph nodes* (*T lymphocyte*) that destroys invading foreign bodies

kilo– prefix: thousand (10^3); symbol: k

kilocalorie see *calorie*

kilogram 1000 grams; abbr. *kg*

–kinesis combining form: motion

Kirschner wire *osteosynthesis* in which wire is used for traction or fixation of bone fragments or implants

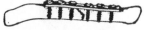

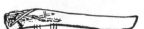

Fig. 266: Kirschner wires

kissing disease *mononucleosis*

KJ abbr. kilojoule

Klatskin tumor malignant tumor of the bile ducts, usually *adenocarcinoma*

Klebsiella pneumonia (Friedländer's pneumonia) *pneumonia* caused by *Klebsiella pneumoniae*, occurring primarily among *immunocompromised* persons

Klebsiella pneumoniae *gram-negative bacterium* that causes *pneumonia*; typical nosocomial pathogen in intensive care units

Kleinert cast bandaging technique for early mobilization in flexor tendon injuries

kleptomania pathological *compulsion* to steal

Klinefelter's syndrome (XXY syndrome) disorder of male reproductive gland development due to a genetic defect (extra *X chromosome*); leads to somatomegaly, diminished *intelligence*, *gynecomastia* and *osteoporosis*, among other things

knee genu

kneecap patella

Kocher clamp *hemostat* according to Kocher, used in *surgery* as a grasping forceps and for various other tasks

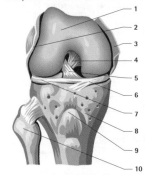

Fig. 267: right knee joint, anterior view
1 Femur 2 Lateral collateral ligament 3 Medial collateral ligament 4 Posterior cruciate ligament 5 Anterior cruciate ligament 6 Medial meniscus 7 Lateral meniscus 8 Tibia 9 Tibial tuberosity 10 Fibula

koilo- combining form: hollow
Koplik's spots spots appearing on the oral mucosa in *measles*
Korsakoff syndrome (anterior superior polioencephalitis) syndrome marked by disorientation as to time, place and identity, learning and attention disorders, as well as tendency to *confabulation*; usually a consequence of *thiamine* deficiency in *chronic alcoholism*
KT abbr. *kidney transplant*
Kuhn system *ventilation* apparatus for anesthetizing children without use of a non-rebreathing system
Kupffer cell cells of the reticuloendothelial system in the liver, whose job it is to filter bacteria and foreign proteins out of the blood

Kussmaul's breathing *acidotic breathing*
kyphoscoliosis combination of *kyphosis* and *scoliosis*
kyphosis convex curvature of the spine; opp. *lordosis*
kytos *cell*

L

L1, L2, etc. abbr. lumbar vertebra 1, 2 etc.
L abbr. *lumbar* segment (of the spine)
L-spine 1) lumbar spine; 2) an x-ray of this area
LA abbr. *local anesthesia*
labia majora larger lips of the female genitalia
labia minora smaller lips of the female genitalia
labial pert. to the lips
labile varying, fluctuating; opp. stable
labium (cheilos) lip; pl. labia
labor contraction of the *uterus* to push out the baby during birth, caused by the hormone oxytocin
labyrinth inner ear, including the cochlea and semicircular canals
labyrinthitis *inflammation* of the inner ear
lac milk
laceration 1) tearing; 2) tearing/crushing wound with ragged irregular edges
lacrim- combining form: tears
lacrima secretions of the *lacrimal glands* that protect the *eye* from drying out and from *infection*
lacrimal bone bone of the viscerocranium
lacrimal caruncle small growth on the *conjunctiva* near the inner canthus
lacrimal gland (glandula lacrimalis) gland in the upper outside corner of the orbit that secretes tears
lact- combining form: milk
lactacidosis *metabolic acidosis* due to increased levels of *lactate* in the blood
lactate salt of lactic acid that forms as an end product of *glucose* metabolism in the absence of *oxygen*, e.g. due to reduced

blood flow to part of the body, *shock* or *hypoxia*

lactation formation of milk in the mammary glands

lactic acidosis *metabolic acidosis* due to increased *lactic acid* in the blood

lactic dehydrogenase *enzyme* of *lactate* metabolism that occurs in almost all types of tissue; important laboratory parameter for detecting organ and tissue damage; abbr. LDH; it can be subdivided in 5 groups of which the most important are *HBDH*, LDH$_1$ in the *heart* muscle, and LDH$_5$ in the *liver* and skeletal muscle

lactose milk sugar

lactose intolerance inability to tolerate *lactose*

lactotropic hormone *prolactin*

lacuna focal loss of brain tissue due to a stroke in a small portion of one of the brain's arteries

LAD abbr. left anterior descending, i.e. the *ramus interventricularis anterior* (part of the left *coronary artery*)

lagophthalmos inability to close the eyelids completely due to pathological open palpebral fissure

lambdoid suture cranial suture between the *occipital* and *parietal* bones

Lambert-Eaton myasthenia syndrome *autoimmune disease* syndrome with *myasthenia*-like muscle weakness in the legs, arms and trunk, as well as weakening of the monosynaptic muscle *reflexes*; 50% of cases are associated with small-cell carcinoma of the lung

lamina thin, flat plate; pl. laminae

laminar pert. to a *lamina*

laminectomy *surgical* removal of the posterior vertebral arch to expose the spinal canal

lancet small double-edged knife for collecting *capillary* blood, e.g.

Landau reflex reflex in which raising an infant in prone position causes it to extend the head and back; present in infants between 3 and 5 months old

Landry's paralysis ascending paralysis due to severe neural disease, e.g. *poliomyelitis*

Langenbeck retractor tissue-preserving *retractor* according to Langenbeck

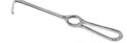

Fig. 268: Langenbeck retractor [A]

Langerhans cells immunocompetent *cells* of the skin

lanugo fine, downy hair covering a fetus

Lanz' point specific testing point for suspected *appendicitis* a tender point located on the rightmost third of the line between the right and left anterior superior spine of the ilium

LAP abbr. *leucine aminopeptidase*

laparatomize to perform a *laparotomy*

laparo– combining form: abdomen, abdominal wall

laparoscope rigid *endoscope* for performing *laparoscopy*

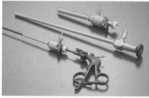

Fig. 269: laparoscope [F]

laparoscopic pert. to *laparoscopy*

laparoscopy *endoscopy* of the abdominal cavity and *organs* with a rigid *endoscope*

laparotomy *surgical* opening of the abdominal cavity

large artery occlusive disease atherosclerosis

large intestine *colon*

larvate hidden

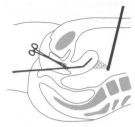

Fig. 270: laparoscopy

laryngeal pert. to the *larynx*
laryngeal mask airway tube assembly for short-term ventilation, e.g. during an operation; the device is equipped with a rubber raft-shaped balloon that, when correctly positioned, closes off the entrance of the esophagus
laryngeal mirror small, angled mirror for examination of the *larynx*

Fig. 271: laryngeal mirror [A]

laryngectomy *surgical* removal of the *larynx* from the *hypopharynx*, where the stump of the *trachea* is sutured to the skin (*tracheostomy*)
laryngeus recurrens, N. *nervus laryngeus recurrens*
laryngitis inflammation of the *larynx*
laryngoscope scope equipped with a light source for examination of the *larynx* or for visually guided *intubation* of the *trachea*
laryngoscope blade blade with a light source, that is attached to the battery grip of a *laryngoscope*; most important types are McIntosh and Foregger
laryngoscopy visual examination of the *larynx*, see Fig. 273

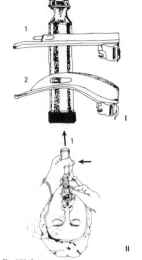

Fig. 272: laryngoscope
I Laryngoscope with attachable blade
1 Straight blade (Miller) 2 Curved blade (McIntosh)
II Oral intubation with laryngoscope
1 Pull in the direction of the handle, do not place lever over the upper teeth

laryngospasm spasmodic contraction of the rima glottidis of the *larynx*, e.g. as part of an *allergic* reaction, leading to significant dyspnea with inspiratory stridor
larynx vocal *organ* in the upper respiratory tract, see Fig. 274
Lasègue's sign sign indicating irritation of the *sciatic nerve* and corresponding *nerve* roots: *passive* elevation of the extended leg causes pain radiating from the buttock into the back of the thight

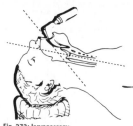

Fig. 273: laryngoscopy
Oral and laryngeal axes are angled into position to facilitate intubation (Jackson position)

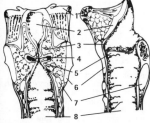

Fig. 274: larynx
1 Hyoid bone 2 Epiglottis 3 Vestibular fold
4 Ventricle 5 Vocal fold 6 Thyroid cartilage
7 Cricoid cartilage 8 Trachea

laser tube heat-resistant *endotracheal tube* that enables laser procedures in the pharyngeal and *tracheal* area

Lassa fever *hemorrhagic fever* caused by the *Lassa virus*; can be transmitted from human to human, but also via dried rodent feces and urine

Lassa virus *virus* that causes *Lassa fever*

late recurrence recurrence of a successfully treated tumor after five years or more

latent concealed; opp. *manifest*

lateral on the side or toward the side; opp. *medial*

lateral cuneiform bone third cuneiform bone; one of the *tarsal bones*

lateral dislocation (dislocatio ad latus) lateral displacement of the bone fragments from a fracture, e.g. bayonet- or fork-shaped

lateral funiculus nerve tracts in the lateral areas of the spinal cord

lateral humeral epicondylitis *tennis elbow*

lateral malleolus lower extremity of the *fibula*

lateral rectus muscle straight ocular muscle that turns the eyeball sideways; *innervation: abducens nerve*

lateral sclerosis disease of the *spinal cord* that leads to paralysis

laterobasal side-to-base

laterolateral side-to-side

lateroterminal side-to-end

latissimus dorsi broad back muscle that pulls the arm downward and turns it slightly inward; innervation: *thoracodorsal nerve*

latissimus dorsi, M. (musculus latissimus dorsi) *latissimus dorsi*

laughing gas *nitrous oxide*

lavage rinsing, flushing

laxa– combining form: loosen, relax

laxative drug used to loosen the bowels

LBBB abbr. *left bundle branch block*

LCA abbr. *left coronary artery*

LD abbr. *lethal dose; lactic dehydrogenase*

LDH abbr. *lactic dehydrogenase*

LDL abbr. low-density lipoprotein; *lipoprotein* with low molecular weight; opp. *HDL*

LDL cholesterol (low-density lipoprotein cholesterol) *cholesterol* bound to *protein*, believed to have damaging effects on the blood vessels; see also *HDL cholesterol*

LE abbr. *lupus erythematosus*

LeFort fracture facial bone fracture involving both sides of the face; classified according to the areas affected: type I (horizontal fracture of the maxilla and palatine bone at the level of the base of the maxillary sinus); type II (maxillary fracture with detachment of the *nasal* and frontal bones); and type III (complete separation of the facial bones from the cranium)

left bundle branch block interruption of electrical conduction in the left *branch* in the heart; abbr. LBBB

left heart failure see *heart failure*

left hepatic veins *veins* that transport blood from the left lobe of the liver to the *inferior vena cava*

left suprerenal vein *vein* that transports blood from the left *adrenal gland* to the *renal vein*

left ventricular hypertrophy enlargement of the left heart, e.g. due to *aortic stenosis*; abbr. LVH

left-to-right shunt pathological connection between *arterial* and *venous* circulation inside or outside the heart

Legionella pneumophila rod-shaped *gram-negative bacterium* that causes *legionellosis*

legionellosis (Legionnaires' disease) *infectious disease* caused by *Legionella pneumophila* that manifests as *Pontiac fever* or *pneumonia*; transmitted mainly via inhalation of contaminated water droplets

Legionnaires' disease *legionellosis*

leio– combining form: smooth

leiomyoma tumor consisting of smooth muscle tissue

Leishmania genus of *parasitic protozoa*

leishmaniasis *infectious disease* caused by *Leishmania* that affects the skin mucosa and internal organs; transmitted mainly by sandflies

lemma (membrana) covering, membrane, skin

–lemma combining form: shell, membrane

lens structure in the *eye* that focuses light rays

lenticular pert. to the *lens* of the *eye*

Leopold's maneuvers series of maneuvers for determining the *intrauterine* position of a baby: 1) check the position of the fundus with the palms; 2) check the sides

of the abdomen to determine the position of the baby's back; 3) determination of vertex or breech presentation; 4) determine position of the foremost part of the baby that has entered the pelvis

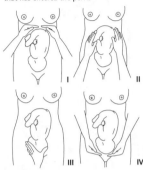

Fig. 275: Leopold's maneuvers I – IV

leproma *nodule* occurring in *leprosy*

leprosy (Hansen's disease) *chronic infectious disease* caused by *Mycobacterium leprae* that manifests in involvement of the skin and *nerves* to the point of limb deformity; transmitted mainly through close physical contact, but also by *droplet infection*

lept(o)– combining form: thin, narrow

leptomeninges *brain* and *spinal cord* membrane consisting of the *arachnoidea* and *pia mater*; sing. leptomeninx

Leptospira genus of motile spiral *gram-negative bacteria* that cause *leptospirosis* and other diseases

leptospirosis (spirochetal jaundice) febrile *infectious disease* caused by *Leptospira* leading to *sepsis* and damage to various *organs*; transmitted mainly through *lesions* on the skin or mucosa, via the cornea of the eye, contact with urine or feces, or with contaminated water droplets

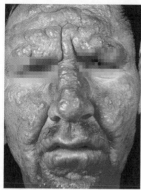

Fig. 276: leprosy

lesion injury; damage

lethal deadly

lethal dose amount of a drug that will cause death; abbr. LD

lethality statistical term indicating the number of deaths from a given disease in relation to the total number of cases of that disease

lethargy sluggishness; sleepiness

leucine aminopeptidase *enzyme* that plays an important role in *protein* metabolism, found primarily in the *intestine*, *kidney*, *bile*, saliva, *gastric* juice and *plasma*; abbr. LAP

leuk(o)– combining form: white

leukapheresis procedure for separating *leukocytes* from donated blood

leukemia malignant disease of the hematogenic system with uncontrolled proliferation of *leukocytes*

leukemia, acute lymphocytic a form of *leukemia*; causes malignant changes in the *lymphocytes*; abbr. ALL;

leukemia, acute myeloid (acute myelogenous leukemia; myelogenous; acute myelogenous leukemia) a form of *leukemia* caused by malignant changes in the immature *granulocytes* or *monocytes*; abbr. AML

leukemia, chronic lymphatic *chronic lymphocytic leukemia*

leukemia, chronic myelogenous *chronic myelocytic leukemia*

leukemia, chronic myeloid *chronic myelocytic leukemia*

leukocoria (leukokoria, cat's eye reflex, amaurotic cat's eye) grayish-white mass behind the lens of the eye, e.g. due to *retinoblastoma*

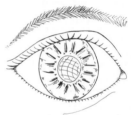

Fig. 277: leukocoria

leukocyte white blood cell; produced in the *bone marrow* and *lymphatic* system; subdivided into *granulocytes*, *lymphocytes* and *monocytes*

leukocyte interferon *interferon* produced by the *leukocytes* (alpha interferon)

leukocytoblast immature *leukocyte*

leukocytoclastic angiitis *cutaneous leukocytoclastic angiitis*

leukocytogenesis *leukopoiesis*

leukocytosis pathological increase in *leukocytes*; opp. *leukopenia*

leukocyturia increased number of *leukocytes* in the urine (> 10/l)

leukodermia lack of pigmentation in the skin, e.g. in *leprosy*

leukoma white opacity on the *cornea*

leukonychia development of white spots on the finger- and toenails, e.g. due to *fungal* infection or *protein* deficiency

leukopenia pathological decrease in *leukocytes*; opp. *leukocytosis*

leukopenic pert. to *leukopenia*

leukoplakia disease of the oral mucosa marked by hardened white patches (*precancerous*)

leukopoiesis (leukocytogenesis) production of *leukocytes*, occurring primarily in the *bone marrow*

leukorrhea discharge from the female external *genitalia*

level concentration of a substance within a fluid, e.g. of a drug in the blood

levo– combining form: left

levulose see *fructose*

LH abbr. *luteinizing hormone*

Lhermitte's sign abnormal tingling sensation along the *spinal column* when flexing the neck; typical of *meningeal* irritation, spinal tumors or *multiple sclerosis*

LHRH abbr. luteinizing hormone-releasing hormone (*gonadotropin-releasing hormone*)

liability responsibility

libido sex drive

lichen nonspecific collective term for skin diseases characterized by development of papules and scaling

lichen ruber planus (lichen planus) skin disease marked by formation of small papules, esp. on the limbs and scalp

lichen sclerosus et atrophicus inflammatory skin disorder mainly affecting the external *genitalia* in older individuals

lichenification skin condition marked by development of small, closely grouped papules

lid retractor *tissue*-preserving surgical instrument according to Desmarres, used for hooking vessels, nerves and wounds, among other tasks

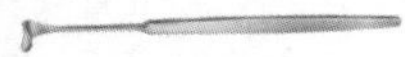

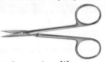

Fig. 278: lid retractor [A]

lien spleen

lienal pert. to the *spleen*

lienalis, A. arteria lienalis

lienalis, V. vena lienalis

lig– combining form: binding

ligament band of fibrous connective tissue that supports or connects body structures e.g. bones

ligamentum cruciatum cruciate ligament

ligate to create a *ligature*

ligature loop of suture for tying off a blood vessel or hollow *organ* during *surgery*, e.g. to arrest bleeding

ligature scissors (suture scissors) small scissors used for cutting surgical sutures

Fig. 279: ligature scissors [A]

lingual veins *veins* that transport blood from the tongue area

limb leads *ECG* leads from the *extremities*; types are bipolar Einthoven-type leads (I, II, III) and unipolar Goldberger-type leads (aVR, aVL, aVF); for electrode positions see *Einthoven*; see also *Wilson chest leads*

limbic system functional unit within the *CNS* that influences numerous *autonomic* and mental functions

limbus corneae border between the *cornea* and *sclera* of the eye

linear in a line

lingu(o)– combining form tongue

lingua (glossa) tongue

linguae, Mm. (musculi linguae) lingual *muscles*

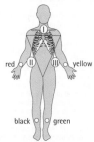

red II   III yellow

black   green

Fig. 280: electrode positioning for limb leads

lingual muscles collective term for the tongue muscles

lingual tonsils lymphoid tissue located at the root of the tongue

linguales, Vv. *venae linguales*

lingualis, A. *arteria lingualis*

Linton-Nachlass (tube) inflatable tube introduced via the nose or mouth for cauterization of bleeding from *varices* in the lower *esophagus* or *cardia*

lipase *enzyme* produced by the *pancreas* that breaks down *fats* for digestion; important laboratory parameter for detection and monitoring of *pancreatitis*

lipemia increased amount of *fat* in the blood

lipid chemical compound of glycerin and fatty acids

lipid reducer drug used to reduce the blood lipid level

lipo– combining form: fat

lipoid *fat*-like substance

lipoidosis nonspecific collective term for diseases marked by excessive storage of fat in the tissues

lipoma benign tumor of *fatty tissue*

lipomatosis presence of multiple *lipomas*

lipoprotein substance composed of *fat* and *protein* that transports water-insoluble lipids in the blood

liposarcoma malignant tumor of fatty tissue

liquid fluid

liquor cerebrospinalis *cerebrospinal fluid*

Lister scissors (bandage scissors) scissors used for cutting off bandages, among other tasks

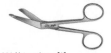

Fig. 281:Lister scissors [A]

Listeria genus of motile rod-shaped *grampositive bacteria*

Listeria monocytogenes *bacterium* of the genus *Listeria* that causes *listeriosis*

listeriosis (listeriosis) *infectious disease* of animals caused by *Listeria monocytogenes*; can also infect immunocompromised humans and cause *flu*-like symptoms or *meningitis*; usually transmitted through contaminated food

–lith, lith(o)– combining form: stone

lithiasis formation of stones in hollow *organs*, e.g. in the *kidneys*, *bladder* or *gallbladder*

lithos stone

lithotomy position a dorsal position assumed for treatment or examination most often in *gynecology* with the patient's hip and knee joints are bent and the legs slightly spread

lithotripsy (ultrasonic lithotripsy) nonsurgical procedure for pulverizing stones in the *kidney*, *bladder* or *gallbladder* using *ultrasonic* waves

live birth any birth in which the newborn infant begins to breathe, or the heart begins to beat, or the umbilical cord pulsates; opp. stillbirth

liver *organ* located in the right upper abdomen, involved in a wide range of metabolic functions

liver biopsy medical procedure using a special biopsy needle, whereby a small sample is taken from the liver and sent to the lab for analysis

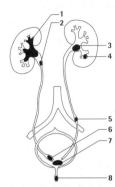

Fig. 282: localization of lithiasis
1 Staghorn calculus 2 Ureteral calculus 3 Kidney stone 4 Caliceal calculus 5 Ureteral calculus 6 Ureteral calculus 7 Urinary calculus 8 Urethral calculus

livor mortis *postmortem lividity*
LLC abbr. limited liability company
LMA abbr. laryngeal mask airway
LMN abbr. lower motor neuron
lob- combining form: lobe
lobar pneumonia pneumonia affecting one or more lobes of the lung
lobe rounded part of an *organ* separated from the body of the organ by boundary structures
lobectomy *surgical* removal of a lobe of an *organ*, e.g. from the *lungs* or *brain*
lobulus auriculae earlobe
local limited to one area; opp. *generalized*
local anesthesia (regional anesthesia) numbing limited to one region for performing *surgery*, e.g. using a local anesthetic agent with patient remaining conscious; abbr. LA; opp. *narcosis*
local anesthetic drug used to achieve *local anesthesia*

local recurrence recurrence of a tumor in its original location
lochia *physiological* discharge from the *uterus* following childbirth
lochiometra retention of *lochia* in the *uterus* following childbirth e.g. due to an obstruction in the *cervical* canal
lockjaw *trismus*
locomotor ataxia *tabes dorsalis*
locus place, location
-log, log(o)- combining form: speech
logoklony (logoclonia) uncontrolled repetition of words or syllables
logopedia (speech therapy) diagnosis, treatment and counseling of patients with vocal, speech and language defects
logorrhea continuous excessive speech
-logy combining form: study, knowledge
long adductor muscle long hip muscle that draws the thigh toward the midline; innervation: *obturator nerve*
long extensor muscle of the great toe lower leg muscle that raises the great toe; innervation: *deep peroneal nerve*
long extensor muscle of the toes long muscle in the lower leg that extends the toes D2-D4; innervation: *deep peroneal nerve*
long thoracic nerve *nerve* arising from the *brachial plexus* that innervates the *anterior serratus muscle*
longissimus, M. (musculus longissimus) *longissimus muscle*
longissimus muscle long back muscle; innervation: *dorsal* branches of the corresponding *spinal nerves*
longitudinal dislocation longitudinal displacement of the fragments of a fracture, e.g. with extension or shortening
loop diuretic drug that promotes excretion of urine by inhibiting reuptake of *primary urine* components in *Henle's loop* in the *renal tubules*
lordosis concave curvature of the spine; opp. *kyphosis*
LOS abbr. length of stay
Lou-Gehrig's disease see amyotrophic lateral sclerosis

louse (pediculus) genus of small insects that can infest the head, pubic area and body of humans; some types can transmit diseases

low blood anemia

lower jaw *mandible*

lower leg *crus*

LPN abbr. licensed practical nurse

LS abbr. *lumbar spine*

LTH abbr. lactotropic hormone (*prolactin*)

LTX abbr. *liver transplant*

lucid interval brief remission of symptoms in psychosis, head injury, or epileptic seizures

Luer Lock connector standard connector for *injection* and *infusion* equipment, e.g. the female connector of a needle into which a *Luer connector* is inserted or screwed

lues *syphilis*

lumbago (lumbalgia) sudden severe back pain in the *lumbar spine* area

lumbalgia *lumbago*

lumbar pert. to the *lumbar spine*

lumbar plexus nerve *plexus* in the lumbar area (branches of the 1st–4th lumbar nerves) that includes the *nervus femoralis* and *nervus obturatorius* et al.

lumbar puncture (spinal puncture, spinal tap) withdrawal of *cerebrospinal fluid* with a hollow needle from the spinal cord at the level of the 3rd/4th *lumbar vertebrae* (below a line connecting the iliac crests), e.g. for examination purposes

lumbar spine (vertebrae lumbales) part of the *spinal column* between the *thoracic spine* and the *sacrum*, consisting of 5 lumbar vertebrae; abbr. LS

lumbar spine syndrome collective term for conditions involving pain in the *lumbar spine*

lumbar vertebrae see *lumbar spine*

lumboischialgia *sciatica*

lumbrical muscles of the foot collective term for the muscles that flex the toes; innervation: *plantar nerve*

lumbrical muscles of the hand collective term for the muscles that flex the fingers and extend the distal phalanges; innervation: *ulnar and median nerve*

lumbrical muscles of the foot collective term for the muscles that flex the toes; innervation: *plantar nerve*

lumbrical muscles of the hand collective term for the muscles that flex the fingers and extend the distal phalanges; innervation: *ulnar and median nerve*

lumbricales manus, Mm. (musculi lumbricales manus) *lumbrical muscles of the hand*

lumbricales pedis, Mm. (musculi lumbricales pedis) *lumbrical muscles of the foot*

lumbus lower back

lumen internal diameter of a hollow structure

lumin– combining form: light

lunate bone (os lunatum) one of the *carpal bones*

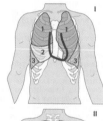

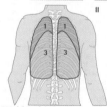

Fig. 283: lobes of the lungs
I Ventral view 1 Superior lobe **2** Middle lobe **3** Inferior lobe
II Dorsal view 1 Superior lobe **2** Inferior lobe

lung paired *organ* located in the thorax, of which the right lung has three *lobes* and the left two; its main function is to facilitate respiration by exchanging *oxygen* and *carbon dioxide* between the bloodstream and the outside environment

lung function *spirometry*

lupus erythematosus (systemic lupus erythematosus) *autoimmune disorder* marked by formation of *antinuclear antibodies*; usually affects the skin or internal *organs*; abbr. *LE*

lute- combining form: yellow

luteinizing hormone *hormone* produced in the *adenohypophysis*; in women, it stimulates the *ovaries* and induces *ovulation*; in men, it stimulates the *testes*; it is inhibited by *progesterone*; abbr. LH

luxate to dislocate, displace

luxated adj. of *luxate*

luxation joint dislocation with complete loss of contact between the ends of the bones that form the joint

Lyell syndrome *toxic epidermal necrolysis*

Lyme borreliosis *Lyme disease*

Lyme disease (Lyme borreliosis) *infectious disease* caused by *Borrelia burgdorferi*, which leads to *flu*-like symptoms, skin changes and severe *inflammation* of the *nerves* and *joints*; transmitted via tick bite, with the classic symptom of *erythema chronicum migrans* (bull's-eye rash)

lymph intercellular fluid that passes from the *capillaries* into the *tissue* spaces and is returned to the bloodstream via the *lymph vessels*

lymph node cherry-sized *organs* that are located along the *lymph vessels*, which filter pathogens, toxins, etc. out of the *lymph*

lymph vessel (vas lymphaticum) fine vessel that returns *lymph* to the bloodstream after passing through the *lymph nodes*

lymphadenectomy *surgical* removal of *lymph nodes*

lymphadenitis *inflammation* of the *lymph nodes*

lymphangiitis *inflammation* of the *lymph vessels*

lymphangioma benign tumor consisting of dilated *lymph vessels*

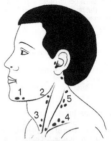

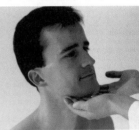

Fig. 284: location and palpation of cervical lymph nodes

lymphatic pert. to *lymph* or the lymphatic system

lymphatic drainage treatment of *lymphedema* using a special massage technique to accelerate the release of *lymph* into the bloodstream

lymphatic system collective term for all lymphatic *tissues* (lymph nodes, spleen, tonsils, thymus)

lymphedema fluid accumulation in the *tissues* due to impaired *lymph* flow usually following *surgical* removal of the *lymph nodes*; see also *Stemmer's sign*

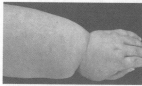

Fig. 285: severe lymphedema

lymphocyte blood cell belonging to the *leukocyte* group; divided into B lymphocytes, which produce *immunoglobulins* for immune defense, and T lymphocytes, which function as *phagocytes*, memory cells and helper cells

lymphogenous pert. to *lymph*

lymphogranulomatosis *Hodgkin's lymphoma*

lymphoma often malignant enlargement of the *lymph nodes*

lymphosarcoma malignant tumor of the *lymphatic tissues*

–lysis combining form: dissolution

lysis gradual reduction of fever

lysosome *cell* organelle involved in the intracellular digestive process

lyssa *rabies*

–lytic pert. to destruction or dissolution

M

M symbol: million (10^6); prefix: mega-

m symbol: thousandth (10^{-3}); prefix: milli-

M. abbr. *muscle*

macerated softened

maceration softening of *tissue*

macro combining form: large, long

macrocyte *erythrocyte* with a diameter > 0.8 μm but of normal thickness

macrocytosis increased presence of *macrocytes* in the blood

macroglobulinemia see *Waldenström's macroglobulinemia*

macroglossia pathological enlargement of the tongue, e.g. in *acromegaly*

macrohematuria visible red discoloration of the urine due to the presence of blood; opp. *microhematuria*

macrophage scavenger cell (*monocyte*); removes debris and *bacteria* in the blood and *tissues*

macroscopic visible to the naked eye; opp. *microscopic*

macula lutea retinae yellow spot on the *retina*; vision is most acute at this point

macular pert. to a macule; spotty

macule (macula) spot; circumscribed change in skin color at epidermal level; one of the *primary efflorescences*

macular degeneration progressive, age-related deterioration of the macula of the retina; types are dry and wet

madarosis loss of the eyebrows and/or eyelashes

Madelung's deformity hereditary growth disorder of the *distal radius* with normal growth of the *ulna*

Magill forceps angled grasping forceps used e.g. to assist in guiding the *endotracheal tube* for *nasotracheal intubation*

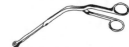

Fig. 286: Magill forceps

magn– combining form: large

magnesium important trace element that activates a variety of *enzymes*; magnesium is found primarily in bones and skeletal muscle tissue; it is taken up by the small intestine and excreted via the *kidneys* in the urine; total amount in the body is ca. 25 g, of which 99% is intracellular and 1% extracellular; chemical symbol: Mg

magnesium sulfate laxative; chemical symbol: $MgSO_4$

magnetic resonance imaging (magnetic resonance tomography) imaging method in which magnetic fields are used to create sectional images of the body; abbr. MRI, MRT, NMRI

magnetic resonance tomography *magnetic resonance imaging*

maidenhead *hymen*

Mainz pouch construction of a substitute *urinary bladder* using the *ileum* and *ascending colon*, which is *anastomosed* with the navel and emptied with a *catheter*

Maisonneuve fracture high *Weber C fracture* marked by crooked fracture line and associated injury to the medial malleolus

major the larger (of two); opp. *minor*

malabsorption impaired intestinal absorption of nutrients

-malacia combining form: softening

malaria mainly tropical febrile *infectious disease* caused by *Plasmodium* protozoa, which leads to damage to numerous organs (*kidneys, lungs, brain, liver*); transmitted via the bite of the *Anopheles* mosquito

maldigestion impaired digestion

Malgaigne fracture combination of anterior and posterior *pelvic ring fractures*, which may be ipsilateral, intersecting or bilateral

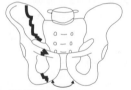

Fig. 287: Malgaigne fracture

malignancy harmfulness; opp. *benignancy*

malignant harmful; opp. *benign*

malignant goiter malignant enlargement of the *thyroid gland*

malignant hyperthermia rare life-threatening *syndrome* marked by acute *hypermetabolic* condition of the muscle *tissues*, usually triggered by *anesthetics*; abbr. MH

malignant tumor harmful neoplasm

malleolar fracture *fracture* of the ankle

malleolus protuberance of the ankle joint

malleus (hammer) one of the three ossicles in the middle ear, located between the *eardrum* and *incus*

Mallory–Weiss syndrome hemorrhage from a tear in the mucosa of the lower esophagus or cardia; usually triggered by a sudden increase in pressure, e.g. during vomiting

malpractice negligent or incorrect medical treatment

Malta fever *brucellosis* caused by *Brucella melitensis*

mammillary line imaginary line passing vertically through the nipple

mamma female breast

mammaplasty *surgical* modification of the breast, e.g. for cosmetic purposes

mammilla nipple

mammography (mammogram) radiography of the breast

mandible (mandibula) lower jaw

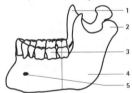

Fig. 288: mandible
1 Coronoid process 2 Condyloid process 3 Teeth
4 Angle of mandible 5 Mental foramen

mandibular prognathism (underbite) *dysgnathia* in which the lower jaw is too far forward with abnormal prominence of the chin (lower front teeth are in front of the upper front teeth); opp. *eugnathia*; see also *prognathism*

mandrin 1) specialized closure for a *Braunula* that fills the interior lumen of the cannula and prevents obstruction; 2) guide for a *catheter* or *endotracheal tube*

-mania combining form: frenzy, drive

mania psychosis characterized by increased drive, euphoria and flight of ideas

manic pert. to mania

manifest clearly visible, evident; opp. latent

manifestation expression, presence

manometer device for measuring pressure

manometry measurement of pressure

manual pert. to the hand

manual therapy chirotherapy

manus hand

MAO abbr. monoamine oxidase

MAP abbr. mean arterial pressure

marasmus (wasting) general physical and mental decline

Marburg fever hemorrhagic fever caused by the Marburg virus; transmitted via contact with green baboons, but also transmissible from human to human

Marburg virus virus that causes Marburg fever

march fracture metatarsal stress fracture due to an unusually long period of walking

Marfan's syndrome hereditary connective tissue disease marked by defects in the skeleton, cardiovascular system and eyes

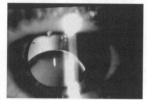

Fig. 289: lens dislocation (Marfan's syndrome)

mariscae anal folds; folds of skin on the anus that cannot be repositioned; a sign of healed perianal thrombosis (but unlike hemorrhoids these do not fill with blood)

masculine characteristic of a male; opp. feminine

mask(like) face facial rigidity seen in conditions like Parkinson's disease or scleroderma

masked covered

masking covering

masseter muscle that raises and moves the lower jaw forward

masseter nerve nerve that innervates the masseter

massetericus, N. nervus massetericus

mastalgia mastodynia

mastectomy surgical removal of the breast, e.g. due to breast cancer

masticatorii, Mm. (musculi masticatorii) masticatory muscles

masticatory muscles collective term for muscles involved in chewing

mastitis inflammation of the mammary glands

mastocarcinoma malignant tumor in the breast

mastodynia painful sensation of tightness in the breasts, usually hormone-related and preceding menstruation

mastoid process of the temporal bone located below the ear

mastoid process mastoid

mastoiditis inflammation of the mastoid

mastopathy disease of the mammary glands

mastos (mamma) female breast

maternal pert. to the mother

mature full-grown, adult; opp. immature

maxill– combining form: upper jaw

maxilla upper jaw; pneumatic bone with four processes in the viscerocranium

maxillaris, A. arteria maxillaris

maxillary sinus sinus located in the maxilla and adjacent to the orbits; see paranasal sinuses

Mb abbr. myoglobin

McBurney's point specific testing point for suspected appendicitis: tender point located in the first third of the line between the right anterosuperior spine of the ilium and the navel

MCH abbr. mean corpuscular hemoglobin

MCHC abbr. mean corpuscular hemoglobin concentration

McIntosh blade curved laryngoscope blade for intubation

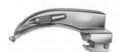

Fig. 290: McIntosh blade [A]

MCL abbr. *midclavicular line*

MCV abbr. mean corpuscular volume

MDI abbr. metered dose inhaler, e.g. albuterol

mean arterial pressure measured or calculated mean arterial blood pressure, consisting of systolic and diastolic arterial blood pressure; abbr. MAP; formula:

$$MAD = \frac{Systole + (2 \times Diastole)}{3}$$

measles (rubeola) *infectious disease* caused by the *rubeola virus*, leading to widespread skin eruptions over the entire body, beginning behind the ears, and in severe cases to *encephalitis*; an attack of measles gives lifelong immunity; transmitted mainly via droplet infection or contact

meatus passage, opening

meatus acusticus auditory canal

meatus acusticus externus external auditory canal

mechanical ileus *ileus* due to blockage of the intestinal lumen

mechanical restraint safety vest; wrist and leg restraints; devices that prevent movement

Meckel's diverticulum finger-shaped protrusion on the *ileum*; can lead to hemorrhages and *inflammation*

meconium infant's first stool, formed during pregnancy

media middle layer of a blood vessel, consisting of muscle

medial in the middle or toward the middle; opp. *lateral*

medial cuneiform bone first cuneiform bone; one of the *tarsal bones*

medial malleolus lower extremity of the *tibia*

median nerve *nerve* that supplies the flexor muscles of the forearm, the ball of the thumb and the palm of the hand, among other things; damage causes *ape hand*; also provides innervation of the *radial flexor muscle of the wrist superficial flexor of the fingers, flexor of the thumb, opposing muscle of the thumb* and *round pronator muscle*

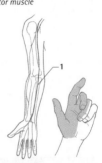

Fig. 291: median nerve
1 Median nerve

median plane body plane that divides the body into right and left halves

mediana antebrachii, V. *vena mediana antebrachii*

mediana cubiti, V. *vena mediana cubiti*

mediastinal emphysema *emphysema* of the *mediastinum* due to air entering the soft tissues of the upper chest and neck area, e.g. from *rupture* of the *trachea*

mediastinal pert. to the *mediastinum*

mediastinitis *inflammation* of the *mediastinum*, e.g. due to *rupture* of the *esophagus*

mediastinoscopy *endoscopy* of the *mediastinum*

mediastinum midthoracic cavity between the *lungs*

medical elastic stockings (TED hose, antithrombosis stockings) tight-fitting hose for prevention of *thrombosis* in susceptible patients via *compression* of the leg *veins,* which results in increased flow rates in the blood vessels

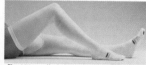

Fig. 292: medical elastic stockings [N]

medicamentous pert. to the medical use of drugs

medication drugs

medicus physician

medull– combining form: (bone) marrow

medulla marrow

medulla oblongata section of the *brain* between the midbrain and *spinal cord*; part of the *brain stem,* see Fig. 293

medullary pert. to *medulla*

medullary cone syndrome (conus syndrome) *radicular compression syndrome* due to damage to the *medullary cone* at the level of the 1st to 2nd lumbar vertebrae; usually associated with urinary and bowel *incontinence, saddle block anesthesia* and preservation of the *Achilles tendon reflex* (in contrast to *cauda equina syndrome*)

medullary menopausal syndrome (climacteric syndrome) *syndrome* occurring during *menopause,* caused by a lack of *estrogen,* with hot flashes, sweats and dizziness

medullary pin *osteosynthesis* of a long bone *fracture* in which a steel rod is used to splint the fragments from the inside, e.g. for a *diaphyseal fracture*

medulloblastoma malignant brain tumor in the area of the posterior cranial fossa

mega– 1) combining form: large; 2) million (10^6), symbol: M

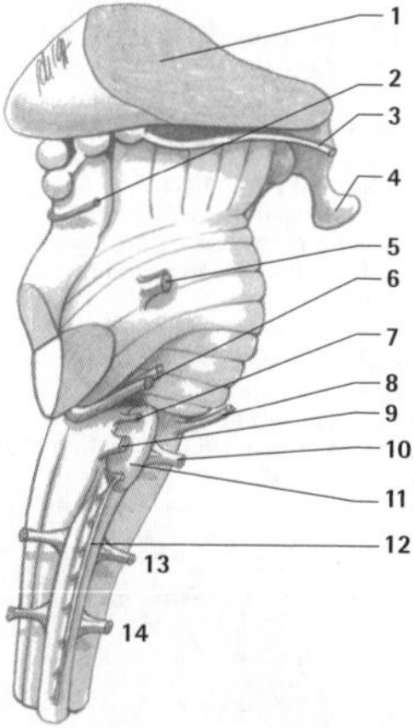

Fig. 293: medulla oblongata with nerve exits
1 Pulvinar **2** Trochlear nerve **3** Oculomotor nerve **4** Pituitary gland **5** Trigeminal nerve **6** Facial and vestibulocochlear nerves **7** Glossopharyngeal nerve **8** Abducens nerve **9** Vagus nerve **10** Hypoglossal nerve **11** Olive **12** Accessory nerve **13** C1 **14** C2

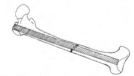

Fig. 294: medullary pin

megacolon extreme enlargement of the *colon*

megakaryocyte *stem cell* of the *thrombocytes,* found in the *bone marrow*

megaloblast abnormally large nucleated *erythrocytes*

megaloblastic anemia *anemia* with enlarged *erythrocytes* due to deficiency of *cyanocobalamin* or *folic acid*

megalocyte abnormally large *erythrocyte*

-megaly combining form: enlargement

meibomian cyst *chalazion*

meibomian glands *tarsal glands*

Meissner's corpuscle *neural receptors* in the skin for collecting and conducting tactile stimuli

melancholia depression

melanin dark pigment, e.g. in the skin *cells*

melano– combining form: black

melanocyte *melanin* cell

melanoma tumor originating in pigment-forming *cells*

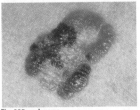

Fig. 295: melanoma

melatonin *hormone* produced in the *pineal gland* that regulates the sleep/wake cycle and inhibits skin pigmentation

melena (tarry stool) feces with black coloration due to blood combined with digestive juices

menarche first *menstruation*, usually occurring around age 12; triggered by *estrogen* and *gestagen* activity

Mendelson's syndrome *aspiration pneumonia* due to *aspiration* of gastric juices

Menière's disease progressive disease of the inner ear with vertigo and hearing impairment

mening(o)– combining form: (brain) membrane

meningeae, Vv. (venae meningeae) *meningeal veins*

meningeal veins *veins* that transport blood from the *dura mater*

meninges outer membranes of the brain and spinal cord, consisting of the *pia mater*, *arachnoidea* and *dura mater*; sing. meninx

meningioma benign tumor originating in the *arachnoidea*

meningism *meningeal* pain due to irritation from *inflammatory* processes, *neoplastic* processes or a *subarachnoid* bleed; test, while patient is supine and relaxed with legs extended, bending the neck causes pain in the nape of the neck and reflexive muscular countertension

meningitis *inflammation* of the *meninges*

meningocele protrusion of the *dura* through a vertebral arch defect with *intact spinal cord* and *spinal nerves*

meningococcal meningitis *meningitis* caused by *meningococci*; transmitted via droplet infection

meningococcus coffee bean-shaped *gram-negative bacterium* that causes *meningococcal meningitis*

meningoencephalitis *inflammation* of the *meninges* and *brain*

meningomyelitis *inflammation* of the *spinal cord* and its *membranes*

meningomyelocele protrusion of the *spinal cord* and *dura mater* through a vertebral arch defect

Fig. 296: meningomyelocele

meniscopathy *degeneration* of the *meniscus*, e.g. due to sports injuries

meniscus disk-shaped cartilage in the knee joint; pl. menisci

menopausal pert. to *menopause*

menopausal syndrome (climacteric syndrome) *syndrome* occurring during *menopause*, caused by a lack of *estrogen*, with hot flashes, sweats and dizziness

menopause (climacteric, change of life) process marking the end of a woman's reproductive years; cessation of regular menstruation

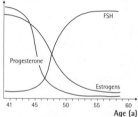

Fig. 297: menopause

menorrhagia prolonged *menstruation* lasting longer than 6 days, usually from *endocrine* or *organic* causes; opp. *brachymenorrhea*

menses *menstruation*

menstrual pert. to *menstruation*

menstrual cycle (endometrial cycle) *cycle* from the first day of *menstruation* to the last day before the next *menstruation*

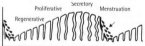

Fig. 298: menstrual cycle

menstruation (period, menses) female cyclic bleeding due to a drop in the *progesterone* level, causing sloughing of the *endometrium* built up during the *menstrual cycle*; duration: 3–5 days; interval: 25–31 days; total blood loss: ½ of a cup

mental block disorder of thought processes with a feeling of one's thoughts being separated or broken off, e.g. in *schizophrenia*

mental retardation below-average intelligence, congenital or acquired in early childhood

mentalis pert. to the chin

mentum chin

–mer(e) combining form: part

mercurialism (hydragyrosis) mercury poisoning

mercury (hydragyrum) metal chemical element with extremely toxic vapors; symbol: Hg

mes(o)– combining form: middle

mesencephalon midbrain; part of the *brain stem*

mesenchyme *embryonic connective tissue*

mesenteric pert. to the *mesentery* or the *mesenteric artery* or *vein*

mesenterica, A. *arteria mesenterica*

mesenterica, V. *vena mesenterica*

mesentery fold of peritoneal *membrane* that attaches the small intestine to the abdominal wall

mesh graft patches of skin intended for transplantation, which are incised in a grid pattern after removal using a special *dermatome* and are then spread out and applied over the graft area

mesial toward the jaw

mesoderm middle *germ layer* in the human blastoderm, from which the supporting structures, musculoskeletal system, blood and *lymph vessels*, and *urogenital system* develop

mesothelioma tumor originating in the *mesothelium*

mesothelium epithelial *cell* layer of the membranes lining the abdominal and thoracic cavities

Messerer fracture typical *fracture* in vehicular accidents, e.g. of the tibia, from contact with the steering column; has a characteristic triangular *fragment* with its base on the side where the force was applied

M

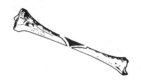

Fig. 299: Messerer fracture

meta– combining form: after, following
metabolic pert. to *metabolism*
metabolic acidosis form of *acidosis* characterized by a decrease in *pH* to below 7.36 and a decrease in *standard bicarbonate*, e.g. due to *lactacidosis*
metabolic alkalosis form of *alkalosis* characterized by an increase in *pH* to above 7.44 and an increase in *standard bicarbonate*, e.g. due to depletion of acid (vomiting or long-term aspiration of stomach contents) or sodium bicarbonate overdose
metabolic disorder disease in which the body's metabolism is impaired, e.g. *diabetes mellitus* or *gout*
metabolism intake, transformation and release of substances for the body's use in energy production, growth or maintenance of functions
metabolite product of *metabolism*
metacarpal pert. to the (bones of the) hand
metacarpals hand bones
metacarpophalangeal joints joints between the hand (metacarpal) bones and the fingers
metacarpus hand
metamorphopsia distorted vision
metamorphosis transformation
metaphyseal pert. to the *metaphysis*
metaphysical beyond the senses
metaphysis growth zone of a long bone, located between the *epiphysis* and *diaphysis*

metastasis appearance of a tumor in another part of the body, e.g. due to transport of malignant *cells* through the bloodstream or *lymphatic system*; pl. metastases
metastasize to spread throughout the body or to another organ (tumors)
metatarsals bones of the foot
metatarsophalangeal joints joints between the foot (metatarsal) bones and the toes
meteorism (flatulence) large amounts of gas in the gastrointestinal tract
meteorotropism (meteorosensitivity) weather-related health conditions
–meter combining form: measuring instrument
metHb abbr. *methemoglobin*
methemoglobin (hemiglobin) *oxidized* form of hemoglobin that is no longer able to transport oxygen due to intoxication or other causes; abbr. metHb
methemoglobinemia increased *methemoglobin* in the blood
methylene blue dye used to stain *bacteria* for microscopic examination
metra (uterus, hystera) womb
metrorrhagia bleeding between *menstrual* periods from *endocrine* or *organic* causes
–metry combining form: measurement
mg abbr. *milligram*
Mg chemical symbol: *magnesium*
$MgSO_4$ chemical symbol: *magnesium sulfate*
MH abbr. *malignant hyperthermia*
MI abbr. *myocardial infarction*; *mitral insufficiency*
micro– combining form: small
microbe *microorganism*
microbial pert. to *microorganisms*
microbiological pert. to the study of microorganisms
microbiology study of *microorganisms*
microcirculation disorder circulation disorder in which the *capillaries* receive a spatially and temporally inconsistent supply of blood
microcyte *erythrocyte* with a diameter < 0.7 μm

microcytosis increased presence of *microcytes* in the blood

microgram 1/1000 mg; abbr. μg

microhematuria presence of *microscopic* amounts of blood in the urine; opp. *macrohematuria*

microlaryngoscopy tube smallbore *endotracheal tube* for performing *surgery* on the *trachea*; abbr. MLT

micromelia abnormally small limbs

micrometer 1/1000 mm; abbr. μm

microophthalmia abnormally small eyeball

microorganism (microbe) smallest type of life form not visible to the naked eye, e.g. *bacteria*

micropsia visual disorder in which objects are seen as smaller than their actual size

microscope lens system for *optical* magnification of specimens

microscopic 1) not visible to the naked eye; 2) pert. to microscopy; opp. *macroscopic*

microscopy *optical* magnification of specimens

microsurgery performing surgical procedures under a *microscope*

micturition urination

MICU abbr. medical intensive care unit

midclavicular line imaginary line used as a thoracic surface landmark; passes through the midpoint of the *clavicle*; abbr. MCL

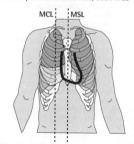

Fig. 300: midclavicular line

migraine (sick headache) sudden, pounding, periodically recurring headaches, usually on one side, lasting 4 to 72 hours; often accompanied by *autonomic* (nausea, vomiting, sensitivity to light and noise), *visual* or *neurological symptoms*

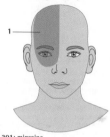

Fig. 301: migraine
1 Pain

miliary tubercle *nodule* caused by *tuberculosis*

miliary tuberculosis form of *tuberculosis* marked by presence of numerous *miliary tubercles* spreading over the entire body; occurs mainly in immunocompromised individuals

milk crust *endogenous eczema* occurring in newborns

milli– combining form: thousandth (10^{-3}); symbol: m

milligram 1/1000 g; abbr. *mg*

mineral inorganic substance

mineralization deposition of mineral substances, e.g. of *calcium* in the bones

mineralocorticoid collective term for *hormones* produced in the *adrenal cortex* with important functions in maintaining the body's water/salt balance, e.g. *aldosterone*

mini-spike plastic cannula for multiple withdrawals of *injection* solutions from storage containers, e.g. *infusion bottles* or *ampules*

M

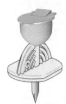

Fig. 302: mini-spike [C]

minute volume amount of air that is inhaled or exhaled in one minute; abbr. MV

miosis contraction of the *pupil*; opp. *mydriasis*

miotic drug that causes contraction of the pupils; opp. *mydriatic*

missed abortion abortion in which the dead *fetus* remains in the *uterus* with little or no *vaginal* bleeding

mite small, spider-like *parasite* that can cause *allergies* and transmit diseases

mitochondrion component of the *cell* that generates energy; pl. mitochondria

mitosis *cell* division

mitral (valve) insufficiency inability of the *mitral valve* to close; abbr. MI

mitral (valve) stenosis *stenosis* of the *mitral valve* orifice, which obstructs blood flow into the left ventricle

mitral valve (left atrioventricular valve, bicuspid valve) bicuspid valve between the left atrium and left ventricle of the heart

MLT abbr. *microlaryngoscopy tube*

Mm. abbr. *musculi*

mobile able to move; opp. *immobile*

mobilization 1) promoting movement, e.g. after surgery; opp. *immobilization;* 2) giving colony-stimulating factors or chemo to help move stem cells from the bone marrow into the bloodstream in order to increase the number of peripheral blood stem cells collected for a stem cell transplant/rescue

modification alteration

Moeller's glossitis superficial inflammation of the *tongue*, e.g. due to *liver* disease

MOF abbr. *multiple organ failure*

mola hydratiosa *hydatid mole*

molar *dens molaris*

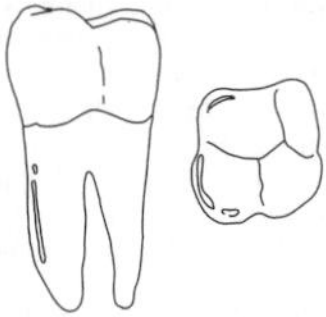

Fig. 303: molars

molded prosthesis removable dental prosthesis molded in one piece and attached to remaining natural teeth with crowns or clamps

molecular pert. to the *molecule*

molecule smallest component of a chemical compound

mollis soft

molluscum soft growth on the skin

molluscum contagiosum (flat wart) skin condition caused by viruses, marked by formation of dimpled flat warts

Monaldi drain *thoracic* drain that is placed in the 3rd *intercostal* space on the *midclavicular line*

mono- combining form: one

monoamine oxidase *enzyme* that promotes breakdown of monoamines; abbr. MAO

monoclonal derived from a single parent *cell* or from a *clone* of a parent cell

monocular periorbital hematoma (black eye) *hematoma* in the upper and lower lids of one eye; classic sign of a *fracture* of the *cranial base*; see also *bilateral periorbital hematoma*

monocyte blood *cell* from the *leukocyte* group; acts as a scavenger cell for immune defense

monocytosis increased *monocytes* in the blood

monomorphic keeping the same appearance; opp. *polymorphic*

mononucleosis (infectiosa) (infectious mononucleosis, Pfeiffer's disease) febrile *infectious disease* caused by the *Epstein-Barr virus* leading to *tonsillitis* and swollen *lymph nodes*, among other things; transmitted mainly through close physical contact ("kissing disease")

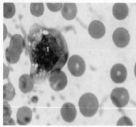

Fig. 304: mononucleosis infectiosa
1 Lymphocyte with vacuolized cytoplasm

monosomy X *Turner's syndrome*

monovette fine tube for collection of blood samples, which can be connected with an adapter to a *venous catheter* or special needle for direct *venipuncture*

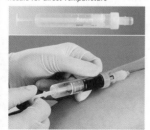

Fig. 305: monovette [L]

mons mound

mons pubis (mount of Venus) pad of fat over the *pubic symphysis*

Monteggia fracture *diaphyseal fracture* of the *ulna* with *dislocation* of the *radial* head, e.g. from falling on a bent arm

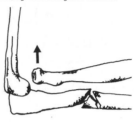

Fig. 306: Monteggia fracture

morb– combining form: disease
morbid diseased
morbid obesity extreme *obesity* with a *body mass index* > 40
morbidity disease rate
morbus disease, illness
moribund dying
Moro reflex (embrace reflex, startle reflex) reflexive embracing motion present in infants up to 3 months old
–morph, morph– combining form: form shape
morphine alkaloid isolated from *opium*
morphology study of forms
mors death
morula embryo at an early stage, consisting of 12-32 cells
Morse Fall Scale method for assessing a patient's risk of falling
morsus bite wound
mort– combining form: death
mortality statistical term for the number of deaths in relation to the total number of the population
morulation division of the fertilized egg up to the 32-cell stage (morula)

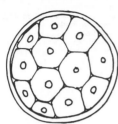

Fig. 307: Morula

mosquito forceps *hemostat* according to Halsted, used for clamping off injured vessels and various other holding tasks

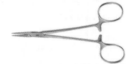

Fig. 308: mosquito forceps [A]

-mot(or), mot(or)- combining form: movement
motility *passive* involuntary movements, e.g. motion of the intestines; opp. *motoricity*
motion sickness illness caused by motion, e.g. seasickness
motor neuron terminal portion of a nerve pathway from the spinal cord to muscles that control active voluntary movement
motoric pert. to *motoricity*
motoricity *active* voluntary movements, e.g. raising an arm; opp. *motility*
mount of Venus *mons pubis*
mouth oral cavity
MRI abbr. *magnetic resonance imaging*
MRSA abbr. methicillin-resistant *Staphylococcus* aureus; patient needs to be placed on contact isolation when diagnosis is confirmed

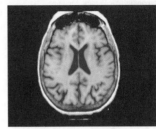

Fig. 309: MRI image of head

MS abbr. *multiple sclerosis*
MSL abbr. *midsternal line*
MSU abbr. *midstream urine*
muc(o)-, muci- combining form: mucus
mucin glyoprotein found in *mucus*
mucocele (mucous cyst) collection of mucus in a cavity, e.g. the *paranasal sinuses*
mucolytic drug used to dissolve *mucus*
mucosa mucous membrane
mucositis inflammation of the *mucosa*
mucous pert. to *mucus*
mucoviscidosis cystic fibrosis
mucus slimy, viscous fluid secreted by mucous glands and membranes
multi- combining form: many
multi-infarct dementia Binswanger's dementia
multifragment fracture *fracture* caused by broad application of force with 44 to 6 bone *fragments*; cf. *comminuted fracture*

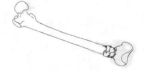

Fig. 310: multifragment fracture

multimorbid suffering from multiple diseases

multipara a woman who has had multiple pregnancies

multiple more than one, numerous; opp. *solitary*

multiple drug dependence *addiction* to several drugs at the same time

multiple myeloma *plasmacytoma*

multiple organ failure failure of several *organs*, e.g. due to *sepsis*; abbr. *MOF*

multiple rib fractures *fracture* of at least 3 ribs at once, usually in connection with *polytrauma*

multiple sclerosis intermittent disease of the *central nervous system* with multiple sites of *inflammation* within the central nervous system, leading to *myelin sheath* destruction with corresponding impairment of *nerve* functions; abbr. MS

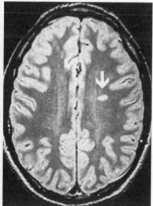

Fig. 311: multiple sclerosis with plaques in MRI

multiple stopcock system assembly comprising several three-way stopcocks mounted together on a holding plate; used to hook up multiple infusion systems to the same *venous catheter*

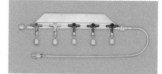

Fig. 312: multiple stopcock system [L]

mummification *gangrene* with drying up and shriveling of *tissue*

mumps *infectious disease* caused by *Rabula inflans* that causes *inflammatory* swelling of the parotid gland and in severe cases also involves other *organs*; transmitted by *droplet* or *smear infection*

Munchausen syndrome repeated or constant simulation of *symptoms* in order to force a hospital stay

mural pert. to the wall of a hollow organ

muscae volitantes *floaters*

muscle compartment syndrome *compartment syndrome*

muscle relaxant drug used to reduce muscle tension, e.g. in the context of *surgery*

muscle tone *tonus* of the muscles

muscular atrophy *wasting away of muscle tissue*

muscular dystrophy hereditary disease characterized by progressive atrophy and muscle weakness; a) **Duchenne** type affects only young males; b) **myotonic dystrophy** may occur anywhere from childhood to late adulthood; c) **Becker** type has an onset in childhood; respiratory and physical therapy needed in all types;

musculocutaneous nerve *nerve* arising from the *brachial plexus* that innervates the *biceps brachii* and *brachial muscles*, et al.

M

Museum forceps long tenaculum forceps used during surgery for holding tasks

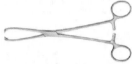

Fig. 313: museum forceps [A]

mutagenic causing changes in the genetic material

mutation 1) change in the configuration of *DNA*; 2) pubertal voice break in males

mutilation disfigurement

mutism speechlessness with no *organic* cause, occurring in the context of a *psychosis*

MVA abbr. motor vehicle accident

MVR abbr. *mitral valve* replacement

myalgia muscle pain

myasthenia gravis *autoimmune* disease marked by muscular weakness related to exertion; caused by formation of *antibodies* to *acetylcholine receptors* of the motor end plate/neuromuscular junction; diagnosis confirmed by Tensilon test and EMG

myasthenic crisis *neurological* crisis with sudden generalized muscle weakness and risk of *respiratory insufficiency, dysphagia* and *aspiration*; usually caused by *acetylcholinesterase* inhibitor overdose, *common cold, surgery* or childbirth

myc(o)- combining form: fungus

mycetes fungi

Mycobacterium genus of acid-fast rod-shaped *bacteria*

Mycobacterium leprae *bacterium* in the *Mycobacterium* group that causes *leprosy*

Mycobacterium tuberculosis (tubercle bacillus) acid-fast rod-shaped *bacterium* in the *Mycobacterium* group that causes *tuberculosis*

Mycoplasma group of *bacteria* that can cause *pneumonia* and other *infections*

mycosis disease caused by a fungus; pl. mycoses

mydriasis dilation of the *pupil*; opp. *miosis*

mydriatic drug used to dilate the pupils; opp. *miotic*

myelin substance in the *myelin sheath* of the *nerves*

myelin sheath sheath around a *neuron* consisting of *myelin*

myelo- combining form: spinal cord; (bone) marrow

myeloablation (ablation) killing of bone marrow by chemo-/radiation therapy

myelocele protrusion of the *spinal cord* through a vertebral arch defect

myeloid pert. to the *bone marrow*

myeloma *bone marrow* tumor

myelon *spinal cord*

myelos (medulla) marrow

myelosarcoma malignant tumor originating in the spinal cord

myelosis nonspecific collective term for forms of *leukemia* originating in the *bone marrow*

myelosis funicular *funicular myelosis*

myo- combining form: muscle

myoarthropathy nonspecific collective term for diseases affecting the muscles and joints

myoatrophy wasting of muscle tissue, e.g. from being bedridden

myocardial pert. to the *myocardium*

Stage	Age	ECG	Criteria
Early Stage	> a few minutes	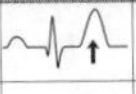	Tall T waves
Stage I	Up to 6 hours	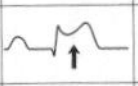	ST elevation R waves No/small Q wave
Intermed. Stage	> 6 hours	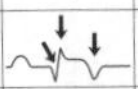	ST elevation with T wave inversion Loss of R wave, infarct Q
Stage II	Days	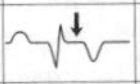	Infarct Q T wave inversion ST normalization
Stage III	Residual	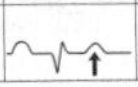	Persistant Q Loss of R wave T normalization

Fig. 314: ECG readings in myocardial infarction

myocardial infarction (heart attack) *necrosis* of heart muscle tissue due to inadequate blood supply in the *coronary arteries*; diagnosis supported by ECG readings; abbr. MI

myocarditis *inflammation* of the *myocardium*, e.g. caused by *streptococci*

myocardium heart muscle

myoclonus sudden brief twitching or spasms of a muscle or muscle group that cannot be voluntarily suppressed, e.g. from *neurological* diseases such as *epilepsy*

myogelosis 1) nodular hardening of muscles, e.g. after overuse; 2) local painfully increased, lingering tension of the muscles usually in the supporting muscles of the back

myogen(et)ic originating in the muscles

myoglobin *protein* related to *hemoglobin* that supplies the muscles with *oxygen* and is released into the blood as a result of muscle damage; abbr. Mb

myoglobinuria presence of *myoglobin* in the urine

myolysis destruction of muscle *tissue*

myoma benign tumor of the *myometrium*

myomectomy *surgical* removal of a *myoma*

myometrium wall of the *uterus*, consisting of smooth muscle

myopathy disease of the muscles

myopia (nearsightedness) visual disorder in which distant objects do not focus clearly due a lengthened eyeball, which causes light rays to focus in front of the *retina*; opp. *hyperopia*

myosarcoma malignant *myoma*

myosin endogenous *protein* important for muscle contraction, which combines with *actin* to form *actomyosin*

myositis *autoimmune inflammatory* disease of the skeletal muscles with *facultative* involvement of the skin and internal *organs*

myospasm muscle spasm

myotomy *surgical* division of a muscle

myotonia congenita congenital lack of muscle tone in early childhood

myotonolytic drug used to reduce muscle tension

myring– combining form: eardrum

myringitis inflammation of the eardrum

mys (musculus) *muscle*

myx(o)– combining form: mucus

myxa (mucus, phlegma) *mucus*

myxadenitis *inflammation* of a *mucus* gland

myxedema doughy swelling of the skin due to *hypothyroidism*

N

n symbol: billionth (10^{-9}); prefix: nano-

N. abbr. *nervus* (nerve)

N$_2$O chemical symbol: *nitrous oxide*

Na chemical symbol: *sodium*

NaCl chemical symbol: sodium chloride

Nagel test test of color perception using color cards

nano– combining form: billionth (10^{-9}); symbol: n

narco– combining form: numbing

narcolepsy pathological need to sleep during the day; attacks last longer than 20 minutes

narcotic drug belonging to a group of strong *analgesics* subject to the controlled substance act (Comprehensive Drug Abuse Prevention and Control Act)

nasal pert. to the *nose*

nasal bone small, square, paired plates of bone at the bridge of the nose

nasal cannula system tubing system that hooks over the ears for delivery of oxygen, with two outlets at the nostrils

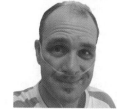

Fig. 315: nasal cannula system

nasal concha turbinate bone; the nasal cavity contains superior, middle and inferior conchae

nasal flaring flaring of the nostrils in synchronization with the breathing; common in dyspnea

nasal speculum *speculum*, e.g. according to Killian, to spread the nostrils for examination and treatment

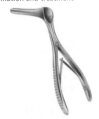

Fig. 316: nasal speculum [A]

nasal tamponade *tamponade* used to arrest bleeding in epistaxis, e.g. *Bellocq tamponade*

nasolabial fold furrow between the corner of the mouth and the edge of the nostril

nasolacrimal duct (ductus nasolacrimalis) connection between the lacrimal sac and the nasal cavity

nasopharyngeal tube *Wendl tube*

nasotracheal through the nose and into the *trachea*; opp. *orotracheal*

nasus *nose*

nat– combining form: birth

nates buttocks

native unaltered; plain

native preparation unstained preparation for *microscopic* examination

nausea queasiness; urge to vomit

navel umbilicus

navicular bone (semilunar bone) one of the *tarsal* bones

navicular fracture *fracture* of the *navicular bone*

NCJ abbr. *needle catheter jejunostomy*

nearsightedness *myopia*

nebulizer inhalation device for nebulizing drugs

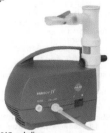

Fig. 317: nebulizer

neck brace padded support collar with a Velcro closure for immobilizing the *cervical spine*, e.g. after a *whiplash injury*

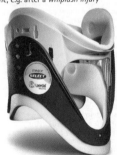

Fig. 318: neck brace [G]

neck dissection *surgical* extirpation of the cervical *lymph nodes* and *tissue* structures in connection with malignant tumors in the neck or head area

necro– combining form: dead
necrophilia sexual attraction to or sexual contact with dead bodies
necropsy *autopsy*
necrosis localized *tissue* death within a living *organism*; one of the *secondary effloresences*
necrotic pert. to *necrosis*
necrotizing causing *necrosis*
necrozoospermia absence of live *sperm* in the *ejaculate*
needle hollow needle for injection, puncture or taking of a blood sample

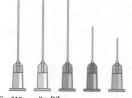

Fig. 319: needles [N]

needle biopsy removal of a small *tissue biopsy* using a needle
needle catheter jejunostomy *intraoperative* insertion of a feeding tube into a segment of the *jejunum* for early postoperative nutrition, usually in connection with prolonged abdominal operations
needle holder *surgical* instrument, e.g. according to Mathieu, used for grasping, holding and guiding a needle for suturing

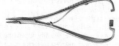

Fig. 320: needle holder [A]

Neer classification classification system for *humeral head fractures*

Neer I *humeral head fracture* with or without minimal *dislocation*
Neer II *humeral head fracture* at the *anatomical neck*
Neer III subcapital *humeral head fracture* that typically occurs in the elderly
Neer IV *avulsion fracture* of the greater tuberosity of the *humerus*
Neer V *avulsion fracture* of the lesser tuberosity of the *humerus*
Neer VI *dislocation fracture* of the humeral head
neglect failure to perceive *visual, tactile* or *acoustic* stimuli on the side opposite to the side damaged by a cerebral *infarction*
Neisseria genus of spherical *gram-negative bacteria*, e.g. *Neisseria gonorrhoeae*, which causes *gonorrhea*
Nelaton catheter *bladder catheter* with a straight tip for *transurethral* placement; see also *Tiemann catheter*

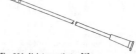

Fig. 321: Nelaton catheter [C]

Nematoda class of roundworms, e.g. pinworms and eelworms; can invade the human body as *parasites*
neo– combining form: new
neologism creation of new words
neonatal pert. to the newborn
neonatological pert. to *neonatology*
neonatologist specialist in *neonatology*
neonatology study of the treatment of diseases affecting newborns
neoplasia new growth; abbr. NPL
neoplastic pert. to *neoplasia*
nephr(o)– combining form: kidney
nephrectomy *surgical* removal of a *kidney*
nephritis acute or chronic inflammation of the *kidney*
nephroblastoma *Wilms' tumor*

nephrogenous pert. to the *kidneys*

nephrohydrosis pathological dilation of the renal tubules

nephrolithiasis presence of stones (usually composed of calcium oxalate or phosphate) in the kidney and urinary tract

nephrological pert. to *nephrology*

nephrologist specialist in *nephrology*

nephrology study of diseases of the kidneys

nephroma *kidney* tumor

nephron smallest functional unit of the kidney; function: production and concentration of urine

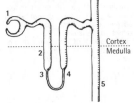

Fig. 322: nephron
1 Bowman's capsule 2 Henle's loop 3 Descending branch (proximal convoluted tubule) 4 Ascending branch (distal convoluted tubule)
5 Collecting tubule

nephropathy disease of the kidneys

nephros *kidney*

nephrosclerosis *arteriosclerosis* of the renal *arteries* and *arterioles*; consequences: renal *hypertension*, renal *failure*

nephrosis (nephropathy) nonspecific collective term for *kidney* disease

nephrostomy surgically created diversion of urine out of the *renal pelvis*

nephrotic syndrome *kidney* disease marked by *proteinuria*, *hypoproteinemia*, *edema* and *hyperlipoproteinemia*

nerve bundle of multiple neurons in parallel alignment within the *nervous system*, which conducts impulses through the system; abbr. N

nervi craniales collective term for the *cranial nerves*

nervi pl. of *nervus*; abbr. *Nn.*

nervous system the system of all the nerves in the body; differentiated into 1) *central nervous system*; 2) *peripheral nervous system*; 3) *autonomic nervous system* and 4) *somatic nervous system*; abbr. NS

nervus gluteus inferior nerve in the buttocks arising from the *sacral plexus*; innervates the *gluteus maximus muscle* et al.

nervus gluteus superior nerve in the buttocks arising from the *sacral plexus*; innervates *gluteus medius* and *gluteus minimus muscles*

nettle rash *urticaria*

neural pert. to the *nerves*

neural therapy treatment using *injections* of *local anesthetics* into the skin to influence the course of a disease

neuralgia pain along the course of a *nerve*

neuralgic pert. to *neuralgia*

neurasthenia "weak nerves"; nervous exhaustion syndrome

neurectomy *surgical* removal of a nerve

neurexeresis *surgical* stripping of a *nerve*

neurilemma (neurolemma, Schwann's sheath) *connective tissue* covering of a *nerve* fiber

neurinoma normally benign tumor originating in the *myelin*-forming *cells* of the *peripheral nerves*

neurite old term for *axon*

neuritis *inflammation* of a *nerve*

neuro- combining form: nerve

neuroblast immature *neuron*

neuroblastoma malignant tumor usually occurring in the abdomen or thorax; usually originates in the *adrenal medulla* or the *sympathetic nerve cells* of the *sympathetic trunk*

neurodermatitis (atopic eczema, atopic dermatitis, endogenous eczema) hereditary *chronic* skin disease, usually appearing in early childhood, marked by itchy, red, scaly, sometimes weeping *eczema*

neuroendocrine system structures involved in the production and secretion of *hormones*

neurofibroma benign tumor originating in the *connective tissue* of the *nerves*

neurofibromatosis (Recklinghausen's disease) genetic disorder marked in particular by the spread of *neurofibromas* over the entire body; abbr. NF

neurogenic originating in the *nerves*

neurohypophysis posterior lobe of the *pituitary gland*; function: storage and release of *hormones* produced by the *hypothalamus*, such as oxytocin or *ADH*

neuroleptic term that refers to the effects of antipsychotic drugs, esp. on cognition and behavior; these drugs lessen confusion and agitation and act as mood stabilizers

neurologic(al) pert. to *neurology*

neurologist specialist in *neurology*

neurology study of diseases of the *nerves*

neuroma benign tumor of a *nerve*

neuromyositis *inflammation* of muscles and nerves

neuron *nerve* cell; consists of a nerve cell body, an *axon* and *dendrites*

neuron–specific enolase important *tumor marker* for small-cell bronchial carcinoma; abbr. NSE

neuropathy noninfectious *nerve* disease

neurosis pathological adaptation disorder based on reactivated subconscious unresolved childhood conflict, or as a self-defense mechanism or an attempt to transform an unresolvable conflict into a more tolerable condition

neurosurgeon specialist in *neurosurgery*

neurosurgery study of the *surgical* treatment of the *nerves*

neurosurgical pert. to *neurosurgery*

neurotherapeutic agent drug used for *neurotherapy*

neurotic pert. to *neurosis*

neurotomy *surgical* division of a *nerve*

neurotoxic pert. to *neurotoxicity*

neurotoxicity poisonous effect on the *nervous system*

neurotransmitter substance that transmits *nerve* impulses among synapses, e.g. *acetylcholine*, *epinephrine*, *norepinephrine*, *serotonin*

neurotropic having an effect on the *nerves*

neurovegetative pert. to the *autonomic nervous system*

neutron neutrally charged subatomic particle

neutropenia decreased *neutrophils* in the blood

neutropenic pert. to *neutropenia*

neutrophilic 1) readily stainable with neutral dyes; 2) consisting of structures or cells endowed with neutrophilic properties

nevus birthmark or mole; skin blemish usually with dark pigmentation

NF abbr. *neurofibromatosis*

NH₃ chemical symbol *ammonia*

niacin (nicotinic acid) water-soluble *vitamin* that the body can manufacture from the *amino acid* tryptophan; niacin deficiency can lead to *pellagra*

nicotinic acid *niacin*

nictitating spasm eyelid spasm causing constant winking

nidation attachment of the *trophoblast* to the *endometrium*, ca. 6 days after *fertilization*

Nissen fundoplication elective surgical procedure to treat gastroesophageal reflux disease (GERD) and hiatal hernia

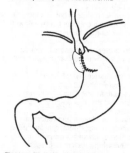

Fig. 323: Nissen fundoplication

nit louse egg

nitrite test test for detecting *bacteria* in the urine; the test is based on the ability of many bacteria to convert *nitrate* taken up with the food into *nitrite*; if the urine is free of bacteria, no nitrite will be formed

nitrous oxide (laughing gas) colorless gas used for *general anesthesia and dentistry*; chemical abbr. N_2O

NMR abbr. nuclear magnetic resonance; see *magnetic resonance imaging*

Nn. abbr. *nervi*

Nocardia genus of rod-shaped *gram-positive bacteria* that cause *nocardiosis*

nocardiosis *infectious disease* caused by *Nocardia* that can lead to *pneumonia* and *abscesses*

noci- combining form: pain

nociceptor receptor for painful stimuli

noctis nights, of the night

nocturia frequent urination during the night

nocturnal emission involuntary ejaculation during sleep

nocturnal at night

nod- combining form: node

nodding spasm nodding motion of the head in adults or upper body in infants, caused by muscle spasms

node (nodule) rounded knot or knob; skin change rising more than 0.5 cm above the epidermis, one of the *primary efflorescences*; see also *papule*

nodular goiter *goiter* marked by nodular *hyperplasias* with normal *thyroid* function

nodule *node*

nodus lymphaticus *lymph node*

non- combining form: not

non-compliant unwilling to cooperate in medical treatment of an illness; opp. *compliant*

non-Hodgkin's lymphoma cancer of *lymphatic tissue*; cytomorphology differs from that of *Hodgkin's lymphoma*

non-rebreathing system (semiopen anesthesia) combination of *anesthetic* gas reservoir and non-rebreathing circuit, such that inspiration is only from the reservoir and expiration is into the atmosphere; opp. *rebreathing system*

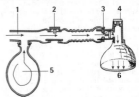

Fig. 324: non-rebreathing system
1 Fresh gas 2 Pressure relief valve 3 Inspiratory valve 4 Expiratory valve 5 Reservoir bag 6 Patient

noni-, nono- combining form: nine

nonproprietary name *generic name*

nonverbal not using speech; opp. *verbal*

noradrenaline *norepinephrine*

norepinephrine circulatory acting *hormone* of the *catecholamine* group produced primarily by the *adrenal medulla*; important *neurotransmitter* in the *autonomic nervous system*

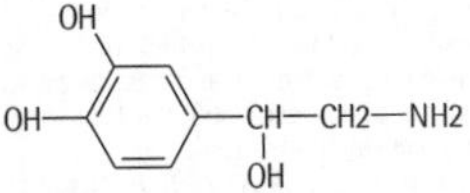

Fig. 325: norepinephrine

norm- combining form: normal

normal bite *eugnathia*

normal weight see *Broca index*

normoblast immature *erythrocyte* in the *bone marrow*

normochromic having a normal color normal stainability or normal *hemoglobin* content

nose organ that perceives smells, also an important part of the upper respiratory tract, which mainly warms, filters and moistens inhaled air

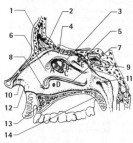

Fig. 326: anatomy of the nose
1 Superior meatus 2 Frontal sinus 3 Middle concha
4 Olfactory epithelium 5 Superior concha
6 Middle meatus 7 Inferior concha 8 Inferior
meatus 9 Sphenoid sinus 10 Limen nasi
11 Pharyngeal ostium of auditory tube 12 Vestibule
13 Hard palate 14 Soft palate

nosebleed epistaxis
noso- combining form: disease
nosocomial infection *infection* acquired
  during a hospital stay, e.g. due to resistant
  germs or inadequate *hygiene*
nosos (morbus, pathos) disease, illness
nov- combining form: new
noxa harmful substance; pl. noxae
NPL abbr. *neoplasm*
NPO nothing per os (by mouth)
NPPL abbr. *nucleus pulposus prolapse*
NPUAP abbr. National Pressure Ulcer
  Advisory Panel; see *decubitus*
NS abbr. *nervous system*
nucha nape of the neck
nuchal pert. to the *nucha*
nuclear medicine use of radioactive
  substances for diagnosis and treatment of
  disease
nucleic acid component of the *cell nucleus*,
  important substance in *protein* synthesis in
  the cell; see also *ribonucleic acid* and
  deoxyribonucleic acid

nucleotide breakdown product of *protein*
  metabolism in the cell *nucleus*
nucleus center; central body of the *cell*
nucleus pulposus gelatinous center of an
  intervertebral disk
nucleus pulposus prolapse *disk prolapse*
nullipara woman who has not yet given
  birth
nutri- combining form: nourishment
nutrition consumption of food and
  utilization of its nutrients by the body
nutritive pert. to *nutrition*
nyct- combining form: night
nyctalgia pain at night
nyctalopia (night blindness) inability of the
  eye to adjust to dim light, e.g. due to
  vitamin A deficiency
nycturia nocturia
NYHA abbr. New York Heart Association
NYHA Classification system for rating the
  degree of severity of *heart failure*
nymphae *labia minora*
nymphomania increased sex drive in a
  female
nystagmus involuntary jerking or pendular
  movements of the eyes, e.g. due to
  neurological disorders

O

O_2 chemical symbol: *oxygen*
O_3 chemical symbol: *ozone*
OAT syndrome combination of
  oligozoospermia, asthenozoospermia, and
  teratozoospermia
ob- combining form: toward, facing
Oberst's method *nerve block anesthesia* by
  injection of a *local anesthetic* into the base
  of a finger or toe, e.g. for *onychectomy*
obesity excessive body weight with a *body
  mass index* between 30 and 40; see also
  overweight; opp. *cachexia*
obesity, morbid (pickwickian syndrome)
  excessive body weight with a *body mass
  index* > 40

objective 1) factual, unemotional; 2)) lower lens of a microscope

objectivity statistical term for the independence of results from the observer

obligate necessary, indispensable; opp. *facultative*

obligatory required, necessary

obliterate to occlude or sclerose

obliteration occlusion or sclerosis of a hollow *organ* or vessel, usually associated with vascular sclerosis, e.g. in *varicosis*

OBS abbr. *organic brain syndrome*

obsessive–compulsive disorder diagnosis for a person who tends to exhibit recurrent, persistent thoughts or actions that intefere with his or her social, occupational or interpersonal functioning, abbr. OCD

obsolete outmoded, outdated

obstetrical forceps type of forceps used for delivery of an infant; see *forceps delivery*

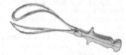

Fig. 327: obstetrical forceps [A]

obstructed blocked

obstruction blockage of a hollow *organ*

obstructive causing blockage

obstructive icterus *jaundice* caused by obstruction of the *bile ducts*

obstructive jaundice (obstructive icterus) *jaundice* caused by disruption of the flow of *bile* in the bile ducts, e.g. due to *cholelithiasis*

obstructive ventilation disorder *ventilation disorder* due to an obstruction in the *lung*

obturation closure or blockage of a hollow organ

obturator nerve *nerve* arising from the *lumbar plexus* that innervates the *short adductor, long adductor* and *gracilis* muscles

occipital bone (occiput) bone at the back of the skull

occipital pert. to the occipital bone

occipital squama (squama occipitalis) bone plate at the back of the head

occiput back of the head; *occipital bone*

occlusion blockage

occlusive arterial disease circulatory disorder of *tissues* that depend on *arteries* affected by *stenosis* or *occlusion*; usually caused by *arteriosclerosis*; see also *peripheral occlusive arterial disease*; abbr. OAD

occlusive dressing dressing that provides a complete seal, e.g. Tegaderm®, Opsite®

occult hidden

oct combining form: eight

ocular bulb eyeball

ocular muscles muscles that move the eye in its socket

ocular tremor *nystagmus*

oculo– combining form: eye

oculocephalic reflex *pathological* polysynaptic *reflex* in which the eyes turn to the opposite side on passive turning of the head (*doll's eyes*); usually due to diffuse brain damage

oculomotor nerve 3rd *cranial nerve*; contains motor and parasympathetic fibers; controls eye movement together with the *trochlear* and *abducens* nerves, with the oculomotor nerve controlling all the eye muscles apart from the *superior oblique muscle* (trochlear) and *lateral rectus muscle* (abducens)

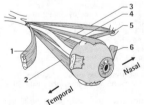

Fig. 328: ocular muscles
1 Lateral rectus 2 Inferior rectus 3 Medial rectus
4 Superior rectus 5 Superior oblique
6 Inferior oblique

oculus eye; pl. oculi
odons tooth
odont– combining form: tooth
odontalgia tooth pain
odontoblast cell that forms *dentin*
odontogenic originating in the *teeth*
odontogenic cyst cyst originating in the *epithelium* of the dental lamina, which is surrounded by *granulation tissue* and has a tendency to grow

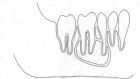

Fig. 329: odontogenic cyst

odontologist *dentist*
odontoma tumor consisting of dental *tissue* with *epithelial* and *mesenchymal* components
odontopathy nonspecific collective term for diseases of the *teeth*
odontorrhagia bleeding after a *tooth extraction*
odontos *teeth*
ohm unit of electrical resistance
-oid combining form: resembling
olecranon large process of the *ulna* at the back of the elbow
olecranon fracture *fracture* of the *olecranon* with dislocation of the *fragment* due to upward traction from the *triceps* muscle
olfact– combining form: smell
olfactory nerve 1st *cranial nerve*; contains exclusively sensory fibers from the periphery to the brain; mainly controls the sense of smell
oligo– combining form: few, small
oligoasthenoteratozoospermia *OAT syndrome*

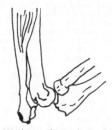

Fig. 330: olecranon fracture

oligodendrocytes *myelin*-forming *cells* of the *central nervous system*
oligodendroglioma *brain* tumor originating in the *oligodendrocytes*
oligohydramnion reduced amount of amniotic fluid in the amnion; opp. *hydramnion*
oligomenorrhea overly infrequent *menstruation*, with an interval of more than 35 days between periods; causes are *endocrine* or *organic*; opp. *polymenorrhea*
oligozoospermia fewer than 20 million sperm per ml of *ejaculate*; opp. *polyzoospermia*
oliguria urinary output of < 400cc per day
oma– combining form: shoulder
-oma combining form: tumor, growth
omalgia shoulder pain
omphal(o)– combining form: navel
omphalitis *inflammation* of the *navel* usually occurring in newborns
omphalocele *umbilical hernia*
omphalolith hard, dark node that develops from the skin around the *navel*
omphalos *navel*
omphalotomy severing and tying off the *umbilical cord* of a newborn
Omsk fever see *viral hemorrhagic fever*
onanism masturbation
onco– combining form: tumor

oncogenic causing tumors
oncologic(al) pert. to *oncology*
oncologist specialist in *oncology*
oncology study of neoplastic diseases
oncotic pressure (colloid osmotic pressure) osmotic pressure of a colloidal solution
onychectomy *surgical* removal of a finger- or toenail
onychia (onychitis) *inflammation* of the nail bed
onychitis onychia
onychophagia nail-biting
onyx finger- or toenail
oocytes egg *cells*
oogenesis ripening of ova in the *ovary*
oon egg cell; see also *ovulation*
oophor- combining form: ovary
oophorectomy *surgical* removal of the *ovaries*
oophoritis *inflammation* of the *ovary*
oophoron *ovary*
oophorosalpingectomy adnexectomy
OP abbr. *operation*
open book (pelvic) injury (symphyseal rupture) separation of the pubic *symphysis*, usually in combination with a posterior *pelvic ring fracture*

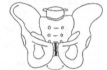

Fig. 331: open book injury

operable able to be treated with an operation; opp. *inoperable*
operate to perform *surgery*
operation *surgical* procedure for medical purposes; abbr. OP
ophthalmia nonspecific collective term for diseases of the *eye*
ophthalmic agent drug for treatment of eye disease

ophthalmica, A. *ophthalmic* artery
ophthalmica, V. *ophthalmic* Vein
ophthalmo- combining form: eye
ophthalmological pert. to eye
ophthalmologist physician who specializes in *diseases of the eye*
ophthalmology study of eye diseases
ophthalmoplegia paralysis of the *ocular* and eyelid muscles
ophthalmos eye
ophthalmoscope instrument for examination of the *ocular fundus* using high illumination and an optical system that largely prevents interfering corneal light reflexes

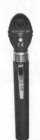

Fig. 332: ophthalmoscope [H]

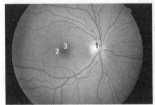

Fig. 333: ocular fundus
1 Papilla 2 Macula 3 Fovea centralis

ophthalmoscopy examination of the *ocular fundus* with an *ophthalmoscope*

-opia combining form: viewing; seeing

opiate narcotic related to *opium*

opistho- combining form: back(wards)

opisthotonos persistent spasm of the back muscles with arching backward extension of the trunk, e.g. due to *tetanus*

opium dried juice of the opium poppy

opportunistic pathogen pathogen that is already present in the body but causes disease only when the immune system is weakened

opposing muscle of the thumb muscle that pulls the thumb into grasping position; innervation: *median nerve*

opposition positioning of the thumb opposite to the other fingers

optic pert. to vision

optic (nerve) atrophy loss of *axons* and *myelin* sheath from the *optic nerve*

optic agnosia form of *agnosia* in which visual impressions cannot be recognized or interpreted despite intact visual field and optic tract

optic chiasm point where the optic nerve fibers cross

optic nerve 2nd *cranial nerve* contains exclusively sensory fibers; mainly controls visual perception

optic papilla (blind spot) point where the optic nerve enters the eye

optimum dose dose of a drug that brings about its full effect

opto- combining form: sight, vision

or- combining form: mouth

ora serrata retinae border between the *retina* and the *ciliary body*

oral pert. to the *mouth*; by mouth

oral contraceptive birth control drug that prevents ovulation; abbr. OC

oral flora normal *bacterial* population of the oral cavity

orbicular muscle of the eye (musculus orbicularis oculi) ring muscle of the eye that closes the eyelid; innervation: *facial nerve*

orbicular muscle of the mouth (musculus orbicularis oris) ring muscle of the mouth that closes the mouth and purses the lips; innervation: *facial nerve*

orbicular oculi reflex (glabella reflex) *pathological polysynaptic reflex* where tapping on the *glabella* leads to *contraction* of the *musculus orbicularis oculi*

orbit bony eye socket in the skull

orchi(o)- combining form: testicles

orchiectomy (castration) *surgical* removal of the *testicles*

orchis *testical*

orchitis (epididymitis) *inflammation* of the *testis*

-orexia combining form: appetite

organ body part; nonspecific term for a functional unit of the *organism*, usually composed of various types of *cells* and *tissues*

organ system functionally related *organs*

organic living; pert. to an *organ* or an entire *organism*; opp. *inorganic*

organic brain syndrome *psychic* disorder caused by brain damage

organism the totality of all *organ systems* in the living body

orgasm sexual climax, e.g. during intercourse

orifice natural opening in the body or an organ

Ormond's disease *retroperitoneal fibrosis*

ornithosis (parrot fever) febrile *flu*-like *infectious disease* caused by *Chlamydia psittaci*; leads to *pneumonia* in severe cases; transmitted to humans mainly by birds (parrots, parakeets, ducks, pigeons) via contaminated dust or droppings

oropharyngeal tube *Guedel tube*

oropharynx mouth and throat area

orotracheal through the mouth and into the *trachea*; opp. *nasotracheal*

orth(o)- combining form: straight, correct

orthodontia area of dentistry concerning alignment of the teeth

orthopedic pert. to *orthopedics*

orthopedics study of diseases of the musculoskeletal system

orthopedist specialist in *orthopedics*

orthopnea labored breathing while lying flat, e.g. in *pulmonary edema*

orthopneic pert. to *orthopnea*

orthostasis upright posture

orthostatic pert. to *orthostasis*

orthostatic hypotension (postural hypotension) circulatory collapse when standing up; determined by taking the patient's BP in a recumbent position, and again after 2 minutes in a standing position; a drop in systolic reading > 20 mmHg is abnormal

orthostatic syndrome *orthostatic hypotension*

orthotopic located or developing in the normal location; opp. *heterotopic*

orthotopic bladder replacement formation of a new *urinary bladder* from the *ileum* with a connection to the *urethra*

orthotopic graft *graft* in which material is taken from and implanted in the same location; see also *isotopic graft, heterotopic graft*

os 1) (stoma) mouth; pl. ora; 2) bone; pl. ossa

oscillating swinging back and forth

oscillation swing, fluctuation

Osgood-Schlatter disease *aseptic osteonecrosis* of the *tibial apophysis*

OSHA abbr. Occupational Safety and Health Administration (federal regulatory agency that monitors worker safety)

-osis combining form: condition

osmolality total number of solute particles dissolved in one kilogram of water; unit: Osm/kg H_2O

osmolarity total number of solute particles dissolved in one liter of water; unit: Osm/L

osmosis equalization of concentrations between two solutions at different concentrations via a semipermeable membrane through which the solvent can pass

osmotic pert. to *osmosis*

osphresi- combining form: smelling

ossa carpi collective term for the eight bones of the wrist, which form two rows of four, *proximal* row: *scaphoid, lunate, triquetral* and *pisiform bones*; *distal* row: *trapezium, trapezoid, capitate* and *hamate bones*

ossa cranii collective term for the bones of the skull

ossa cruris collective term for the bones of the lower leg (*tibia* and *fibula*)

ossa digitorum manus collective term for the finger bones

ossa digitorum pedis collective term for the toe bones

ossa metacarpalia hand bones

ossa metatarsalia midfoot bones

ossa tarsi collective term for the seven ankle bones, which are larger than the *carpal bones* but less neatly arranged: *talus, calcaneus, navicular, cuneiform* (three of these) and *cuboid bones*

osseous pert. to the bones

ossification formation of bone; transformation into bone

ostase bone-specific *alkaline phosphatase*

osteitis deformans *Paget's disease*

osteo- combining form: bone

osteoblast bone-forming *cell*; opp. *osteoclast*

osteocalcin bone protein; made by the *osteoblasts*

osteocarcinoma carcinoma in a bone, or a carcinoma that contains foci of osseous tissue

osteochondromatosis formation of *hyaline* cartilage in the *synovium* with development of free bodies

osteoclast cell that breaks down bone; opp. *osteoblast*

osteocyte bone-forming *cell*

osteodensitometry *radiological* procedure to measure bone density

osteofibroma tumor consisting of bone and fibrous *tissue*

osteogenesis bone formation

osteolysis destruction of bone *tissue*

osteolytic pert. to *osteolysis*
osteoma benign bone tumor
osteomalacia generalized softening of bone due to reduced amounts of minerals in the bone
osteomyelitis *acute* or *chronic inflammation* of the *bone marrow*
osteonecrosis *necrosis* of bone tissue
osteoporosis bone loss due to decreased bone density
osteoporotic pert. to *osteoporosis*
osteoradionecrosis osteo*necrosis* following excessively high dose in *radiation therapy*
osteosarcoma malignant bone tumor

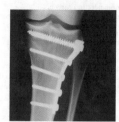

Fig. 335: plate osteosynthesis, left tibia

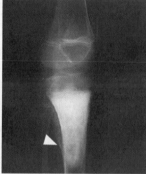

Fig. 334: osteosarcoma of the knee

osteosynthesis *surgical* joining and fixation of the *repositioned* bone fragments, e.g. after a *fracture*
osteotomy incision into a bone
ostitis *acute* or *chronic inflammation* of bone tissue, clinically indistinguishable from *osteomyelitis*
ostium entrance; opening
ostium uteri external *cervical os*
otalgia (otodynia) *ear pain*

otitis externa *inflammation* of the external ear
otitis media *inflammation* of the middle ear, e.g. due to *measles*
oto– combining form: ear
otologic 1) drug used to treat disease of the ear; 2) pert. to diseases of the ear
otologist specialist in diseases of the ear
otopharyngeal tube *eustachian tube*
otorrhea discharge from the ear
otosclerosis hearing impairment due to bony growth in the middle ear, causing damage to the acoustic nerve
otoscope (ear speculum) instrument for examination of the external auditory canal and eardrum, equipped with a light source, cone-shaped speculum and integrated magnifying lens

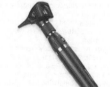

Fig. 336: otoscope

O

otoscopic pert. to *otoscopy*

otoscopy examination of the external ear and eardrum with an *otoscope*

ototoxic damaging to the ear

outpatient treated without admission to a hospital unit; opp. *inpatient*

output substance excreted or expelled

ovarian pert. to the *ovary*

ovarian carcinoma malignant tumor in the *ovary*

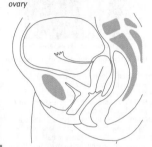

Fig. 337: ovarian carcinoma

ovarian cystadenoma benign tumor of the *ovary* originating in the glandular tissue

ovarica, A. *ovarian artery*

ovariectomy (oophorectomy) *surgical* removal of one or both ovaries

overbite maxillary *prognathism*

overflow incontinence emptying disorder of the *bladder* with involuntary loss of urine; usually caused by disorder of the bladder musculature with *passive* overextension

overweight increase in body weight to a *body mass index* between 24 and 30 for females, or between 25 and 30 for males; see also *obesity*; opp. *underweight*

ovotestis gonad comprising both *testis* and *ovary* tissue, occurring in hermaphrodites

ovulation release of a mature egg cell from the *ovary* following the rupture of a *follicle*

ovum egg; see also *ovulation*

ox- combining form: oxygen

Oxford tube right-angled *endotracheal tube* for *oral intubation*

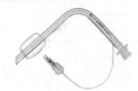

Fig. 338: Oxford tube [K]

-oxia combining form; oxygen

oxidation chemical reaction with *oxygen*

oxidize to react with *oxygen*

oximeter device for measuring *oxygen saturation*, e.g. *pulse oximeter*

oximetric pert. to *oximetry*

oxy- combining form: sharp, acute, acid

oxygen element that is vitally important for most of the body's metabolic processes; enters into the blood via the *lungs* through breathing; chemical symbol for the molecule: O_2

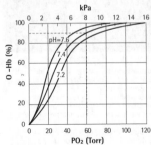

Fig. 339: oxygen binding curve

oxygen binding curve (oxygen dissociation curve) relationship of *oxyhemoglobin* to total *hemoglobin* and *partial pressure of oxygen*; curve moves left with *alkalosis* and lowered body temperature, or right with *acidosis* and elevated body temperature

oxygen concentrator device for concentrating *oxygen* out of room air

oxygen dissociation curve *oxygen binding curve*

oxygen mask face mask for delivery of *oxygen*; used for patients for whom delivery via *oxygen tube* or *nasal cannula* is not sufficient, or who breathe through the mouth

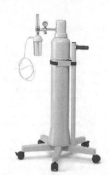

Fig. 341: oxygen tank [H]

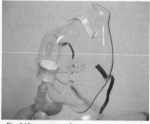

Fig. 340: oxygen mask

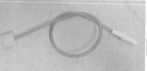

Fig. 342: oxygen tube

oxygen saturation *abbr.* sO_2

oxygen tank portable tank holding oxygen, equipped with a *regulator* and *flowmeter* for oxygen delivery

oxygen tube tube with foam rubber padding that is inserted into the nose for delivery of *oxygen*

oxyHb *abbr. oxyhemoglobin*

oxyhemoglobin *hemoglobin* saturated with *oxygen*; abbr. oxyHb

oxitocin hormone formed by the hypothalamus; function: stimulates uterine contractions in labor and milk secretion

Oxyuroidea family of nematodes that includes the pinworms

ozena abnormally broad nose due to atrophy of the mucosa and bones, with deterioration of the mucus glands

ozone form of oxygen present in the stratosphere, comprising 3 oxygen atoms; chemical symbol O_3; when ozon is depleted, there is increased exposure to ultraviolet light, which favors the development of skin cancers

P

P 1) *pulse*; 2) symbol: quadrillion (10^{15}); prefix: peta-

p symbol: trillionth (10^{-12}); prefix: pico-

P wave atrial excitation wave as seen in the *ECG*; duration 0.05 to 0.10 seconds

p.o. abbr. *per os*

PA catheter (pulmonary artery catheter) used for monitoring right and left intracardiac pressures, cardiac output and venous oxygen saturation, as well as to measure pulmonary capillary wedge pressure (PCWP); certification needed to insert and read

PAC abbr. *pulmonary artery catheter*

pacemaker artificial device or specialized cells that trigger heart contractions with electrical impulses

pacer *pacemaker*

pachy- combining form: thick, solid

pachyderma congenital thickening of the skin

pad *compress*

Paget's disease (osteitis deformans) bone disease, usually occurring in older males, with uncontrolled bone destruction followed by excessive bone growth, resulting in thickened, unstable bones; mostly affects the pelvis, *femur*, *tibia*, skull and *lumbar spine*

palatine bone bone forming the roof of the mouth

palatine tonsils lymphoid tissue masses located on either side of the oral pharynx

palatinum, os (os palatinum) *palatine bone*

palatoschisis *cleft palate*

palatum palate, arched roof of the mouth

paleo- combining form: old

palin- combining form: repetition

pallanesthesia impaired ability to sense *vibration*

pallesthesia (vibratory sense) perception of *vibration*

palliative giving relief; opp. *curative*

pallium *cerebral cortex* and its white matter

palma palm of the hand

palmar pert. to the palm of the hand

palmar erythema rash on the palm of the hand, e.g. due to *cirrhosis*

palmomental reflex *pathological* polysynaptic *reflex* in which stimulation of the palm of the hand leads to contraction of the chin muscles on the same side, usually occurring with diffuse brain damage

palmuria strong bifurcated urine stream, e.g. due to *stricture* of the *urethra*

palpatio cordis palpitations

palpation examination of the body by feeling

palpebra (blepharon) eyelid

palpebra- combining form: eyelid

palpebral glands *tarsal glands*

pan- combining form: total, everything

panaris (paronychia) purulent *infection* of the fingers or toes, usually caused by *streptococci* or *staphylococci*

panarthritis *inflammation* of all joints

pancarditis *inflammation* of the entire heart (all layers of the cardiac wall and all valves)

Pancoast's tumor special form of *peripheral bronchial carcinoma* near the apex of the lung

pancrea- combining form: pancreas

pancreas organ in the left upper abdomen whose functions include production of digestive *enzymes*, *insulin* and *glucagon*

pancreatectomy *surgical* removal of the *pancreas*

pancreatic carcinoma malignant tumor of the *pancreas*

pancreatic pert. to the *pancreas*

pancreatic duct *ductus pancreaticus*; duct leading out of the *pancreas*

pancreatitis *acute* or *chronic inflammation* of the *pancreas*

pancreozymin *enzyme* produced in the small intestine that promotes *pancreatic* function

pancytopenia decrease in *erythrocytes*, *granulocytes* and *thrombocytes* in blood, e.g. in *aplastic anemia*

pandemic *epidemic* encompassing nations and continents

Pándy's test test for the presence of *protein* in the *cerebrospinal fluid*

panniculitis *inflammation* of the subcutaneous fatty tissue of the abdomen

panplegia complete paralysis of the entire body

pansinusitis *inflammation* of all the *paranasal sinuses*

pantothenic acid water-soluble *vitamin*; component of *coenzyme A* with an important role in general metabolism

PAOD abbr. *peripheral arterial occlusive disease*

PAP abbr. *pulmonary artery pressure*; *prostatic acid phosphatase*

Pap test (Pap smear, Papanicolaou's smear) smear taken from the *vaginal* and *cervical* mucosa for the purpose of *microscopic* examination for malignant *cells*

papilla of Vater (duodenal papilla, papilla vateri) opening of the *bile* ducts into the *duodenum*

papillary muscles muscles whose tendons connect the *endocardium* with the *heart valves*

papilledema (choked disk) inflammation of the *optic nerve* where it enters the *retina*, creating a visible swelling at the *papilla*

papillitis *papilledema*

papilloma *epithelial* tumor of the skin or mucosa

papillomavirus *virus* that causes *condyloma acuminatum*

papillotomy incision of the *bile* duct opening into the *duodenum*, usually in connection with an *endoscopy*, e.g. for stones in the bile ducts

papule bump or pimple; skin eruption rising less than 0.5 cm above the epidermis; one of the *primary effloresences*; see also *nodule*

par(a)– combining form: near, deviating from the norm

paracentesis *surgical* incision of a body cavity to remove fluid; usually performed on the abdomen

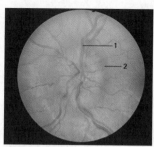

Fig. 343: papilledema
1 Dilated veins 2 Mushroom-shaped papillary prominence

paracolpium *connective tissue* surrounding the *vagina*

paradoxic(al) seemingly illogical, unexpected

paradoxical breathing condition caused by multiple rib *fracture* in which the fractured rib area is retracted during *inspiration* and pushed outward during *expiration*

paragrammatism inability to produce grammatically correct sentences

paralysis complete loss of movement

paralytic ileus absence or decrease of intestestinal peristalsis (bowel sounds); usually occurs after abdominal surgery and can have serious consequences

parameter measured quantity

parametrium *connective tissue* around the *uterus*

paramnesia deceptive memory in which the patient remembers events that never happened in reality, e.g. in *psychosis*

paramyxovirus group of *RNA viruses* that cause various *infectious diseases*, incl. *measles* and *mumps*

paranasal sinuses collective term for the *frontal* and *maxillary sinuses*; air-filled mucosa-lined cavities of the *viscerocranium*

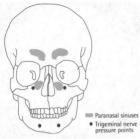

Paranasal sinuses
Trigeminal nerve pressure points

Fig. 344: paranasal sinuses

paranasal sinusitis see *(pan-)sinusitis*

paraneoplastic syndrome signs associated with a neoplastic disease that are triggered by *metastases* rather than the original tumor

paranoia personality disorder marked by mistrust, dogmatism and vengefulness; the patient believes himself misunderstood and persecuted by others and shows increased egotism

paraphimosis (Spanish collar) strangulation of the *glans penis* caused by a narrow foreskin

paraphrasia pathological jumbling and invention of words due to mental illness

paraplegia complete paralysis below an injury or lesion of the spinal cord; affects both legs (low injury) or both arms and legs (higher injury); also called *quadriplegia, tetraplegia*

paraprotein abnormal *protein* body

parasit- combining form: parasite

parasite organism that lives off a host

parasitology study of *parasites*

parasternal beside the *sternum*

parasternal line imaginary line used as a thoracic surface landmark; passes along the lateral border of the *sternum*; abbr. *PSL*; see also *midsternal line*

parasympathetic nervous system part of the *autonomic nervous system* that controls eating, digestion, excretion, relaxation; antagonist: *sympathetic nervous system*

parasympatholytic (cholinolytic) drug used to inhibit the *parasympathetic nervous system*; opp. *parasympathomimetic*

parasympathomimetic (cholinergic) drug used to activate the *parasympathetic nervous system*; opp. *parasympatholytic*

parasystole *cardiac dysrhythmia* caused by impulses from two different excitation centers

paratenon *tissue* surrounding the tendons

paratenonitis *inflammation* of the *paratenon*

parathymia expression of inappropriate emotions, e.g. laughing at a funeral due to *schizophrenia* et al.

parathyroid- combining form: parathyroid gland

parathyroid hormone *hormone* produced by the *parathyroid gland* that raises *calcium* levels and reduces *phosphate* levels in the blood and breaks down mineral substances from the bones; abbr. PTH; antagonist: *calcitonin*

parathyroidectomy *surgical* removal of the *parathyroid*

paratyphoid fever febrile *infectious disease* caused by *Salmonella paratyphi* that leads to *diarrhea*, among other things; the clinical picture is similar to that of *typhoid fever* but is less severe; transmitted mainly via contaminated food and water, as well as by *smear infection*

paravascular near a blood vessel

paravenous near a *vein*

paravertebral line imaginary line used as a body surface landmark; passes along the back parallel to the spinous processes of the *vertebrae* abbr. *PVL*

pareidolia sensory deceptions combined with real perceptions, e.g. due to fatigue

parenchyma essential *cells* and *tissues* of an *organ*

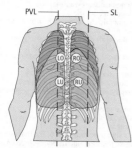

Fig. 345: paravertebral line
PVL Paravertebral line **SL** Scapular line
UL Upper left **UR** Upper right **LL** Lower left
LR Lower right

parenteral circumventing the *gastrointestinal tract*
-paresis combining form: weakness, partial paralysis
paresthesia abnormal sensation not caused by touch, e.g. tingling or burning
paresthetic nocturnal brachialgia *Wartenberg's disease*
parietal pert. to a wall
parietal bone one of the cranial bones
parietal pleura *pleura* that lines the chest wall; see *pleura*
Parkinson's disease (parkinsonism; paralysis agitans) common neurological disease in elderly persons due to the *degeneration of dopaminergic neurons*, marked by movement disorders, resting tremor and *rigidity*
parotid gland salivary gland
parotitis *inflammation* of the salivary glands
parotitis epidemica *mumps*
-parous combining form: having children
paroxysmal sudden, in the form of an attack
paroxysmal supraventricular tachycardia sporadically occurring *tachycardia* visible in an ECG, with a *frequency* of 130–250 per

minute; caused by *ectopic* impulse generation in the atrial area or *atrioventricular node*, or by *reentry*; abbr. PSVT

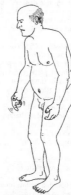

Fig. 346: Parkinson's disease (typical posture)

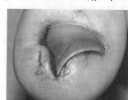

Fig. 347: paronychia due to ingrown toenail

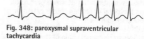

Fig. 348: paroxysmal supraventricular tachycardia

parrot fever *ornithosis*

partial crown tooth-preserving variant of a *crown*, covering only the mastication surface of the *tooth*

partial denture removable denture that is attached to remaining natural *teeth* by means of *crowns* or clamps

partial pressure of carbon dioxide abbr. pCO_2

partial pressure pressure exerted by a given component in a gas mixture

partial pressure of oxygen abbr.is pO_2

partial remission incomplete remission

partial thromboplastin time group test of blood coagulation that encompasses *Factors I, II, V, VIII, IX* and *XI*; important as a screening test in patients with tendency to bleed, during *surgery*, and in therapy with anticoagulants (e.g. heparin) or *thrombolytics*; abbr. PTT, aPTT

-partum combining form: birth

partus birth

partus immaturus *abortion*

partus prematurus *premature birth*

parvus small

passage transit through a hollow organ

passive without active participation; opp. *active*

passive immunization administration of *antibodies* for *immunization*

Pasteurella collective term for a group of rod-shaped *bacteria*

patch 1) area of skin differing from the rest of the surface; 2) flat, adhesive piece of material used to deliver a drug through the skin

patell- combining form: kneecap

patella kneecap

patellar pert. to the *patella*

patellar dislocation *dislocation* of the kneecap from its natural position

patellar reflex (kneejerk reflex) monosynaptic *reflex* in which percussion on the *patellar* tendon causes extension of the knee joint

path(o)- combining form: disease, pain

pathogenesis causal chain of the course of a disease

pathogenic disease-causing; opp. *apathogenic*

pathognomic characteristic of a particular disease

pathologic(al) diseased, disease-related; opp. *physiological*

pathological fracture spontaneous fracture

pathology study of disease

pathophysiological pert. to *pathophysiology*; opp. *physiological*

pathophysiology study of *pathological* body functions; opp. *physiology*

pathos disease, illness

-pathy combining form: disease, pain

pavor fear

Payr's sign pain in the sole of the foot under passive pressure; sign of *phlebothrombosis*

pCO_2 partial pressure of *carbon dioxide* in the blood; measured as part of *blood gas analysis*; normal values for arterial blood: 35 mmHg

PCP abbr. *Pneumocystis carinii pneumonia*; *primary care provider*

PCR abbr. *polymerase chain reaction*

PCWP abbr. pulmonary capillary *wedge pressure*

peak and trough terms used to specify when to collect blood samples for determination of blood level of a drug; **peak draw** should be done 30 minutes after drug is given; **trough level** should be taken 30 minutes prior to the next dose of medicine; drug and route of administration may alter the timing for peak level and trough level

Péan forceps *hemostat* according to Péan

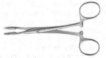

Fig. 349: Péan forceps [A]

pector- combining form: chest

pectoral pert. to the chest

pectus chest; breast

pectus carinatum (pigeon breast) thoracic deformity due to a keel-like protrusion of the sternum, usually as a consequence of *rickets*

pectus excavatum (funnel breast, pectus recurvatum) congenitally concave chest due to depressed *sternum*

ped– combining form: foot

pedal spasm foot cramp

pederasty form of *pedophilia* characterized by a sexual relationship between an adult male and an underage boy

pedia– combining form: child

pediatric pert. to *pediatrics*

pediatrician specialist in *pediatrics*

pediatrics study of children's diseases

pedicul– combining form: lice

pediculosis itchy skin disease due to infestation with lice

pediculus louse

pediculus humanis capitis head louse

pedis feet

pedophilia sexual attraction to children

PE abbr. *pulmonary embolism*

peeling removal of the uppermost layer of the skin, e.g. to treat skin disease

PERRLA abbr. pupils equal, round, reactive to light and accommodation

PEG abbr. *percutaneous endoscopic gastrotomy*

pella skin

pellagra disease caused by *vitamin B₂* deficiency, characterized by diarrhea, *dementia* and *dermatitis*

peloid mudlike substance for external application

pelvi– combining form :pelvis

pelvic diaphragm muscular pelvic floor

pelvic presentation *breech presentation*

pelvic ring bone ring formed by the pelvic bones and *sacrum*

pelvic ring fracture *fracture* of the *pelvic ring* due to significant force, e.g. in connection with *polytrauma*

pelvis lower portion of the trunk of the body, see Fig. 352

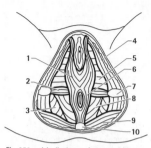

Fig. 350: pelvic diaphragm (pelvic floor)
1 Bulbospongiosus m. 2 Superficial transverse perineal m. 3 Internal obturator m.
4 Ischiocavernous m. 5 Deep transverse perineal m. 6 External sphincter m. of anus 7 Ischial tuberosity
8 Levator ani m. 9 Gluteus maximus m. 10 Coccyx

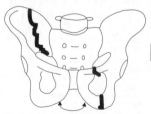

Fig. 351: pelvic ring fracture

pen pen-like reusable *syringe* with integrated drug *reservoir*, e.g. for self-*injection* of *insulin* by diabetic patients

penetrate to pierce or enter

penetration piercing; entering into

–penia combining form: lack, deficiency

penicillin *antibiotic* for treatment of *infections* caused by *bacteria*

penicillinase *enzyme* produced by *bacteria* that renders *penicillin* ineffective

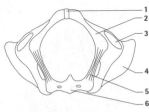

Fig. 352: pelvis
1 Symphysis pubis 2 Ischial tuberosity
3 Acetabulum 4 Ilium 5 Sacrotuberal ligament
6 Sacrum

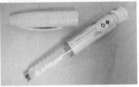

Fig. 353: pen

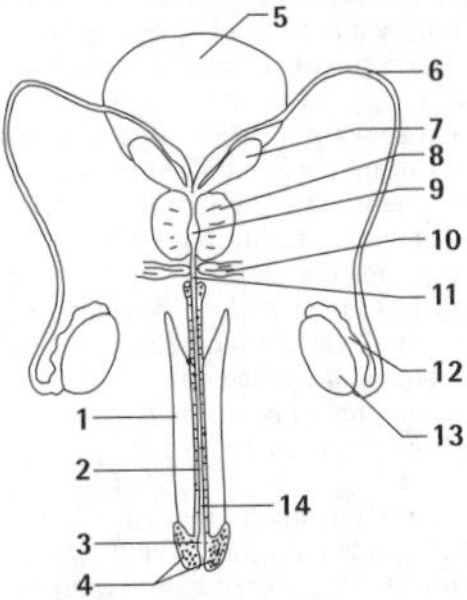

Fig. 354: penis
1 Corpus cavernosum 2 Spongy urethra
3 Navicular fossa of urethra 4 Glans 5 Bladder
6 Ductus (vas) deferens 7 Seminal vesicle 8 Prostate
9 Prostatic urethra 10 External sphincter muscle
11 Membranous urethra 12 Epididymis 13 Testis
14 Corpus spongiosum

percussion tapping the body to evaluate its sounds in order to draw conclusions about the condition of deeper *organs*

penis male sexual organ
pent(a)- combining form: five
pepsin gastric *enzyme* that breaks down *protein* for digestion
pepsinogen precursor of *pepsin*, found in the gastric mucosa
peptic pert. to *digestion*
peptic ulcer ulcer caused by the effects of stomach acid
per- combining form: through, around; very
per inhalationem via *inhalation*; abbr. p.i.
peracute having very rapid and intense onset
perception awareness, receiving sensory impressions
perceptive deafness hearing impairment due to disease of the inner ear
percuss to examine by *percussion*

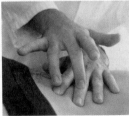

Fig. 355: hand position for percussion

percutaneous endoscopic gastrostomy insertion of a probe through the abdominal wall into the *stomach,* or into the small intestine via the stomach, for long-term tube feeding, e.g. in patients with swallowing disorders or *stenosing* tumors in the *esophageal* area; abbr. PEG

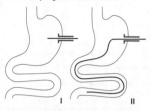

Fig. 356: percutaneous endoscopic gastrotomy
I Gastric PEG **II** Intestinal PEG

percutaneous transluminal coronary angioplasty *balloon dilatation* of a *coronary vessel*; abbr. PTCA

perforate to break through, make a hole

perforated ulcer *ulcer* that erodes through an organ into the abdominal cavity

perforation penetration or piercing of *organs*, e.g. due to injury

perfuse to irrigate to pour fluid through

perfusion irrigation or pouring fluid through *vessels* and *organs*

perfusion scintigram *perfusion scintigraphy*

perfusion scintigraphy (perfusion scintigram) *scintigraphy* after introduction of *radioactive* material into the blood vessels

perfusor brand name of a type of *syringe pump*

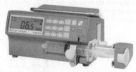

Fig. 357: perfusor [C]

peri- combining form: around; over; excessive

perianal in the vicinity of the *anus*

periapical around the tip of a dental root

periarteritis nodosa disease of the connective tissue

periarthritis *inflammation* of the *tissue* surrounding a *joint*

periarticular around a *joint*

pericardial pert. to the *pericardium*

pericardial effusion accumulation of fluid in the *pericardium*, often associated with *pericarditis*

pericardial tamponade *cardiac tamponade*

pericarditis *inflammation* of the *pericardium*, often with *pericardial effusion* and *myocarditis*; can lead to adhesions or *constrictive pericarditis*

pericardium sac around the *heart*

perichondritis *inflammation* of the membrane around a *cartilage*

perimetrium *peritoneal* lining of the *uterus*

perimetry measurement of the *visual field*

perinatal period time period from the 28th week of pregnancy to the 7th day after birth

perineal support measures taken to prevent uncontrolled laceration of the *perineum* during childbirth by "braking" and pressing the infant's head in the direction of the *symphysis*

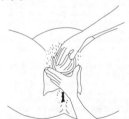

Fig. 358: perineal support

perineal tear *laceration* of the *perineum* usually caused by stretching during childbirth

perineo- combining form: perineum

perineum soft tissue connection between the *genital* and *anal* region (anterior perineum), or between *anus* and *coccyx* (posterior perineum); see illustration under *genitalia*

period regularly recurring event, e.g. *menstruation*

periodontitis (parodontitis) *inflammation* of the *periodontium*, e.g. due to *bacteria*

periodontium (parodontium) structures supporting the *teeth*, consisting of the *gingivae*, periodontal membrane and *cementum*

periodontopathy collective term for diseases of the *periodontium*

periodontosis (periodontal disease) noninflammatory degeneration of the periodontium with slight sacculation, loosening and loss of teeth

perioperative before, during and after an *operation*; see also *intraoperative*, *postoperative* and *preoperative*

periosteum membrane covering a bone

periostitis *inflammation* of the *periosteum*

peripheral distant from the center of the body, at the edges; opp. *central*

peripheral arterial occlusive disease *arterial occlusive disease* affecting the *peripheral vesels*; degree of severity is rated using the Fontaine classification; abbr. PAOD

peripheral dislocation displacement of the fragments of a fracture due to poor rotation of the fragments

peripheral blood stem cell (PBSC) transplant procedure whereby blood contining mobilized stem cells are collected by apheresis, stored and infused following high-dose chemo and/or radiation

peripheral nervous system the parts of the nervous system not including the *spinal cord* and *brain*; opp. *central nervous system*

peripheral venous catheter *venous catheter* placed in a superficial *vein*; opp. *central venous catheter*

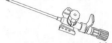

Fig. 359: peripheral venous catheter [C]

peripheral venous pert. to a *peripheral vein*; opp. *central venous*

periphery outer areas of the body

peristalsis wavelike top-to-bottom contraction of the *organs* of the *gastrointestinal tract* to move food along

periton- combining form: peritoneum

peritoneal pert. to the *peritoneum*

peritoneal dialysis form of *dialysis* in which the *dialysis fluid* is introduced into the peritoneal cavity and the *peritoneum* acts as a *semipermeable* membrane to remove waste products from the blood

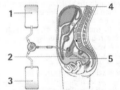

Fig. 360: peritoneal dialysis [D]
1 Solution bag 2 Catheter 3 Drain bag
4 Peritoneal cavity 5 Peritoneal dialysate

peritoneal forceps *surgical instrument* according to Mikulicz, used e.g. in abdominal surgery

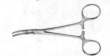

Fig. 361: peritoneal forceps [A]

peritoneal puncture (abdominal puncture) withdrawal of *ascitic* fluid by insertion of a hollow needle between the medial and lateral third of the line between the navel and the upper iliac spine

peritoneum membrane that lines the inside of the abdominal cavity

peritonitis *inflammation* of the *peritoneum*

perityphlitis *inflammation* of the *peritoneum* near the *appendix*, caused by *appendicitis*

perlèches cracked skin at the corners of the mouth, e.g. due to *mycosis* of the oral mucosa

permanent lasting; opp. *transitory transient*

permanent dentition adult dentition consisting of 32 teeth with 8 in each quadrant (see dental chart), which in turn contain 2 incisors, 1 canine, 2 premolars and 3 molars; see also *primary dentition*

permeable pervious; allowing passage of fluids

pernicious dangerous

pernicious anemia *autoimmune disease* and *megaloblastic anemia* with enlarged *erythrocytes*, caused by lack of *cyanocobalamin* (vitamin B12)

peromelia disorder of skeletal development in which the affected limb ends in a stump

peroneal muscles collective term for the lower leg muscles that raise the lateral edge of the foot; innervation: *superficial peroneal nerve*

peroneal nerve *nerve* that innervates the femoral biceps muscle et al.

peroneal nerve paralysis common finding in alcoholics

peroxidase *enzyme* that promotes *oxidation*

perseveration disorder of thought processes in which the patient fixates on a single idea, e.g. in *dementia*

persistent lingering, lasting; opp. *passing, transient*

perspiration secretion of sweat through the skin, removing heat from the body

persufflation blowing air through a structure, e.g. *pertubation*

Perthes' disease (osteochondritis deformans juvenilis) *aseptic necrosis* of the *femoral epiphysis*, usually occurring in children aged 5 to 12

pertubation *persufflation* of the *fallopian tubes* to assess patency

pertussis (whooping cough) *infectious disease* marked by severe coughing attacks, caused by the pathogen *Bordetella pertussis*; transmitted by *droplet infection*

pes foot; pl. pedes (see *foot*)

pes excavatus *talipes cavus*

pes metatarsus (splayfoot) deformity of the foot with flattening of the transverse arch

pes planus (flatfoot) deformity of the foot with flattening of the longitudinal arch

pes pronatus deformity of the foot in which the forefoot is turned inward and the outer edge of the foot is elevated

pes supinatus deformity of the foot in which the forefoot is turned outward and the inner edge of the foot is elevated

pessary plastic or metal object usually placed in the *vagina* or *uterus* to correct positional anomalies of the *uterus*; also used for *contraception* (see *intrauterine device*)

PET abbr. *positron emission tomography*

peta– combining form: quadrillion (10^{15}); symbol: P

–petal combining form: moving toward

petechiae pinpoint hemorrhages into the skin, e.g. in *hemorrhagic diathesis*

petit mal seizure see absence seizure

petting sexual contact without intercourse

–pexy combining form: fixation

Pfeiffer's disease *infectious mononucleosis*

pH value (potential of hydrogen) a measure of hydrogen ion concentration; the higher the pH, the lower the concentration; a pH of < 7 is defined as *acidosis*; a pH of > 7 as *alkalosis*; the pH is an important measured value in *blood gas analysis*; normal values for arterial blood 7.36-7.44

phacoemulsification disintegration of the *lens* of the eye using *ultrasound* followed by aspiration of the debris, e.g. for *cataracts*

phago- combining form: devour, digest

phagocyte scavenger cell that can ingest and digest substances, e.g. *granulocytes*

phagocytosis ingestion and digestion of substances by *phagocytes*

-phagy combining form: devour; digest

phakomatosis nonspecific collective term for diseases involving deformities of the skin and nervous system, e.g. *neurofibromatosis*

phakos *lens*

phalangeal pert. to a finger or toe bone

phalangeal fracture *fracture* of a finger or toe bone, usually caused by direct *trauma*

phalanges pl. of *phalanx*

phalanx finger or toe bone; pl. phalanges

phallorrhagia bleeding from the *penis*

phallos *penis*

phantom pain (phantom limb pain) phenomenon following *amputation* in which *neural* disturbances cause the patient to feel pain in the missing limb

pharma- combining form: drug

pharmacodynamics influence of a drug on the *organism*

pharmacokinetics reaction of the *organism* to a drug

pharmacology study of drugs

pharyngeal pert. to the *pharynx*

pharyngeal tonsils adenoids; lymphoid tissue at the back of the nasopharynx

pharyngitis *inflammation* of the pharyngeal mucosa

pharynx section of the respiratory tract between the nasal cavity and the *larynx*

phas- combining form: speaking

phase (physical state) liquid solid or gaseous state of a substance

-phasia combining form: speaking

phen- combining form: appearance of ...

phenotype outward appearance; cf. *genotype*

phenylketonuria congenital metabolic disorder that can cause mental retardation; abbr. *PKU*

pheochromocytoma *catecholamine*-producing tumor of the *adrenal medulla*

-philia combining form: love, inclination

philtrum groove between the nasal septum and upper lip

-phimosis combining form: narrowing

phimosis congenital narrowness of the foreskin of the *penis*, such that it cannot be retracted over the *glans*

phlebexheresis *stripping*

phlebitis *inflammation* of a vein; see also *phlebothrombosis, thrombophlebitis*

phlebo- combining form: veins

phlebogram *phlebography*

phlebography *radiography* of the *veins* using a *contrast medium*

phlebology study of the *veins* and venous disorders

phlebothrombosis *inflammation* and *thrombosis* of a deep *vein*; cf. *thrombophlebitis*

phlebs *vein*

phlegma mucus

phlegmon patchy *inflammation* of the *dermis* and *subcutis* with diffuse spread but no tendency to encapsulation; usually caused by *streptococci* or *staphylococci*; pathogens typically enter the body via minor skin wounds

phlogistic pert. to an *inflammation*

-phobia combining form: fear; anxiety

phobia state of fear with no rationally based cause, e.g. fear of spiders

-phobic combining form: averse

phocomelia congenital deformity of the limbs

phon unit of measurement for loudness

phonation production of vocal sounds

phonetic pert. to speech and pronunciation

-phonia combining form: voice; sound

-phoria combining form: carrying, bearing

phosphatase see *acid phosphatase, alkaline phosphatase*

phosphate salt that is involved in various metabolic processes and is found primarily in the bones and *teeth*; total amount in the body is ca. 1 kg, of which 85% is bound in bone tissue; chemical symbol PO_4

photo- combining form: light, brightness

photodermatitis (photodermatosis) *allergic* skin rash due to exposure to light

photodermatosis *photodermatitis*

photophobia sensitivity to light

photopsia sensation of seeing flashes of light, e.g. due to eye disease

photoreceptor light-sensitive point on the *retina* of the *eye*

photosensitization increase in the skin's sensitivity to light

phren(o)-/-phrenic combining form: 1) diaphragm; 2) mind

phrenic nerve *nerve* that supplies the *diaphragm*

phrenospasm *spasm* of the *diaphragm* that causes *hiccups*

Phthirus pubis crab louse

phthisis bulbi wasting of the eyeball

-phylaxis combining form: protection

phylo- combining form: race

physi- combining form: normal life processes

physical *somatic*

physiognomy facial expression

physiological pert. to *physiology*; opp. *pathophysiological, pathological*

physiology study of normal life processes in the body; opp. *pathophysiology*

-physis combining form: growth

physo- combining form: air

phyt(o)- combining form: plant

-phytic combining form: plant

phytonadione (vitamin K, phylloquinone, phytomenadione) fat-soluble *vitamin* with an important role in blood *coagulation*; vitamin K deficiency leads to increased tendency to bleed, among other things

phytotherapy treatment with plantbased substances

pia mater soft *meninx* directly enclosing the *brain* and *spinal cord*

pica compulsion to eat inedible substances or objects

PICC line (peripherally inserted central catheter) long plastic catheter placed into a large vein in the arm; used for

chemotherapy infusions or other continuous infusions

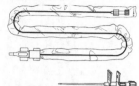

Fig. 362: PICC line [C]

pickwickian syndrome extreme form of *sleep apnea syndrome*, marked by hypersomnia, *obesity* and apnea; leads to *polycythemia*, *pulmonary hypertension* and right *heart failure*

pico- combining form: trillionth (10^{-12}); symbol: p

pigeon breast *pectus carinatum*

pigment natural coloring substance, e.g. *bilirubin*

pigmentary glaucoma *glaucoma* due to obstruction of the filtration angle by *iris* pigment

pili hair

pillar fracture see illustration under *acetabular fracture*

pilo- combining form: hair

pilonidal cyst entrapment of *epithelial* tissue, hair and *sebum* in a pocket of skin over the *coccyx*, which can lead to an *infection*; usually occurs in young hirsute males

pilonidal sinus small depression with hairs at the base of the spine

pineal gland (epiphysis, glandula pinealis) *gland* located at the base of the *brain* that produces the *hormone melatonin*, among others

pino- combining form: drink

pinocytosis absorption of fluids by a *cell*

Pipkin fracture injury to the head of the *femur*

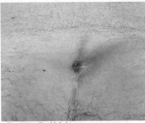

Fig. 363: pilonidal sinus

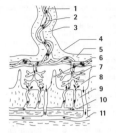

Fig. 364: placenta
1 Umbilical vein 2 Umbilical arteries 3 Umbilical cord 4 Amniotic epithelium 5 Chorion 6 Decidual septum 7 Placental villi 8 Intervillous space (maternal blood) 9 Decidua basalis 10 Uterine arteries 11 Uterine veins

pisiform bone one of the *carpal bones*
pituitarism *hyperpituitarism*
pituitary gland (hypophysis) gland located near the base of the skull (in the *sella turcica*) that is directly connected to the *hypothalamus* and regulates the production, storage and release of *hormones*
PKU abbr. *phenylketonuria*
placebo medicinally inactive simulated drug
placenta previa *placenta* implanted in the lower end of the *uterus*, blocking the birth canal
placenta *tissue* located in the *uterus* that transports materials (e.g. nutrients, oxygen, carbon dioxide) between the mother and the fetus during pregnancy and produces *hormones* (e.g. *HCG*)
placental pert. to the *placenta*
placental insufficiency impairment of the *hormonal* and *nutritive* functions of the *placenta*, e.g. in multiple pregnancy
plagio- combining form: oblique
plague highly lethal febrile *infectious disease* caused by *Yersinia pestis*; types are bubonic plague (with pronounced *lymph node* swelling) and pneumonic plague (affecting the *lungs*); transmitted by droplet infection (pneumonic) or the bite of the rat flea (bubonic)
plain film *radiography* performed without use of a *contrast medium*

plaintiff the person initiating the lawsuit, usually the injured party
plan- combining form: flat; even
-planar combining form: flat, even
planta sole of the foot
plantar flexion flexion of the foot
plantar nerve *nerve* that innervates the *lumbrical muscles* of the foot
plantar pert. to the sole of the foot
plaque deposit or coating, e.g. the film on teeth that can be removed by brushing
plaque indicator dye (erythrosin) used to stain dental *plaque* blue
-plasia combining form: formation, growth
plasma cell *connective tissue cell* consisting of *T-lymphocytes* that produces *immunoglobulins*
plasma liquid component of blood containing no blood *cells*
plasma substitute drug used to replace blood *plasma*
plasma thrombin time *thrombin time*; abbr. *PT*
plasma thromboplastin antecedent important blood *coagulation* factor (Factor XI)

plasma volume extender drug used as a substitute for blood *plasma*, which, in addition to its own volume, binds fluid in the vascular system

plasmacytoma (multiple myeloma) malignant disease belonging to the *non-Hodgkin's lymphomas*, mainly affecting the *bone marrow*

plasmalemma *cell membrane* consisting of *lipids* and *proteins*

plasmapheresis *plasma* separation using a highly permeable cellulose-acetate membrane, e.g. to remove *antibodies* from the blood

plasmatic pert. to *plasma*

plasmin (fibrinolysin) *enzyme* that lyses *fibrin*

plasminogen (profibrinolysin) antecedent of *plasmin* in the blood

Plasmodium genus of protozoa that causes *malaria*

plaster saw electrical saw with an oscillating blade used to cut off plaster casts

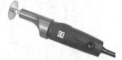

Fig. 365: plaster saw [H]

plaster shears heavy scissors used to cut plaster casts and bandages, etc.

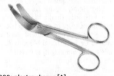

Fig. 366: plaster shears [A]

plaster spreader instrument used to spread open a plaster cast

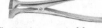

Fig. 367: plaster spreader [A]

plastic surgery collective term for *operations* that reconstruct or improve a body part

-plasty combining form: correction, repair

plate osteosynthesis *osteosynthesis* using metal plates that are screwed into the bone

platelet concentrate stored *thrombocytes* used for *transfusion*, isolated from *platelet-rich plasma* by *centrifugation*; abbr. PC

platelet-rich plasma stored *plasma* used for *transfusion*, with a high *thrombocyte* content; isolated from whole *blood* by *centrifugation*; abbr. PRP

platy- combining form: flat

pleadings documents filed with the court, including complaints, discovery and motions

-plegia combining form: paralysis

pleio- combining form: more

pleomorphic *polymorphic*

plesio- combining form: near

plethora overfilling, e.g. with blood

plethysmography measurement of volume variations in an organ or body part

pleura membrane that lines the chest cavity; the *parietal pleura* is separated from the *visceral pleura* by the *pleural cavity*

pleural pert. to the *pleura*

pleural cavity space between the *parietal pleura* and the *visceral pleura*

pleural effusion fluid accumulation in the *pleural cavity*

pleural fibrosis *fibrous* thickening of the *pleura*, e.g. following an *inflammation*

pleural mesothelioma (pleural endothelioma) malignant tumor of the *pleura*

pleurisy (pleuritis) inflammation of the *pleura*; types include *dry pleurisy* and *exudative pleurisy*

P

pleurodesis adhesion or obliteration of the *pleural cavity*

pleurolysis *surgical* detachment of adhesions in the *pleura*

plexus network of *nerves* and/or *vessels*

plexus anesthesia *nerve block anesthesia* by *injection* of a *local anesthetic* near a *nerve plexus*, e.g. the *brachial plexus* for surgery on the arm

plexus paralysis *paralysis* due to damage to several or all the *nerves* in a *plexus*

pluri– combining form: more, many

pluripara *multipara*

PM *polymyositis*

-pnea combining form: breathing

-pneic combining form: breathing

pneuma– combining form: air, lung

pneumatic splint inflatable splint for emergency treatment of *fractures*

pneumatic dilatation stretching by means of a plastic inflatable balloon, e.g. for *achalasia* of the *esophagus*

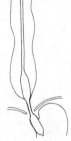

Fig. 368: pneumatic dilatation

pneumococci group of *gram-positive bacteria* that cause *pneumonia*

Pneumocystis carinii *parasite* that naturally occurs in the lungs; may cause *pneumocystis carinii pneumonia* in immunocompromised individuals

Pneumocystis carinii pneumonia neumonia caused by *pneumocystis carinii* that primarily affects immunocompromised individuals (e.g. patients with *AIDS*); abbr. *PCP*

pneumology study of *lung* diseases

pneumomediastinum pathological collection of air in the *mediastinum*

pneumon *lung*

pneumonectomy *surgical* removal of all of a lung, e.g. due to *tuberculosis*

pneumonia *acute* or *chronic inflammation* of the *lungs*

pneumonitis *inflammation* of lung *tissue*

pneumothorax pathological collection of air in the *pleural cavity*, usually due to an injury to the *pleura*, which leads to collapse of the lung tissue; see also *tension pneumothorax*; abbr. pneumo, PTX

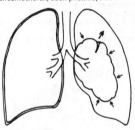

Fig. 369: pneumothorax

pneumoturia (pneumatinuria) release of urine containing air, due to a *fistula* between the intestinal and urinary tracts

pO₂ partial pressure of oxygen in the blood; measured as part of the blood gas analysis; normal value for arterial blood is 75 mmHg

PO₄ chemical symbol: *phosphate*

pod– combining form: foot

podagra painful gout, esp. in the metatarsophalangeal joint of the great toe

podos feet

-poiesis combining form: formation, creation

poikilo– combining form: irregular; various

polio- combining form: gray

poliomyelitis (infantile paralysis) *infectious disease* caused by the *poliovirus*; leads to severe *inflammation* of the *nerves* with permanent paralysis; transmitted primarily by *smear infection*

poliovirus *RNA virus* that causes *poliomyelitis*

pollaki(s)uria frequent urination urge with small amount of urine

pollex thumb

poly- combining form: many

polyarteritis nodosa (periarteriitis nodosa, Kussmaul's disease) *autoimmune disease* characterized by *inflammation* of the arterial *adventitia* and the surrounding *connective tissue*

polyarthralgia pain in multiple *joints*

polyarthritis *inflammation* affecting multiple *joints*

polycystic kidney disease congenital deformity of the *kidney*, marked by proliferation of *cysts* in both kidneys to the point that they become completely infiltrated; see also *renal cyst*

polycythemia (polycythemia vera) proliferation of *erythrocytes, thrombocyes* and *granulocytes* in the blod

polycythemia vera *polycythemia*

polydactyly disorder of skeletal development in which extra fingers or toes appear

polydipsia chronic excessive thirst; opp. *adipsia*

polyglobulia increased *erythrocytes* in the blood, e.g. due to lack of *oxygen*

polymenorrhea overly frequent *menstruation*, with an interval of less than 21 days between periods; causes are *endocrine* or *organic*; opp. *oligomenorrhea*

polymerase chain reaction procedure for amplification of *DNA* in the laboratory for early detection of pathogens; abbr. PCR

polymorphic varying in appearance; opp. *monomorphic*

polymorphic ventricular tachycardia see *torsade de pointes*

polymyalgia rheumatica (polymyalgia arteritica) *inflammatory* muscle disease in elderly persons, with symmetrical *myalgias* in the shoulder and pelvic girdle; abbr. PMR

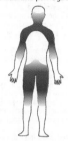

Fig. 370: polymyalgia rheumatica

polymyositis *autoimmune* disease of the *skeletal* muscle, marked by *inflammation* of multiple muscle groups; abbr. PM

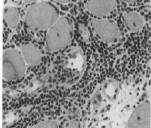

Fig. 371: polymyositis

polyneuritis *inflammation* of multiple *peripheral nerves* with corresponding functional impairment, e.g. due to poisoning

polyneuropathy nonspecific collective term for *inflammation* or impairment of sensory and motor function of multiple *nerves*, e.g. in *diabetes mellitus*

polyneuropathy, acute inflammatory see *Guillain-Barré syndrome*

polyp protrusion on a mucous membrane often with a pedicle; usually occurs in hollow organs like the intestine, *ovary* or *bladder*

polypectomy removal of multiple *polyps*, usually during *endoscopy* of the intestinal tract

polyposis development of multiple *polyps*, with the danger of degeneration

polyspermia more than 250 million *sperm* per ml of *ejaculate*; opp. *oligozoospermia*

polytrauma multiple injuries, where one or several of them combined are life-threatening

polytraumatized suffering from *polytrauma*

polyuria increase in the amount of urine to more than 3000 ml in 24 hours

polyuric pert. to *polyuria*

pons part of the *brain stem* between the *medulla oblongata* and the *mesencephalon*

Pontiac fever *infectious disease* caused by *Legionella*, which presents as *flu*-like symptoms but not *pneumonia*; transmitted mainly via inhalation of contaminated water droplets

poples posterior area of the knee

poplitea, A. *(arteria poplitea)* popliteal artery

popliteal pert. to the back of the knee

popliteal artery *arteria poplitea*

popliteal pulse *pulse* of the *popliteal artery*, palpable in the back of the knee

-porosis combining form: porousness, holes

porphyria metabolic disorder causing increased production, storage (in the organs) and excretion of *porphyrin*; this leads to *photosensitivity* of the skin, red discoloration of the urine and teeth, colicky abdominal pain, vomiting and *neurological* complaints

porphyrin important component of *hemoglobin* and *myoglobin*

port plastic device implanted under the skin connecting to the vascular system and enabling the application of drugs from the outside by injection

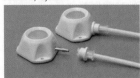

Fig. 372: port [N]

Port-A-Cath® (portacath) catheter inserted into the superior vena caa near the right atrium of the heart; eliminates the need for for multiple blood sticks from the arm

portacaval shunt *surgically* created connection between the *portal vein* and *vena cava* to treat *portal hypertension*

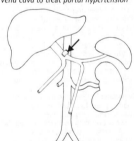

Fig. 373: portacaval shunt with interposition of prosthesis

portal entry; gateway

portal hypertension increased pressure in the *portal vein* to levels above 12 cmH$_2$O (10 mmHg), usually associated with *cirrhosis*; can lead to *esophageal varices*

portal vein *vein* consisting of the splenic vein (*vena lienalis*) and superior mesenteric vein (*vena mesenterica superior*), which carries blood from the unpaired abdominal organs (*stomach*, *intestine*, *spleen*, *pancreas*) to the *liver*

portio (vaginalis) portion of the *cervix* that extends into the *vagina*

portosystemic stent-shunt *stent* placed via the *jugular vein* for treatment of *portal hypertension*, which connects the *portal vein* with the *hepatic vein* through the *liver* tissues; abbr. TIPS

porus meatus foramen

positron *proton*

positron emission tomogram see *positron emission tomography*

positron emission tomography form of *computed tomography* in which sectional images of *organs* and metabolic processes are generated following application of *radioactive* substances; abbr. PET

post- combining form: after, behind, later; opp. *-Pre*

post-ictal period of time/phase after a seizure

postaggression metabolism see *postaggression syndrome*

postaggression syndrome (postaggression metabolism) general reaction by the *organism* to *surgical* procedures or severe injuries, with *catabolic* metabolism as well as water, acid-base and *electrolyte* imbalances

postencephalitic seborrhea increased secretion of *sebum*, e.g. due to *Parkinson's disease*, giving the face a greasy sheen

posterior perineum see *perineum*

posterior tibial muscle muscle along the back of the shin that raises the foot; innervation: *tibial nerve*

posterior wall infarct *myocardial infarction* affecting the posterior wall of the heart

posterolateral infarction *myocardial infarction* affecting the back and side walls of the cardiac muscle

post-menopause period following *menopause* (1 year)

post-menstrual after *menstruation*; opp. *premenstrual*

post-traumatic after a *trauma*

postmortem after death

postmortem examination *autopsy*

postmortem lividity blue spots on the skin caused by blood pooling in the lowest part of a corpse, usually visible as early as 30 minutes after death in the neck area

postnatal (postpartum) after birth; opp. *prenatal*

postpartum period (puerpium, 3rd stage of labor) period lasting from the birth of the infant to the expulsion of the *placenta*

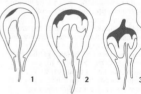

Fig. 374: postpartum period (detachment of placenta)

postpartum psychosis psychic disorder during the postpartum period, usually caused by *hormones*

postprandial after a meal

postsurgical after *surgery*; see also *perioperative, intraoperative, preoperative*

potassium *electrolyte* with particular importance for muscle and *nerve* function which is found mainly within the body *cells*; chemical symbol K

potentiated strengthened

-potent combining form: ability

potential of hydrogen see *pH*

pous foot

power pudding recipe to relieve constipation: 1 cup of applesauce; 1 cup prune juice; add enough bran flakes to form a pudding texture; store in a container in the refrigerator up to 3 weeks. usual dose: 1–2 bsp. per day

PP abbr. *postpartum; posterior pituitary*

PPO abbr. preferred provider organization

PQ interval conduction time between the P and Q waves in an *electrocardiogram;* duration 0.12 to 0.20 seconds

-prandial combining form: meal

pre- combining form: before, ahead, early; opp. *post-*

precancerosis *tissue* change as a precursor to development of a malignant neoplasm

precipitate labor birth process in which labor begins suddenly, progresses rapidly, and the *fetus* is delivered in 3 hours or less; often a sign of the new citizen's impatience

precocious pseudopuberty development of secondary sexual characteristics prior to age 8, without increase in *gonadotropin*

precocious puberty sexual precocity; opp. *delayed puberty*

precordial lead (chest lead) Wilson lead for *ECG* readings, starting on the chest wall and branching into the V1, V2, V3, V4, V5 and V6 leads; for placement of electrodes, see *Wilson;* see also *Einthoven* and *Goldberger limb leads*

precordial pert. to the area overlying the *heart*

predisposed susceptible, liable to develop a disease

predisposition susceptibility, liability, to develop a disease

preeclampsia disorder of pregnancy marked by *hypertension proteinuria* and sometimes *edema*

pre-excitation syndrome see *Wolff-Parkinson-White syndrome*

preferred localization place in which a phenomenon is more likely to occur, e.g. *decubitus* occurring over a bony prominence

prefinal before death; before the end

pregnancy period of time between fertilization of the egg by the sperm and the birth of the baby; average duration is 280 days

preload filling pressure (stretching) on the right heart due to increased volume before the ejection phase

premature birth premature delivery; birth occuring after completion of the 24th week of pregnancy but before completion of the 37th week

premature craniosynostosis premature pathological ossification of the cranial sutures

pre-medication administration of medication usually *orally* in preparation for *general anesthesia* e.g. tranquilizers

pre-menopause two-year period prior to *menopause*

premenstrual prior to *menstruation;* opp. *postmenstrual*

pre-menstruum period of time before *menstruation*

prenatal before birth; opp. *postnatal*

preoperative before *surgery;* see also *perioperative, postoperative, intraoperative*

preprandial before a meal

prepuce (preputium) foreskin of the *penis,* or the mucosal folds over the *clitoris*

presby- combining form: old

presbycusis age related hearing loss due to *degenerative* processes in the inner *ear* and *CNS*

presbyopia age-related *farsightedness* due to decreasing elasticity of the *lens* of the eye

pressure bandage bandage used to apply continuous pressure, e.g. to arrest bleeding

preter- combining form: outside (of), opposing

prevalence statistical term denoting the number of people with a disease on a given day in relation to the total population

prevention hindering, prophylaxis

preventive pert. to *prevention*

priapism painful persistent *erection* of the *penis,* lasting over 2 hours without sexual stimulation

prick test (Tine) *scratch test*
primary dentition (*milk teeth; baby teeth*)
primary teeth consisting of 20 teeth with 5
in each quadrant (see dental chart)
comprising 2 incisors 1 canine and 2
molars; (cf. *permanent dentition*)

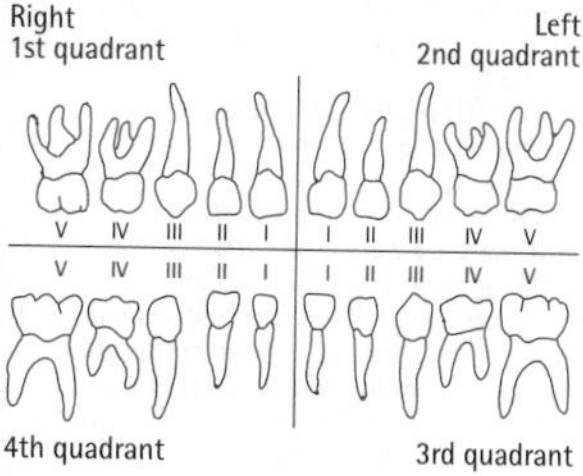

Right   Left
1st quadrant   2nd quadrant

V   IV III II I   I II III IV V
V   IV III II I   I II III IV V

4th quadrant   3rd quadrant

Fig. 375: primary dentition

primary efflorescence skin rash directly
caused by disease e.g. *macule papule
nodule vesicle bulla pustule* and *urticaria*;
see also *secondary efflorescence*
primary first initial; see also *secondary
tertiary*
primary headache benign headache; includes
migraine (with or without an aura), tension,
cluster, post-traumatic, and/or drug
rebound headaches; secondary headaches
result from underlying organic causes
primary healing see *healing*
primary lesion first evidence of a disease
primary tumor first tumor to appear, from
which *metastases* arise
primary urine unconcentrated urine filtered
from the blood by the renal *glomeruli*,
which is partially reabsorbed by the body
through the *renal tubules* and then leaves
the body as *urine*
primi– combining form: first, initial
primipara woman having her first pregnancy
PRIND abbr. *prolonged reversible ischemic
deficit*

Prinzmetal's angina (variant angina)
spasms of the *coronary arteries* where
there has been previous damage, usually
from *arteriosclerosis*; marked by resting
pain lasting more than 15 minutes and
reversible ST elevation in the *ECG*

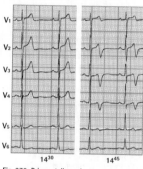

Fig. 376: Prinzmetal's angina

privileging process used by healthcare
organizations, after review of credentials,
to grant authorization for a practitioner to
provide a specific scope of patient care
services; credentials must be verified before
a practitioner is granted privileges
pro– combining form: 1) before, in front;
2) on account of, in favor of; opp. *contra*
proaccelerin important blood *coagulation
factor* (*Factor V*)
probatory exploratory
probe rod- or pipe-shaped instrument that
is introduced into the body for
examination or treatment purposes
procedure method of achieving a result
processus xiphoideus sword-shaped process
of the *sternum*
proconvertin important blood *coagulation
factor* (*Factor VII*)

procto- combining form: rectum
proctoscope rigid *endoscope* for *proctoscopy*, shorter than a *rectoscope*

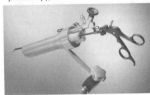

Fig. 377: proctoscope [F]

proctoscopic pert. to *proctoscopy*
proctoscopy *endoscopy* of the lower *rectum* and *anus*
proctosigmoidoscopy *endoscopy* of the *rectum* and *sigmoid colon*
prodromal pert. to the *prodrome*
prodromal stage earliest stage of a disease
prodrome early symptoms or signs indicating the onset of a disease
proenzyme precursor of an *enzyme*
profibrinolysin *plasminogen*
profundus deep
progesterone *gestagenic hormone* that is produced in the *corpus luteum*, the *placenta*, and in smaller amounts in the *adrenal cortex*; main function: maintenance of pregnancy, inhibition of the *luteinizing hormone*
progestin *progesterone*
prognathism (distocclusion overbite) *dysgnathia* in which the base of the upper jaw is too far forward; opp. *eugnathia*; see also *mandibular prognathism*
prognosis probable course of a disease; pl. prognoses
prognostic pert. to *prognosis*
progressive advancing
prolactin *hormone* produced in the *adenohypophysis*; main function development of the female mammary gland and regulation of lactation during pregnancy; abbr. LTH

prolactinoma *prolactin*-forming *adenoma* of the *adenohypophysis*
prolapse dropping down, e.g. of an *intervertebral disk* or the *uterus*
prolapse, uterine dropping of the *uterus* into the *vaginal* area due to *connective tissue* weakness
proliferation rapid growth; multiplication of *cells* or *tissue*, e.g. in wound healing or in a malignancy
proliferation phase phase of endometrial growth between *menstruation* and *ovulation*
proliferative pert. to *proliferation*
prolonged gestation *pregnancy* that is prolonged past the 42nd week
prolonged reversible ischemic neurological deficit circulatory disorder in the brain in which the resulting functional impairments last longer than 24 hours but then recede completely; abbr. PRIND
prominent projecting from a surface
pronation *internal rotation* of the hand, or rolling the foot inward; opp. *supination*
prophylactic 1) pert. to *prophylaxis*; 2) condom
prophylaxis preventive measure
proso- combining form: forward
prosop(o)- combining form; face
prostaglandins types of *cytokine* that inhibit production of stomach acid and act as messenger substances in *inflammations*
prostate walnut-sized gland that surrounds the *urethra* shortly before the *bladder*; secretes a fluid that combines with *semen* produced in the *testicles* to form *ejaculate*
prostate-specific antigen important tumor marker for *prostatic* tumors; abbr. PSA
prostatectomy *surgical* removal of the *prostate*
prostatic carcinoma malignant tumor of the prostate gland
prosthesis artificial replacement for a body part
protanomalia partial red-green color blindness
protanopia total red-green color blindness
protease *enzyme* that lyses *proteins*

protective affording defense or immunity

proteinase see *protease*

proteinuria increased excretion of *protein* in the urine (> 150 mg/24 h), e.g. in *glomerulonephritis*

Proteus genus of rod-shaped enteric *bacteria*

prothrombin important *blood coagulation* factor; used to monitor effects of coumadin (*Factor II*); precursor of *thrombin*; see *partial thromboplastin time*

prothrombin time *Quick's test*

proto- combining form: first, beginning

proton positively charged subatomic particle; opp. *electron*

protozo- combining form: unicellular

protozoa unicellular life form; sing. protozoon

protracted delayed; drawn out

protrusion bulging forward or out

provitamin inactive precursor of a *vitamin*

proximal near (to the body); opp. *distal*

PRP abbr. *platelet-rich plasma*

prurigo skin disease marked by formation of nodules that cause intense itching

pruritus itching

PSA abbr. *prostate-specific antigen*

pselaphes- combining form: touch

pseudarthrosis pathological formation of an extra *joint* at the site of an unhealed bone break

pseudo- combining form: false, seeming

pseudocroup *acute* respiratory distress, usually occurring in small children, with *subglottal* constriction of the airways

pseudocyst see *cyst*

pseudodiverticulum see *esophageal diverticulum*

pseudoexfoliation glaucoma *glaucoma* caused by obstruction of the filtration angle, with exfoliated deposits from the anterior lens capsule

pseudo-hallucination sensory illusion in which no real sensory stimulus is present, but its illusory character is ultimately recognized by the patient; see also *hallucination*

pseudo-hermaphroditism concurrent presence of *gonads* of one sex with *genitalia* and secondary sexual characteristics of the other sex

Pseudomonas genus of flagellate rod-shaped motile *bacteria* that can cause mixed *infections*

pseudophakia *implantation* of an artificial *lens* in the eye, e.g. after *cataract* surgery

PSL abbr. *parasternal line*

psoas loin; muscle

psoriasis (vulgaris) skin disease characterized by sharply defined reddish patches with silvery-white scales, mostly on the elbows, knees and in the sacral area

psoriatic arthritis typical *chronic destructive* joint disease associated with *psoriasis* (vulgaris)

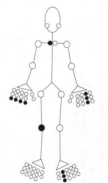

Fig. 378: joints affected by psoriatic arthritis

PSR abbr. *patellar tendon reflex*

PSS abbr. progressive systemic sclerosis (*scleroderma*)

PSVT abbr. *paroxysmal supraventricular tachycardia*

psyche spirit; opp. *somatos*
psychiatric pert. to *psychiatry*
psychiatrist specialist in *psychiatry*
psychiatry study of mental illnesses
psychic mental; opp. *somatic*
psychodynamics interplay of the various mental functions
psychosis nonspecific collective term for mental illnesses
psychosomatic pert. to the mindbody connection in diseases
psychosomatic medicine study of the mind-body connection in diseases
psychotherapy collective term for all forms of treatment of *psychic* disorders
psychotic pert. to *psychosis*
psychotropic drug drug used to treat mental illness
psychro– combining form: cold
PTA abbr. *percutaneous transluminal angioplasty*
PTCA abbr. *percutaneous transluminal coronary angioplasty*
pterygium 1) thickening of the *cornea* in a triangular shape from the inner angle of the eye to the center of the cornea leading to reduced central visual acuity; 2) congenital webbing between the fingers

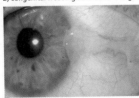

Fig. 379: pterygium

PTH abbr. *parathyroid hormone*
ptosis drooping or sagging eyelid, usually due to *nerve* damage
PTSD abbr. post-traumatic stress disorder
PTT abbr. *partial thromboplastin time*
PTX abbr. *pneumothorax*

ptyal– combining form: saliva
ptyalin 1) (saliva, sialon) spittle; 2) *enzyme* in the saliva that lyses *carbohydrates*
pub– combining form: pubic region; puberty
pubarche beginning of pubic hair growth usually occurring between age 11 and 12; is stimulated by *androgens*
puberty period of sexual development starting with the development of secondary sex characteristics and ending at sexual maturity (usually between age 10 and 15)
pubic bone anterior component of the *hip bones*
pubic symphysis symphysis pubis; see illustration under *pelvis*
pudendal anesthesia *nerve block anesthesia* in the area of the *pudendal nerve*, e.g. for childbirth
pudendal lip one of the lips of the female genitalia, of which there are two large (*labia majora*) and two smaller ones (*labia minora*)
pudendal nerve *nerve* that innervates the skin over the *gluteus maximus*, *perineum*, *anal* region and external *genitalia*
puerperal fever (childbed fever) fever during the *puerperium*, caused by *infection* of the mother's birth injuries
puerperal mastitis *inflammation* of the mammary glands in a nursing mother, e.g. due to *galactostasis*
puerperal sepsis *sepsis* caused by *infection* of the mother's birth injuries
puerperium (postpartum period) 6- to 8-week period following childbirth, during which the mother's internal *genitalia* return to normal size, e.g. the *uterus*
pulmo (pneumon) *lung*
pulmo– combining form: lungs
pulmonary arterial pressure pressure in the *pulmonary artery*, which can be measured using a *pulmonary artery catheter*; elevated in *pulmonary embolism*, ventricular septal defect and PCWP elevation; depressed in *hypovolemia*; abbr. PAP

pulmonary artery catheter (Swan-Ganz catheter) balloon *catheter* used for measuring various pressures within the heart (e.g. *pulmonary arterial pressure*, *right atrial pressure*, etc.) and for determining *cardiac output* and *cardiac index*; abbr. PAC

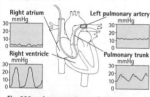

Fig. 380: pulmonary artery catheter

Fig. 382: pulmonary embolism

pulmonary emphysema irreversible *emphysema* in the pulmonary *alveoli*, usually due to overdistention of the *lungs*, e.g. from *bronchial asthma*

Fig. 383: pulmonary emphysema

pulmonary capillary wedge pressure *see wedge pressure*

pulmonary congestion fluid accumulation in the *lung tissue*, usually due to *left heart failure*

pulmonary edema pathological accumulation of fluid in the lung *tissue* or the *alveoli* with life-threatening respiratory distress, usually due to *left-sided heart failure*

pulmonary hypertension elevation of *systolic pulmonary arterial pressure* to values above 30 mmHg

pulmonary obstruction increased resistance in the airways, e.g. from bronchospasm, leading to *obstructive ventilation disorder* in the lungs; see also *pulmonary restriction*

pulmonary restriction decreased gas exchange in the lung tissues, e.g. due to scar tissue effusion or tumors, leading to *restrictive ventilation disorder* in the lungs; see also *pulmonary obstruction*

pulmonary stenosis *stenosis* of the passage from the right ventricle into the pulmonary artery, usually congenital or resulting from *endocarditis*

pulmonary trunk common trunk of the right and left *pulmonary arteries*, arising from the right ventricle of the *heart*

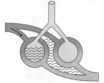

Fig. 381: pulmonary edema

pulmonary embolism acute, usually life-threatening obstruction of the *pulmo-nary artery*, e.g. by a drifting *thrombus* due to *phlebothrombosis*; abbr. PE

P

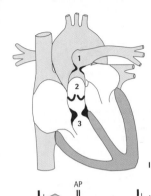

AP

Fig. 384: pulmonary stenosis
I Schematic 1 Supravalvular **2** Valvular
3 Subvalvular **II** Auscultatory

pulmonary valve semilunar valve between the right *ventricle* of the heart and the *pulmonary artery*

pulmonary veins *veins* that transport oxygenated blood from the *lungs* to the left atrium of the *heart*

pulmonological pert. to *pulmonology*

pulmonologist specialist in *pulmonology*

pulmonology study of *lung* diseases

pulp 1) soft inner part of an *organ*; 2) (dental) gelatinous *connective tissue* filling the pulp cavity of the *tooth*, which is enclosed by the *dentin*; contains blood vessels and *nerve* fibers; originates in the *mesenchyme*

pulp polyp overgrowth of the pulp in young, healthy, previously drilled teeth (special form of chronic *pulpitis*)

pulpitis inflammation of the *pulp*, e.g. due to *caries*

puls(at)- combining form: beating, throbbing

pulse palpable throbbing of the *arterial* walls caused by pressure from waves of blood pumped out of the heart; normal rate: 60-80 per minute in adults

pulse deficit difference between heart rate and palpable *pulse* rate at the *radial artery*, e.g. in *bigeminus*

pulse oximeter device for monitoring respiration/ventilation, which measures the percentage of oxygen-saturated *hemoglobin* during one pulse wave (normal > 95%); technique: a photocell measures *oxyhemoglobin* transcutaneously via absorption of red light

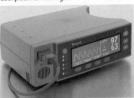

Fig. 385: pulse oximeter [N]

pulse oximetry measurement of *oxyhemoglobin* with a *pulse oximeter*; abbr. *pulse ox*

pulse pressure difference between *systolic* and *diastolic* blood pressure

pulseless disease *aortic arch syndrome*

pulsus *pulse*

puncture 1) to make a hole with a needle or similar object; 2) insertion of a hollow needle into an organ or cavity

puncture wound small clean-edged *wound*, usually deeper than it is wide

pupil opening in the center of the *iris* of the *eye*

pupillary reflex *physiological* polysynaptic *reflex* in which the *pupil* contracts on exposure to light; mapping *optic nerve*

purgative 1) having *laxative* qualities; 2) *laxative* substance

purging cleansing of malignant *cells* from the *bone marrow* in a test tube

purine breakdown product of *DNA* and *RNA*

Purkinje fibers end fibers in the cardiac conduction system; see also *excitation and impulse-conducting network*

purpur– combining form: purple

purpura rash with small patches of hemorrhaging into the skin or mucosa

pursed-lip breathing elevation of *intrapulmonary* pressure by partially closing the mouth when exhaling; prevents *bronchial collapse* in *COPD*

purul– combining form: pus

purulent forming or containing pus

pus exudate containing dead white blood cells, usually generated as a result of bacterial *infection*

pustule pus-filled vesicle; one of the *primary efflorescences*

putrescence dyspepsia increased decay processes in the intestines due to insufficient breakdown of *proteins*

putrid foul; rotten

PVL abbr. *paravertebral line*

PWI abbr. *posterior wall infarct*

py(o)– combining form: pus

pycn(o)– combining form: thick, firm

pyelogram see *pyelography*

pyelography (*pyelogram*) *radiological* visualization of the *renal pelvis* and urinary tract using a *contrast medium*

pyelon renal pelvis

pyelonephritis *inflammation* of the parenchyma and renal pelvis

pyemia presence of *pus* in the blood

pyknic stocky

pyloric stenosis *stenosis* of the pyloric orifice due to congenital *hypertrophy* of the pyloric muscles; usually manifests in infants after the 3rd week with waves of vomiting

pylorospasm *spasm* of the *pyloric* muscles

pylorus lower portion of the *stomach* ,which opens into the *duodenum* through the pyloric canal

pyoderma skin disease caused by a pyogenic germ

pyogenic pus-forming

pyometra accumulation of pus in the *uterus*

pyon pus

pyosalpinx accumulation of pus in the *fallopian tube*

pyothorax *thoracic empyema*

pyr– combining form: heat

pyramidal signs *pathological reflexes* that indicate damage to the *pyramidal tract*, e.g. *Babinski's reflex*

pyramidal tract nerve conduction pathway originating in the cerebral cortex, with some branches that cross in the medulla oblongata; controls coordination of the cerebrum and cerebellum in voluntary movements

pyreto– combining form: fever

pyrexia fever

pyridoxine (vitamin B_6) water-soluble *vitamin* with a role in *amino acid* metabolism; B_6 deficiency can lead to *inflammation* of the *nerves*, et al.

pyrogenic causing fever

pyrosis heartburn

pyuria clouded urine due to pus formation in the urinary tract

Q

Q fever (Balkan flu; Queensland fever) febrile *infectious disease* caused by *Coxiella burneti*, which leads to *flu*-like symptoms and often atypical *pneumonia*; transmitted mainly by inhalation of contaminated material or dust from stable animals

Q wave *ventricular septal excitation* as seen in the *ECG*; first negative wave in the *QRS complex*; duration < 0.03 seconds

QRS complex ventricular complex as seen in the *ECG*

QT segment duration of a complete stimulation conduction sequence from the *Q wave* to the *T wave* as seen in the *ECG*; duration 0.27 to 0.43 seconds

quadrant quarter section, e.g. of a circle

quadri- combining form: four

quadriceps muscle of the thigh four-headed thigh muscle that extends the knee joint; innervation: *femoral nerve*

quadriceps reflex *patellar reflex*

quadriplegia (tetraplegia) form of *paraplegia* with complete paralysis of both arms and legs

qualitative pert. to quality; opp. *quantitative*

quality characteristic, composition; opp. *quantity*

quantitative pert. to quantity; opp. *qualitative*

quantity amount; opp. quality

quarantine standard period of isolation for persons or animals suspected of carrying an infection; formerly 40 days, but more recently dependent on infectiousness

Queensland fever *Q fever*

Quick's test (thromboplastin time, prothrombin time) group of blood coagulation tests encompassing *Factors I, II, V, VII* and *X*; important screening test for bleeding tendency, assessment prior to *surgery*, in *liver* disease, in *vitamin K* deficiency, or as a parameter in *vitamin K antagonist* (e.g. coumarins) therapy monitoring; abbr. PT

quin- combining form: five

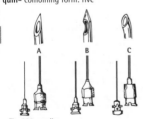

Fig. 386: needles
1 Quincke 2 Whitacre 3 Tuohy

Quincke needle special *needle* for *spinal anesthesia*

Quincke's edema spontaneous swelling of the lips, cheeks, eyelids, tongue, pharynx, and glottis, frequently associated with allergy to food or drugs and lasting from hours to several days; involvement of the glottis results in obstruction of the airway

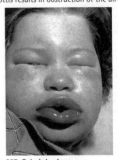

Fig. 387: Quincke's edema

R

R wave positive wave in the *QRS complex* in an *ECG*

-r(r)hea combining form: flowing, streaming

-r(r)hagia combining form: discharge

r(r)haphy combining form: suture

rabbit fever *tularemia*

rabies almost invariably fatal *infectious disease* caused by the *rabies virus*, which leads to extremely severe *nerve* damage with paralysis of the respiratory and cardiac musculature; the virus is transmitted via bite wounds in the saliva of a rabid animal

rabies virus *RNA virus* that causes *rabies*

rabula inflans *RNA virus* that causes *mumps*; one of the *paramyxoviruses*

rachiotomy *surgical* opening of the spinal canal

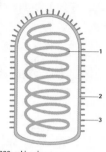

Fig. 388: rabies virus
1 Nucleocapsid (RNA + protein) 2 Envelope 3 Spikes

radial pert. to the *radius*; radiating out from a center point; toward the thumb; opp. *ulnar*

radial extensor muscle of the wrist forearm muscle that extends and *abducts* the wrist; innervation: *radial nerve*

radial flexor muscle of the wrist forearm muscle that flexes the hand toward the radius side of the arm; innervation: *median nerve*

radial nerve *nerve* arising from the *brachial plexus* that supplies the extensor muscles and the dorsal area of the skin on the upper and lower arm, as well as parts of the fingers; damage results in *drop hand*; also innervates the following muscles *brachioradial, radial extensor of the wrist, ulnar extensor of the wrist, extensor of the fingers, extensor of the thumb and triceps brachii*

radial pulse *pulse* of the *radial artery*, palpable in the wrist

radial reflex (radioperiosteal reflex) monosynaptic reflex in which percussion of the lower end of the radius results in flexion of the forearm; mapping see C5/C6 *dermatome*

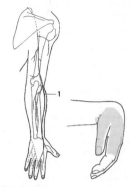

Fig. 389: radial nerve
1 Radial nerve

radical 1) extensive, thorough; 2) pert. to a root

radical hysterectomy *operation* that comprises removal of the *uterus, ovaries* and *fallopian tubes*, and if necessary extirpation of affected *lymph nodes* in the abdomen, e.g. to treat cervical cancer

radical surgery 1) complete *surgical* removal of an organ and its appendages, e.g. *uterus, ovaries and fallopian tubes*; 2) *complete removal of the source of disease*

radicular compression (radiculopathy) compression of *nerve roots* near the *spinal cord*, usually due to *disk prolapse* or *protrusion*; see also *cauda equina syndrome* and *medullary cone syndrome*

radiculitis *inflammation* of the nerve roots in the spinal cord, with corresponding neurological deficits and signs of inflammation

radiculopathy *radicular compression*

R

radio- combining form: radiation, x-rays

radioactive pert. to *radioactivity*

radioactivity quality exhibited by certain substances, in which atoms disintegrate with accompanying release of energy in the form of rays

radiocarpal joint *joint* between the *radius* and *carpal* bones

radiodermatitis skin *inflammation* due to exposure to strong x-rays

radioepidermitis *radiodermatitis*

radioimmunoassay examination procedure using *radioactive* substances to detect *antibodies* or *antigens* in the blood; abbr. RIA

radioiodine therapy radiotherapy of *thyroid* tumors or their *metastases* by application of *radioactive* iodine

radiological pert. to *radiology*

radiologist specialist in *radiology*

radiology study of the use of radiation for diagnosis and treatment of disease

radionuclide unstable atom (*isotope*) that converts to a stable state after emitting radiation

radiopharmaceutical drug that emits radiation

radius lower arm bone on the thumb side, opposite the *ulna*

radix root

radix dentis *dental root*

radix linguae *root of the tongue*

rales (crackles) crackling sound heard in the lungs on auscultation

ram- combining form: branch

ramus branch

ramus circumflexus *circumflex artery*

ramus interventricularis anterior *anterior interventricular artery*

RAP abbr. *right atrial pressure*

raphe seam; ridge

rapid eye movements cyclical eye movements during sleep abbr. REM

raptus sudden burst of movement

rash transient skin eruption, e.g. due to *multiple causes*

ratbite necrosis fingertip *necroses* that classically occur in *scleroderma*

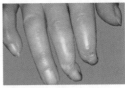

Fig. 390: ratbite necrosis

ratio 1) relationship between two numbers; 2) reason, rationality

rational based on reason or fact

raucedo (raucitas) hoarseness

Raynaud's disease disorder affecting the fingers, causing to paroxysmal arterial spasms that result in painful *ischemias* in the fingers or toes

RBBB abbr. *right bundle branch block*

RCA abbr. *right coronary artery*

RCX abbr. *circumflex artery*

RDS abbr. *respiratory distress syndrome*

re- combining form: back, again

reactive 1) responsive to a stimulus; 2) opposing or counteracting

reanimate to resuscitate or revive

reanimation resuscitation procedures after respiratory or circulatory arrest, e.g. *defibrillation*, ventilation, *cardiac massage*

rebound pain *Blumberg's sign*

rebound phenomenon exaggerated contrary motion when resistance is removed (see *rebound test*); associated with diseases of the cerebellum

rebound test test in which the patient is to extend the elbow with fist clenched working against resistance placed on the joint by the examiner; in diseases of the cerebellum, removal of the resistance results in uncontrolled movement upwards (caution: risk of injury)

rebreathing system (circle system) rebreathing apparatus for use during general anesthesia, in which the exhaled air is passed through a CO_2 absorber and partly reinhaled by the patient; opp. *non-rebreathing system*

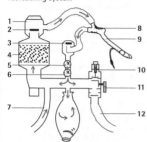

Fig. 391: rebreathing (closed) system
1 Oxygen probe 2 Inspiratory valve 3 Expiratory valve 4 CO_2 absorber (absorbent lime)
5 Volumometer 6 Pressure gauge 7 Fresh gas inflow
8 Y-piece 9 Tube 10 Pressure relief valve 11 Manual switch 12 Anesthesia gas exhaust system

Fig. 392: rectal prolapse

Fig. 393: rectal speculum [A]

recanalization reopening of an occluded blood vessel
receptor 1) sensory nerve ending; 2) cell structure that receives chemical or physical stimuli
recessive less strong, hidden, e.g. pert. to heredity; opp. *dominant*
reciprocal mutual; interchangeable
Recklinghausen's disease *neurofibromatosis*
reclination bending the *cervical*, *thoracic* or *lumbar spine* backwards; opp. *inclination*
reconstruction rebuilding
rect– combining form: rectum
rectal pert. to the *rectum*
rectal carcinoma malignant tumor of the *rectum*, usually an *adenocarcinoma*
rectal prolapse (proctocele) prolapse of all the layers of the *rectum*, usually due to pelvic floor *insufficiency*; cf. *anal prolapse*
rectal speculum *speculum*, e.g. according to Sims, inserted into the *rectum* for *proctological* examination or treatment

rectal temperature body temperature measured in the *rectum*
rectoscope rigid *endoscope* for *rectoscopy* longer than a *proctoscope*

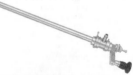

Fig. 394: rectoscope [F]

rectoscopic pert. to *rectoscopy*
rectoscopy *endoscopy* of the *rectum*
rectum last section of the *intestine* before the *anal sphincter*
rectus straight
rectus abdominis muscle muscle of the anterior abdominal wall that lowers the ribs and lifts the pelvis; innervation: *costal nerves*

recurrent laryngeal nerve branch of the *vagus nerve*, controls the vocal cords

recurrent nerve paresis paresis of the vocal cords and hoarseness due to damage to the *recurrent laryngeal nerve*, e.g. after *thyroid surgery*

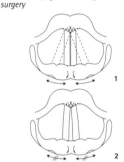

Fig. 395: recurrent nerve paresis
1 Normal vocal cord mobility
2 Bilateral recurrent nerve paresis

redon bottle vacuum bottle used to suck off blood and other secretions from the wound area after surgical operations

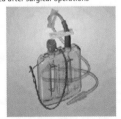

Fig. 396: redon bottle [J]

reduce to perform a *reduction*
reduced lessened

reduction restoring an *organ* or body part to its normal *anatomical* position, e.g. after a *fracture* or *hernia*

Reed-Sternberg cell (Sternberg-Reed cell; Sternberg's giant cell) type of *cell* consisting of merged *Hodgkin cells,* typical of *Hodgkin's lymphoma*

reentry cycling of an electrical impulse, usually associated with cardiac dysrhythmias, e.g. *paroxysmal supraventricular tachycardia*

refertilization *surgical* restoration of *fertility*

reflex involuntary reaction to a given stimulus

reflex arc chain of neurological events involved in a *reflex*

reflex hammer hammer for testing reflexes by percussion of muscles and tendons, e.g. *patellar reflex*

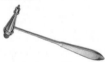

Fig. 397: reflex hammer [A]

reflex incontinence involuntary loss of urine due to abnormal *spinal detrusor reflex* activity, e.g. in *paraplegia*

reflex rating scale 0 = absent, despite reinforcement; 1 = sluggish; hypoactive; 2 = active; 3 = very lively; 4 = pathologically brisk; 5 = sustained clonus

reflexive pert. to a *reflex*

reflux backward flow

reflux cystogram *reflux cystography*

reflux cystography (*reflux cystogram*) *radiography* of the bladder, and sometimes also of the *ureters,* using a *contrast medium*; performed by filling the bladder directly with CM and then emptying it by pressing

reflux esophagitis *esophagitis* caused by reflux of gastric juice into the *esophagus*

refraction deflection of light rays, e.g. by the eye or an eyeglass lens

refractory resistant, unable to be influenced; disease that has not responded to initial therapy

regeneration recovery or renewal, e.g. of *tissue* from previous damage

regional anesthesia (local anesthesia) *anesthesia* limited to a region of the body, e.g. using a *local anesthetic* for performing *surgery* without loss of consciousness; opp. *general anesthesia*

regression return or relapse to a previous state, e.g. to childish behavior patterns

regulator device with a pressure gauge that is connected to a gas tank (e.g. an *oxygen tank*); regulates the flow of gas as it leaves the tank; some regulators are combined with a *flowmeter*

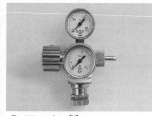

Fig. 398: regulator [H]

regurgitation backward flow, e.g. of stomach contents into the oral cavity

rehabilitate to reintegrate

rehabilitation occupational or social reintegration

rehydration replacement of lost body fluids, e.g. via *infusion*

Reiter's syndrome *inflammatory* disorder of the joints that results from *gastrointestinal* or *urogenital bacterial infection*; affects primarily the knee and ankle joints

rejection reaction defensive reaction of the body against a transplanted *organ*

relaps- combining form: relapse

relapse reappearance of a disease after apparent healing

relapsing recurring

relapsing fever *infectious disease* characterized by cyclic recurrence of febrile episodes, caused by the pathogens *Borrelia recurrentis* (louse-borne relapsing fever) or *Borrelia duttoni* (tick-borne relapsing fever); leads to circulatory collapse, spleen damage and joint inflammations; transmitted by the body louse (louse-borne type) or tick bites (tick-borne type)

relaxant *muscle relaxant*

relaxation slackening of a muscle, e.g. due to use of a *muscle relaxant* for surgery

releasing hormone hormone produced by the *hypothalamus* that controls the formation or release of other *hormones* in the *pituitary gland*

reliability statistical term for the reproducibility of measured results

REM abbr. *rapid eye movements*

remineralization replacement of mineral substances, e.g. of *calcium* in the bones

remission temporary abatement of disease symptoms

remitting improving temporarily

ren- combining form: kidney

ren kidney; pl. renes

renal pert. to the *kidneys*

renal agenesia failure of the *kidneys* to develop

renal aplasia *rudimentary* development of the *kidneys*

renal colic sudden pain in the *kidneys*, usually due to *nephrolithiasis*

renal cyst *cyst* in the kidney *tissues*; see also *polycystic kidney*

renal duplication presence of two renal calices with two *ureters* branching off of one kidney; see also *uretur fissus, ureter duplex*

R

renal failure insufficient *kidney* function marked by insufficient formation of urine, resulting in an increase in blood levels of substances normally excreted in the urine and imbalances in water and *electrolytes*; see also *nephrotic syndrome*

renal hilum point where the renal vessels enter the *kidney*

renal hypoplasia (contracted kidney) *kidney* weighing less than 50 g

renal tubule tubule that carries *primary urine* from the *glomerulus* toward the *renal pelvis*; along the way the *primary urine* is partially reabsorbed by the body

renal vein (vena renalis) *vein* that transports blood from the kidney to the *inferior vena cava*

Rendell–Baker mask *ventilation* mask with no inflatable ring, specifically intended for noninvasive ventilation in children

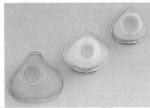

Fig. 399: Rendell–Baker masks [H]

renin *hormone* produced by the *kidneys* that regulates the water and *electrolyte* balance, as well as *blood pressure*

reparable able to be restored or repaired; opp. *irreparable*

replacement transfusion *exchange transfusion*

repolarization restoration of an electrical voltage gradient

RES abbr. *reticuloendothelial system*

rescue grip underarm hold used in first aid to drag a person to safety

resect to perform a *resection*

resection *surgical* removal of *tissue*

reservoir place of storage, container

residual left behind, remaining afterward

residual urine urine remaining in the *bladder* after seemingly complete evacuation

residual volume amount of air remaining in the lungs after a maximal expiration; abbr. RV; see illustration under *spirometry*

resistance ability to oppose or fight off

resistant able to oppose or fight off

resonance resounding

resorb to absorb, draw up

resorption absorption or drawing up of substances

respir- combining form: breathing

respiration breathing

respirator ventilation device

respiratory pert. to *respiration*

respiratory acidosis form of *acidosis* caused by respiratory disturbances, characterized by a decrease in the *pH* to below 7.36 and an increase in the pCO_2 to above 45 mmHg, e.g. due to *hypoventilation*

respiratory alkalosis form of *alkalosis* caused by respiratory disturbances, characterized by an increase in the *pH* to above 7.44 and a decrease in the pCO_2, e.g. due to *hyperventilation*

respiratory arrhythmia harmless *dysrhythmia* caused by respiratory influences, often occurring in children

respiratory center respiratory regulation system located in the *medulla oblongata*

respiratory depression lessened respiration e.g. due to a drug

respiratory distress syndrome (of the preterm infant) *syndrome* marked by *cyanosis*, *dyspnea* and/or *tachypnea* in a newborn, e.g. due to lack of *surfactant*; abbr. RDS

respiratory failure impairment of external respiration that leads to reduced levels of *oxygen* in the *arterial* blood; types are: partial failure, marked by decreased oxygen but normal or slightly low *carbon dioxide* levels in the blood, and global failure, marked by low oxygen and high carbon dioxide levels

respiratory rate number of breaths per minute

respiratory tract respiratory organs

responsive disease disease that responds to therapy

resting tremor trembling of the fingers while at rest, e.g. due to overactivity of the *thyroid gland*

restitution restoration

restless legs syndrome itching or creeping sensation in the legs, usually occurring at night, that improves when the legs are moved; e.g. associated with *polyneuropathy*

restriction limitation

restrictive ventilation disorder *ventilation disorder* due to *pulmonary restriction*

retardation slowing delay

retention keeping, retaining

reticular cell carcinoma malignant tumor of the *reticuloendothelial system*

reticular cells star-shaped *connective tissue* cells that form into networks; important element of the *reticuloendothelial system*

reticulocyte immature *erythrocyte* containing fragments of *cell* organelles

reticulocytosis increase in *reticulocytes* in the blood; sign of increased *erythropoiesis*

reticuloendothelial system body system that controls various metabolic processes and plays a role in the *immune system* via *phagocytosis* and *antibody* formation; abbr. RES

retin- combining form: retina

retina inner membrane of the *eye* where *optic nerve* stimuli are received

retinal detachment pathological separation of the *retina* of the eye

retinitis *inflammation* of the *retina*

retinoblastoma malignant tumor of the *retina* occurring during childhood

retinoids derivatives of *retinol*

retinol (vitamin A) fat-soluble *vitamin* with an important role in *cell* growth; formed from the *provitamin beta-carotene*; vitamin A deficiency leads to *night blindness* and *corneal* clouding, among other things

retinopathy noninflammatory disease of the *retina*, see Fig. 403

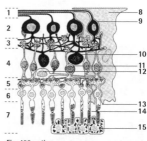

Fig. 400: retina
1 Nerve fiber layer 2 Ganglion cell layer 3 Inner plexiform layer 4 Inner nuclear layer 5 Outer plexiform layer 6 Outer nuclear layer 7 Receptors 8 Müller cell (glia) 9 Ganglion cell 10 Amacrine cell 11 Bipolar cell 12 Horizontal cell 13 Cone 14 Rod 15 Pigment epithelium

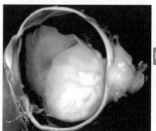

Fig. 401: retinoblastoma

retract- combining form: withdraw, pull back

retractor (bone hook) *surgical* instrument with a single hook used for various holding tasks during surgery

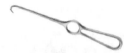

Fig. 402: retractor [A]

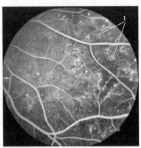

Fig. 403: microaneurysms (1) in diabetic retinopathy (fluorescent angiogram)

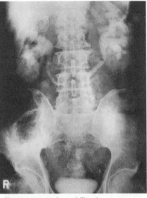

Fig. 404: retroperitoneal fibrosis
Excretion urogram

retro- combining form: backward, behind, back

retrobulbar behind the eyeball

retroflexion backward flexion; opp. *anteflexion*

retrograde moving backward in space or time; from behind; opp. *anterograde*

retrograde amnesia *amnesia* in which the loss of memory relates to events that occurred prior to the traumatic event

retromandibular vein *vein* running from the ear toward the lower jaw, which joins the *facial vein*

retroperitoneal pert. to the *retroperitoneum*

retroperitoneal fibrosis (Ormond's disease) *usually idiopathic* form of *retroperitoneal fibrosis* with urinary obstruction due to compression of the *ureters*

retroperitoneum space behind the abdominal cavity between the *diaphragm* and *spinal column*

retrosternal behind the *sternum*

retroversion tendency to rotate the arm backward in the *sagittal plane*; opp. *anteversion*

retrovirus *RNA virus*

reversible able to be reversed; opp. *irreversible*

RF abbr. *rheumatoid factor*; *rheumatic fever*; risk factor

Rh factor surface property of *erythrocytes* that is determined along with the *blood group* prior to a *transfusion*; the presence or absence of the factor (also called antigen D) on the erythrocytes is the main determinant: antigen D present = Rh positive; antigen D absent = Rh negative

rhabdomyolysis destruction of skeletal muscle, e.g. due to *compartment syndrome*

rhabdomyoma benign tumor of skeletal muscle

rhabdomyosarcoma malignant tumor of skeletal muscle

rhagades fissures in the skin; one of the *secondary efflorescences*

rheology study of the flow properties of blood

Rhesus factor *Rh factor*

rheumatic disease collective term for painful conditions of the *joints*, muscles, *nerves* and tendons

rheumatic fever *inflammatory* disorder that mainly affects the major joints; usually appears 1 to 4 weeks after *infection* with group A *beta-hemolytic streptococci*; abbr. RF

rheumatism *rheumatic disease*

rheumatoid pert. to *rheumatic disease*

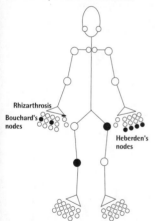

Rhizarthrosis

Bouchard's nodes

Heberden's nodes

Fig. 405: joints affected in rheumatoid polyarthritis

rheumatoid arthritis (chronic polyarthritis) form of *arthritis* triggered by immune reactions; affects primarily the joints of the musculoskeletal system, as well as the tendon sheaths and synovial *bursae*; classical manifestations include *ulnar deviation, boutonnière deformity* and *swan neck deformity* of the hands; abbr. RA

rheumatoid factor *autoantibody* that appears as a result of *rheumatic* disease, e.g. *polyarthritis*; abbr. RF

-rhexis combining form: rupture

rhin(o)- combining form: nose

rhinitis (coryza) *inflammation* of the nasal mucosa

rhinolalia nasal-sounding speech

rhinologic agent drug used to treat diseases of the nose

rhinology study of diseases of the nose

rhinomanometry measurement of pressure and volume for assessing patency of the nasal passages

rhinophyma bulbous swelling of the nose

rhinoscopy *endoscopy* of the nasal cavity; methods are anterior rhinoscopy (visualization through the nostril using a *nasal speculum*) and posterior rhinoscopy (visual. via the *pharynx* using a mirror)

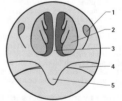

Fig. 406: rhinoscopy
1 Tubal orifice 2 Nasal conchae 3 Nasal septum
4 Soft palate 5 Uvula

rhis nose

rhizo- combining form: root

rhodo- combining form: red, rosy

rhonchus wheezing, squeaking or snoring breath sounds

rhythm regularly repeating sequence of beats or impulses, e.g. heart rhythms

R

RIA abbr. *radioimmunoassay*

rib flat, hollow bones that originate at the *spinal column* and arch around to enclose the chest cavity; most attach to the *sternum* in front

rib bone bony part of a *rib*

riboflavin (lactoflavin, vitamin B₂); water-soluble vitamin with a role in various chemical reactions in the body; vitamin B₂ deficiency can lead to *pellagra*

ribonucleic acid messenger molecule where the genetic information from *DNA* is transcribed; abbr. RNA

rice-water stool watery, cloudy stools occurring in *cholera*

rickets disease caused by *vitamin D* deficiency, leading to softening of the bones

Rickettsia genus of rod-shaped or spherical *gram-negative bacteria*

Rickettsia prowazekii *bacterium* of the *Rickettsia* genus that causes *epidemic typhus*

Rift Valley fever *viral hemorrhagic fever*

right atrial pressure pressure in the right atrium of the *heart*, which can be measured using a *pulmonary artery catheter*; normal value: 45 mmHg; elevated in right heart failure, e.g. due to right-side *myocardial infarction, pulmonary embolism, hypervolemia, tricuspid valve insufficiency,* or *cardiac tamponade*; depressed in *hypovolemia*; abbr. RAP

right bundle branch block (Wilson Block) interruption in electrical conduction in the right *Tawara branch* of the heart; abbr. RBBB

right coronary artery *coronary artery* that supplies the right *ventricle* posterior wall of the left ventricle and the posterior third of the *septum*; abbr. RCA

right heart failure see *heart failure*

right hepatic veins veins that transport blood from the right lobe of the liver to the *inferior vena cava*

right suprarenal vein *vein* that transports blood from the right *adrenal gland* to the *inferior vena cava*

right-to-left shunt pathological connection between the *arterial* and *venous* circu-lation occurring inside or outside the heart

rigid stiff; inflexible

rigor heightened muscular tension, e.g. in *Parkinson's disease*

rigor mortis stiffening of the *joints* beginning after death, which reverses as putrefaction processes begin; depending on the ambient temperature, rigor can begin just 2 hours after death, starting in the lower jaw and spreading downward

rima fold, split

rima ani cleft between the buttocks

ringworm *microsporosis*

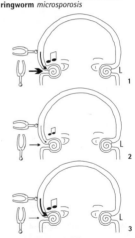

Fig. 407: Rinne test, right ear
1 Normal hearing: air conduction (AC) > bone conduction (BC)
2 Perceptive deafness, right ear: AC > BC
3 Conduction deafness, right ear: AC < BC

Rinne test hearing examination in which bone conduction is tested using a vibrating *tuning fork* (which is placed against the mastoid process of the ear), as well as air conduction (holding the tuning fork in front of the ear); normally air conduction exceeds bone conduction

risus sardonicus distortion of the facial muscles due to *tetanus*

RIVA abbr. *ramus interventricularis anterior*

RNA abbr. *ribonucleic acid*

RNA virus (retrovirus) *virus* with a single strand of *RNA* as its genetic material

roeteln *rubella*

Rolando fracture Y- or T-shaped *fracture* of the first metacarpal, with *joint* involvement; see also *Winterstein fracture* and *Bennett fracture*

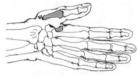

Fig. 408: Rolando fracture

Romberg's maneuver neurologic assessment of cerebellar function; see *Romberg test*

Romberg test *neurological* test in which the patient stands with eyes closed, arms extended and feet together; if he sways or falls, the test is positive, e.g. in sensory *ataxia*

rooming-in keeping an infant and mother together in the same hospital room

root of the tongue posterior part of the tongue extending to the *epiglottis*

rosacea chronic skin disease that primarily affects the cheeks, forehead, chin and nose

roseola dilation of blood vessels caused by toxins, appearing on the skin as small bright red spots that turn white when depressed with a finger or instrument

rotat- combining form: turning

rotation turning

rotavirus common type of *virus* that can cause *gastroenteritis;* found worldwide

round lesion rounded opacity on an *x-ray* image

round pronator muscle flexor muscle of the arm that enables adduction of the forearm; innervation: *median nerve*

rounds physician's visit to patients

Roux retractor tissue-preserving double-ended *retractor* according to Roux

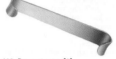

Fig. 409: Roux retractor [A]

Roux-en-Y anastomosis Y-shaped *surgical anastomosis* between the *resected* stomach and immobilized, *jejunum* e.g. in *gastric carcinoma*

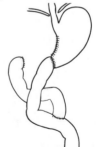

Fig. 410: Roux-en-Y gastrojejunostomy

RR abbr. respiratory rate

rubella (German measles) *infectious disease* caused by the *rubivirus*, which leads to a skin rash beginning on the face and spreading to the entire body, with medium-sized spots (larger than in *scarlet fever* but smaller than *measles*); can lead to *arthritis* or *meningitis* in some cases; transmitted by droplet infection

rubella embryopathy damage to the *embryo* caused by *rubella infection* in the mother; usually results in severe deformities

rubeola *measles*

rubeola virus virus that causes *measles*; one of the *paramyxoviruses*

rubivirus *RNA* virus that causes *rubella*

rubor redness; see also *signs of inflammation*

rubr- combining form: red

ructus belching

rudiment underdeveloped, remnant or vestige

rudimentary un(der)developed, vestigial

rule of nines Wallace's rule for estimating the *body surface area* by percentages; used for quick estimation of the extent of *burns*

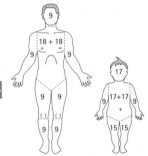

Fig. 411: rule of nines for estimating body surface area (percentages include front and back of body)

rumination voluntary regurgitation of *stomach* contents to be chewed again

rumor noise; sound

Rumpel-Leede test test for bleeding tendency, in which constriction of the upper arm for 5 minutes results in *petechiae* on the forearm

runny nose *rhinitis*

rupture tearing apart of *tissue* or *organs* (as *in a hernia*)

rupture of (fetal) membranes rupture of the *amnion* during the birth process

Russian spring-summer encephalitis *infectious disease* affecting the brain (*encephalitis*) caused by the *CEE virus;* transmitted via bites from infected lice

RV abbr. *residual volume*

S

S wave negative wave in the *QRS complex* as seen in an *ECG*; duration < 0.06 seconds

s.c. abbr. *subcutaneous*

s.l. abbr. *sublingual*

S.P. abbr. *status post*

SA block abbr. *sinoatrial block*

SAB abbr. *subarachnoid bleed*

Sabin vaccine oral vaccine for *poliomyelitis*

saccharo- combining form: sugar

sacculated kidney *hydronephrosis*

sacculus small sac

saccus sac

saccus lacrimalis lacrimal sac

sacral pert. to the *sacrum*

sacral plexus nerve *plexus* in the *sacral* area (branches of the L4-S4 spinal nerves) that includes the *nervus gluteus inferior* and *nervus gluteus superior*, et al.

sacrodynia pain in the *sacral* area

sacroiliac joint *articulation* between the *sacrum* and *ilium*

sacrum part of the *spinal column* between the *lumbar spine* and the *coccyx*, consisting of 5 fused *vertebrae*; see illustration under *pelvis*

sacrum, os *(os sacrum)* sacrum

saddle block anesthesia *sensory* disorder in the external *genitalia*, *anus*, *perineum* and inner thigh (the areas that would be in contact with the saddle when riding horseback) due to damage to the *caudal spinal cord*, e.g. in connection with *cauda equina syndrome*

sadism sexual gratification resulting from causing *mental* or *physical* pain to the partner

SAE abbr. *subcortical arteriosclerotic encephalopathy* (Binswanger's dementia)

sagittal plane body plane extending back to front, from the crown of the head through the center of the body and down between the feet; used in the context of imaging procedures

sagittal suture suture between the *parietal bones* of the skull

saliva spittle; *secretions* of the *salivary glands*

salivation secretion of *saliva*

Salmonella genus of motile rod-shaped *gram-negative bacteria* that produce *endotoxins* and cause *infectious diseases* such as *typhoid fever* (S. typhi) *paratyphoid fever* (S. paratyphi) *acute gastroenteritis* (S. enteritidis) or *enteric fever* (S. typhimurium)

salmonellosis collective term for *infectious diseases* caused by *Salmonellas*

salpingectomy *surgical* removal of a *fallopian tube*

salpingitis *inflammation* of the *fallopian tube* mucosa, e.g. due to *gonorrhea*

salpingopalatine fold mucosal fold in the lateral wall of the *pharynx*

salpinx *fallopian tube* or *eustachian tube*

Salter I *Aitken 0*
Salter II *Aitken I*
Salter III *Aitken II*
Salter IV *Aitken III*
Salter V *Aitken IV*

Salter–Harris classification classification system for epiphyseal growth plate injuries; see *Aitken*

saluretic drug used to increase excretion of *electrolytes* in the urine

sample excision excision of a tissue sample for examination

sanctions penalties, especially for violating a moral principle or international law

sanguis blood

sanitation taking measures to ensure hygienic conditions and prevent disease

sapro– combining form: decay, putrescence

saprogenic causing putrefaction

saprophytes *bacteria* that live and thrive on dead *tissue*

sarco– combining form: decay

sarcoidosis (Boeck's sarcoid) disease affecting the entire body, marked by formation of *granulomas* in the *lungs*, internal *organs*, skin and *lymph nodes*

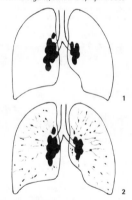

Fig. 412: sarcoidosis

sarcoma malignant tumor of the *connective* and supporting *tissues*

sarcomatosis *metastasis* of a *sarcoma* through the entire body

Sarcoptes scabiei (itch mite) species of mite whose female causes *scabies*

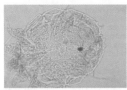

Fig. 413: Sarcoptes scabiei

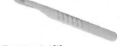

Fig. 415: scalpel [A]

SAS abbr. *sleep apnea syndrome*
scab *crust*
scabbard trachea indentation of the *trachea* due to a tumor or *goiter*
scabies *infectious disease* caused by *Sarcoptes scabiei* mites, leading to skin disease marked by rash, severe itching and mite burrows in the skin; transmitted by skin or sexual contact, or infested clothing

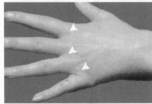

Fig. 414: scabies mite burrows

scald *burn* caused by moist heat, e.g. boiling water)
scale *squama*
scalenus syndrome (costocervical syndrome) damage to the *subclavian artery* and *brachial plexus* due to compression, marked by impaired circulation, pain and numbness
scalp avulsion tearing away of the *scalp*
scalpel fixed-blade surgical knife with variously shaped blades, used for diverse cutting tasks in *surgery*

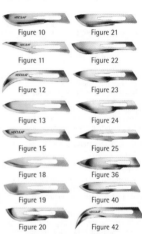

Figure 10	Figure 21
Figure 11	Figure 22
Figure 12	Figure 23
Figure 13	Figure 24
Figure 15	Figure 25
Figure 18	Figure 36
Figure 19	Figure 40
Figure 20	Figure 42

Fig. 416: scalpel blades (Feather) [A]

scan sectional image of the body created with *ultrasound*
scapha (scaphoid fossa) furrow in the external *ear* between the *helix* and *antihelix*
scaphoid bone one of the *carpal bones*
scapul- combining form: shoulder blade
scapula (shoulder blade) flat, triangular bone of the upper back
scapular fracture rare *fracture* of the *scapula*, usually occurring in connection with *polytrauma*

scapular line imaginary line used as a body surface landmark; passes along the back into the inferior angle of the *scapula*; abbr. *SL*; see illustration under *paravertebral line*

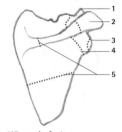

Fig. 417: scapular fractures
1 Coracoid process 2 Acromion 3 Glenoid fossa
4 Scapular neck 5 Fracture lines

scarlatina *scarlet fever*
scarlet fever (scarlatina) febrile *infectious disease* caused by *toxin*-forming *beta-hemolyzing* group A *streptococci*; usually begins with *angina* and leads to a pinpoint rash (smaller than in *rubella*) over the entire body, as well as the classic mucosal rash ("strawberry tongue"); in severe cases there may be diarrhea, vomiting and *myocarditis*, caused by the toxins; transmitted mainly by *droplet* and *smear infection*
scato- combining form: feces; stool
SCCA abbr. *squamous cell carcinoma antigen*
Schanz cervical collar (neck brace) padded supportive collar for immobilization of the *cervical spine*, e.g. after a *whiplash injury*
Schellong test circulation test to detect *orthostatic dysregulation* (e.g. in *autonomic neuropathy*) by measuring *pulse* and *blood pressure* in supine and standing positions, as well as before and after exertion

Scheuermann's disease *aseptic necrosis* of the vertebral laminae and end plates with development of structural *kyphosis*
Schick test skin test to check *diphtheria immunity*
Schilling test test to assess intestinal absorption of oral *vitamin B_{12}*
Schirmer's test test for reduced tear production by laying a strip of paper in the conjunctival sac for 5 minutes, followed by assessment of the wet area: < 15 mm = *pathological*, e.g. in *Sjögren's syndrome*

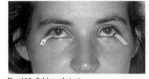

Fig. 418: Schirmer's test

–schisis combining form: split
schist– combining form: split
Schistosoma genus of tropical parasitic blood flukes that cause *schistosomiasis*
Schistosoma haematobium tropical parasitic blood fluke that causes urinary *schistosomiasis*
Schistosoma japonicum tropical parasitic blood fluke that causes Oriental *schistosomiasis*
Schistosoma mansoni tropical parasitic blood fluke that causes intestinal *schistosomiasis*

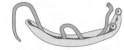

Fig. 419: Schistosoma mansoni

schistosomiasis *infectious disease* caused by *Schistosoma haematobium* (urinary schistosomiasis), *Schistosoma mansoni*

S

(intestinal schistosomiasis) or *Schistosoma japonicum* (Oriental schistosomiasis) that results in damage to various organs; *infection* usually occurs in stagnant water where the larvae of the intermediate host snail are excreted and picked up by the final human host through the skin

schizo- combining form: split

schizophrenia *psychosis* characterized by an abnormal relationship to the external world with regard to perception, experience and thought, but which does not limit the patient's intellectual abilities

Schmorl's nodes breaks in the vertebral end plates and laminae with prolapse of the *nucleus pulposus* into the vertebral body; classic sign of *Scheuermann's disease*

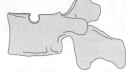

Fig. 420: Schmorl's nodes

Schönlein's disease *idiopathic thrombocytopenic purpura*

Schröder's sign sign of placental abruption in which the *fundus* of the *uterus* is elevated and the transverse diameter of the *uterus* is reduced

sciatic nerve (nervus ischiadicus) large nerve running along the back of the thigh; provides *innervation* for the *semitendinous* and *semimembranous muscles*, et al.; irritation leads to *sciatica*

sciatica inflammation of the sciatic nerve; characterized by pain from the lower back to the ankle; travels the length of the sciatic nerve and is usually posterior; relieved by trigger point injections into buttocks and by physical therapy

scint- combining form: sparkle, glitter

scintigram *scintigraphy*

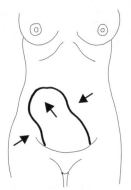

Fig. 421: Schröder's sign

scintigraphic pert. to *scintigraphy*

scintigraphy (scintigram) examination procedure in *nuclear medicine* for visualizing *organs* and organ functions using *radioactive* substances

scintillating scotoma vision impairment marked by sudden lightning-like flashes, e.g. in *migraines*

scler(o)- combining form: hard

sclera outer layer of the *eye*; thick white *connective tissue* coating, containing elastic fibers with an outer layer of connective tissue (*episclera*)

scleral staphyloma protrusion of the *sclera*, such that the blue *choroid* can be seen through it

scleral venous sinus *canal of Schlemm*

scleroderma (progressive systemic sclerosis) *autoimmune disease* of the vascular system and *connective tissue*; classical symptoms are, e.g., *ratbite necrosis*, mask-like face and *Raynaud's syndrome*; abbr. PSS

sclerose to harden

-sclerosis combining form: hardening

sclerosis hardening e.g. of *varices*

sclerotherapy treatment by sclerosing diseased veins or cavities, either surgically or via *injection* of a sclerosing agent, e.g. for treatment of *varicose veins*

sclerotic hardened

scolio- combining form: curved

scoliosis lateral curvature of the spine

-scope combining form: viewing instrument

-scopy combining form: visual examination

scotoma reduction or complete loss of the *visual field*

scratch test (prick test) *allergy* test in which an *allergen* is applied to a scratch on the skin

screening mass testing of a population for investigative purposes

Scribner shunt *tube* used to create a *shunt* between an *artery* and a *vein* in the forearm for *dialysis*

scrotal pert. to the *scrotum*

scrotal hernia complete inguinal hernia located in the scrotum

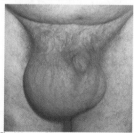

Fig. 422: scrotal hernia

scrotum pouch of skin containing the male's *testicles* and *epididymis*

scurvy disease caused by *vitamin C* deficiency characterized by tooth loss, impaired wound healing and bleeding diathesis

se- combining form: away, apart

seasonal illness illness connected with the season, e.g. hayfever or the *common cold*

sebaceous cyst *atheroma*

sebaceous glands (glandulae sebaceae) *sebum*-producing glands that open into the hair follicles of the skin

sebo- combining form: fat

seborrhea increased production of *sebum* by the skin; opp. *sebostasis*

sebostasis decreased production of *sebum* by the skin; opp. *seborrhea*

sebum collective term for fatty substances solid at normal temperature, that are produced by the body's *sebaceous glands* to protect the skin

second-look operation followup *operation* performed after extirpation of a malignant tumor in order to remove any subsequent *metastases* as early as possible

secondary second in a sequence, second in importance; see also *primary*, *tertiary*

secondary efflorescence skin condition developing from a *primary efflorescence*, e.g. *squama*, crust erosion, excoriation, *rhagades*, ulceration, *cicatrix*, *necrosis* and atrophy

secondary healing see *healing*

secondary hemorrhage bleeding after an *operation*, childbirth or normal *menstruation*

secrete to discharge a *secretion*

secretin *hormone* that stimulates *bile* flow, produced in the *duodenal* mucosa under the influence of *gastric acid*; inhibited by *gastrin*

secretion fluid discharge, e.g. from the respiratory tract or a *wound*

secretion bag (ostomy bag) plastic bag for collection of *secretions* from a *stomach tube* or other type of *drainage* via an integrated tubing system

secretolytic drug used to liquefy *secretions*

sect- combining form: cutting

sectio cut; *section*

section 1) process of cutting; 2) area or division of an organ

S

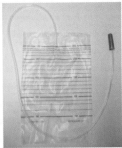

Fig. 423: secretion bag

secund- combining form: two
sedat- combining form: calming
sedate to tranquilize
sedation administration of a tranquilizer
sedative tranquilizer; having tranquilizing qualities
sediment precipitate or residue from *centrifugation* or deposition, e.g. *urine sediment*
seeds *radioactive* capsules placed inside the body for irradiation of tumors
segment portion; area; piece
segmental spinovertebral syndrome disease marked by pain in the *dermatome* of one or more *spinal nerves*, e.g. due to *disk prolapse*
seizure sudden, excessive discharge of cerebral neurons; a) **partial** (focal): begins in one or more cortical areas; aura, déjà-vu, and clonic movements of a limb are the hallmarks of this type seizure; b) **generalized**; begin simultaneously in both hemispheres; grand mal seizures are the hallmark of this type
selective proximal vagotomy see *vagotomy*
self-retaining retractor (wound retractor) surgical instrument; e.g. according to Weitlaner, for holding wound edges apart during minor procedures or for wound care

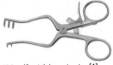

Fig. 424: self-retaining retractor [A]

sella saddle
sella turcica depression on the sphenoid bone where the pituitary gland sits
semen combination of *sperm* cells and seminal fluid

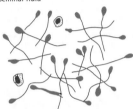

Fig. 425: semen

semi- combining form: half
semimembranous muscle muscle that flexes the knee; innervation: *sciatic nerve*
semin combining form: seed; sperm
seminoma malignant *testicular* tumor originating in the spermatogenic *tissues*
semiopen anesthesia system *nonrebreathing system*
semipermeable partially permeable
semitendinous muscle muscle that flexes the knee; *innervation sciatic nerve*
senex (geron) elderly person
Sengstaken-Blakemore tube inflatable probe inserted into the nose or mouth to stop bleeding from *esophageal varices*
senil- combining form: old, elderly
senium old age
sensation perception of sensory stimuli, physical feeling

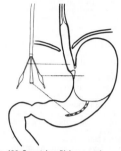

Fig. 426: Sengstaken–Blakemore tube

sensi- combining form: sensitive, sensation
sensibilization *sensitization*
sensitive 1) pert. to *sensitivity*;
    2) susceptible
sensitivity ability to perceive emotional and
    sensory impressions
sensitization (sensibilization) increase in the
    sensitivity of the body's *immune system* to
    foreign, potentially *allergenic* substances;
    opp. *desensitization*
sensory pert. to the senses
sensory disturbance disorder of perception
    or sensation, e.g. due to disease or injury to
    the *nerves*
sensory nervous system part of the *nervous
    system* that receives and conducts stimuli
sentinel event an unexpected occurrence
    involving death or serious injury in a
    healthcare setting, requiring immediate
    investigation and response (per Joint
    Commission on Accreditation of Healthcare
    Organizations)
sepsis *inflammatory* reaction affecting the
    entire body, caused by *bacteria* and/or
    their toxins in the blood; can lead to
    multiple organ failure
sepsis lenta insidious *sepsis*

sept(i)- combining form: seven
septic shock *shock* that can be triggered by
    sepsis
septicemia *inflammatory* reaction affecting
    the entire body, caused by *bacteria* and/or
    their toxins in the blood
septum partition or dividing wall; pl. septa
sequence series of events
sequential occurring in *sequence*
sequestration formation of a *sequestrum*
sequestrum dead section of an *organ* or
    tissue that has become separated from the
    remaining tissue inside the body
serial fractures multiple *fractures* of bones
    or bone groups, e.g. *serial rib fracture*

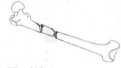

Fig. 427: serial fractures

serological pert. to *serum*
seroma accumulation of *serum* or *lymph* in
    the *tissues*
serosa collective term for membranes that
    line body cavities, e.g. the *pleura* or
    peritoneum
serotonin important *hormone* in the
    nervous system, formed from tryptophan
serous resembling *serum*
serum incoagulable fluid portion of blood,
    lacking *fibrinogen* and blood *cells*; pl. sera
sesqui- combining form: one and a half
sex- combining form: six
sexual pert. to sex
sexually transmitted disease disease that is
    transmitted through sexual intercourse, e.g.
    AIDS; abbr. STD
shaking palsy *Parkinson's disease*
shear fracture *fracture* caused by direct
    application of force at the borderline
    between supported and unsupported bone

S

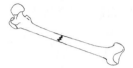

Fig. 428: shear fracture

Sheehan's syndrome disease caused by overactivity of the *adenohypophysis*

shift to the left increase in the number of young *leukocytes* in the blood count, e.g. due to *inflammation*

Shigella genus of nonmotile rodshaped gramnegative *bacteria* that cause *dysentery*

shigellosis *infectious disease* caused by *Shigella*, e.g. bacillary dysentery

shinbone *tibia*

shingles (herpes zoster, zoster) painful *infectious disease* caused by the *varicella-zoster virus*, usually occurring in immunosuppressed persons; it spreads in a beltlike pattern along a *dermatome* by affecting a *spinal nerve*; usually affects the chest area, with vesicles on a red background; usually transmitted via *droplet infection* by children who have *chicken pox*, by *smear infection*, or by reactivation of varicella-zoster virus lying dormant in the *glia* after recovery from chicken pox

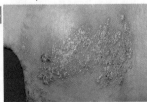

Fig. 429: shingles

shivering *chills*

shock serious circulatory disturbance with impaired circulation to the *tissues*, leading to *oxygen* deficiency in the tissues and metabolic disturbances; see also *hypovolemic shock, anaphylactic shock, cardiogenic shock, septic shock*

shock kidney *renal failure* caused by lack of circulation due to *shock*

shock lung *adult respiratory distress syndrome*

short adductor muscle short hip muscle that draws the thigh toward the midline; innervation: *obturator nerve*

short extensor muscle of the toes short muscle in the lower leg that extends the toes D2-D4; innervation: *deep peroneal* and *accessory nerve*

shoulder blade *scapula*

shunt 1) abnormal connection into the bloodstream; 2) artifical device to connect to the bloodstream, e.g. for *dialysis*

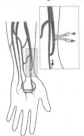

Fig. 430: shunt

sial(o)- combining form: saliva

sialoadenitis inflammation of a *salivary gland*

sialolith (salivary stone) solid object in a *salivary gland* or duct, leading to pain when eating

sialon (saliva, ptyalin) spittle

sicc- combining form: dry

SICU surgical intensive care unit

sick sinus syndrome sinus node syndrome

sickle cell anemia *anemia* marked by sickle-shaped *red blood cells*

side effect effect that accompanies a treatment

sidero- combining form: iron

sideroachrestic anemia *iron-deficiency anemia*

sideropenia *iron* deficiency

siderosis bulbi deposition of *iron* in the *eye*

sigmatism lisp; inability to produce the S sound and other sibilants, associated with *dyslalia*

sigmoid pert. to the *sigmoid colon*

sigmoid colon S-shaped final section of the large intestine, before the *rectum*

signet ring cell carcinoma form of *adenocarcinoma* with visible *intracellular* storage of mucin; usually in the *stomach*, *colon* and *rectum*

significant meaningful; of importance

signs of inflammation the five classic signs of inflammation according to Galen: redness (*rubor*), swelling (*tumor*), pain (*dolor*), heat (*calor*) and impaired function (*functio laesa*)

silic- combining form: quartz; silica

silicosis (black lung) *lung* disease caused by inhalation of dust containing silicic acid, e.g. among miners

silver-fork fracture (silver-fork deformity) malposition typical of radial extension fracture marked by dorsal displacement of the distal *radial* fragment

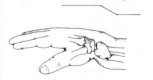

Fig. 431: silver-fork fracture

simplex simple
simulate mimic; pretend
simultaneous at the same time

sinciput presentation abnormal birth presentation in which the baby enters the birth canal with the front upper part of the head foremost

single button suture special *surgical* suturing technique for closing a wound

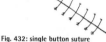

Fig. 432: single button suture

singultus *hiccups*

sinist(r)- combining form: left; opp. *dext(r)*

sinister left; opp. *dexter*

sinoatrial block conduction disorder between the *sinus node* and atrium, visible in an *ECG*; abbr. *SA block*

sinoatrial node (sinus node) primary impulse generator in the right atrium of the *heart*, which acts as a natural *pacemaker* and generates *impulses autonomically*; see also *excitation and conduction system*

sinus arrhythmia *cardiac dysrhythmia* in which the heart rate increase upon inspiration and decreases during expiration; common in children

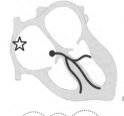

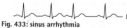

Fig. 433: sinus arrhythmia
I Schematic II ECG

S

sinus bradycardia *cardiac rhythm* originating in the *sinoatrial node* with a frequency of less than 60 per minute, visible in an *ECG*

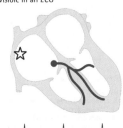

Fig. 434: sinus bradycardia
I Schematic II ECG

sinus cavernosus venous structure near the *sella turcica*; part of the *cranial sinus*

sinus cavity; hollow, channel

sinus coronarius *coronary sinus*

sinus frontalis *frontal sinus*

sinus node syndrome (sick sinus syndrome) *cardiac dysrhythmia*, visible in an *ECG*, caused by *sinoatrial node* malfunction; abbr. SSS

sinus rhythm (normal sinus rhythm) physiologic *cardiac rhythm* originating in the *sinoatrial node*, with a *frequency* of 60100 per minute, visible in an *ECG*

sinus tachycardia *cardiac rhythm* originating in the *sinoatrial node*, with a frequency of 100220 per minute, visible in an *ECG*

sinus thrombosis *thrombosis* in a *venous* sinus, e.g. in the brain, due to purulent *otitis media*

sinusitis *inflammation* of the *paranasal sinuses*

SIRS abbr. *systemic inflammatory response syndrome*

situs position, location, e.g. of the *organs* within the body

situs inversus viscerum mirror-image displacement of internal *organs*

Sjögren's syndrome *autoimmune* disease that affects the *lacrimal* and *salivary glands*, et al.; usually occurs in post*menopausal* women

skeleton bony framework of the body

SL abbr. *scapular line*

SLE abbr. *systemic lupus erythematosus*

sleep apnea syndrome cessation of breathing lasting more than 10 seconds and occurring more than 30 times per night; common in obese men; abbr. SAS

sleeping sickness (African trypanosomiasis, trypanosomiasis) tropical *infectious disease* caused by *Trypanosomes*, which leads to severe *central nervous system* damage, among other things; transmitted to humans by the *tsetse fly*

slide small rectangular glass plate for *microscopy*, onto which the specimen is placed or smeared

slit compress compress with slits for care of *drain* or *catheter* sites

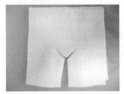

Fig. 435: slit compress

small intestine section of the intestine between the pylorus and the large intestine; comprises the *duodenum*, *jejunum* and *ileum*

small saphenous vein *vein* that takes blood from the outer edge of the foot to the *great saphenous vein* along the back of the leg

smallpox (variola) febrile *infectious disease* caused by the *variola virus*, considered eradicated since 1977 the *variola virus*; leads to vesicle formation over the entire body with severe scarring; transmitted by contact or dust, but also by *droplet infection*

smear method of obtaining specimens for examination from the skin or mucosa

smear infection transfer of disease-causing agents by smearing of contaminated material onto other parts of the body and direct contact, e.g. anus-finger-mouth

smegma thick *sebaceous* secretion found under the foreskin of the *penis* or under the *labia minora* around the *clitoris*

Smith fracture (Colles fracture) *distal fracture* of the *radius* with displacement of the distal *fragments* on the palmar side, usually from falling onto the back of the hand

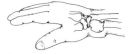

Fig. 436: Smith fracture

Snellen test test to assess ability to see letters at a distance of 20 feet using a Snellen Chart

sO₂ oxygen saturation of *hemoglobin*; determined as part of *blood gas analysis* or via *oximeter*; normal values for arterial blood 94 to 98%

SOB abbr. shortness of breath

socio– combining form: society

SOAP documentation format used in many hospitals, which includes subjective, objective, assessment and plan data

sodio– combining form: sodium

sodium chloride chemical name for *salt*; abbr. *NaCl*

sodium citrate anticoagulant additive used in measuring *erythrocyte sedimentation rate*

sodium *electrolyte* with particular importance for the body's water balance;

found throughout the body outside of the *cells*; chemical symbol: Na

sodomy anal or oral intercourse

sole plantar surface of the foot

solid firm

solitary individual, isolated; opp. *multiple, ubiquitous*

solu– combining form: solution

soma (corpus) body

somat(o)– combining form; body

somatic (physical) of the body; opp. *psychic*

somatic nervous system part of the nervous system that controls voluntary active muscle movement; opp. *autonomic nervous system*

somatos body; opp. *psyche*

somatostatin *hGH-releasing hormone*

somatostatinoma *somatostatin*-producing tumor, usually malignant

somatotropic hormone *somatotropin*

somatotropin (human growth hormone, somatotropic hormone) growth hormone produced by the adenohypophysis; abbr. hGH, GH, STH

somn– combining form: sleep

somnambulism sleepwalking

somnolence type of altered mental status in which the patient is sleepy but able to be roused at any time

son– combining form: sound, tone

sono abbr. sonography; see *ultrasound*

sonogram *ultrasound*; abbr. *sono*

sonograph to examine by *ultrasound*

sonographic pert. to *ultrasound* examination

sonography *ultrasound*; abbr. *sono*

sopor stupor

sound conduction disorder hearing impairment due to poor air conduction of sound (bone conduction is not subject to failure); see *Rinne test*

sound conduction transmission of sound waves through the air or the skull bones to the inner ear

SPA abbr. *spinal anesthesia*

Spanish collar *paraphimosis*

–spasm, spasm– combining form: seizure, twitching

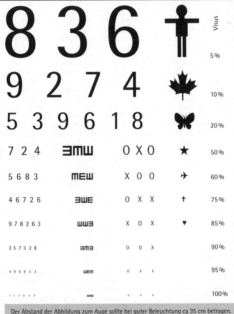

The chart contains, from top to bottom with Visus percentages on the right:

8 3 6 — 5%
9 2 7 4 — 10%
5 3 9 6 1 8 — 20%
7 2 4 ЗMШ 0 X 0 ★ — 50%
5 6 8 3 MEШ X 0 0 — 60%
4 6 7 2 6 ЗШE 0 X X † — 75%
9 7 8 2 6 3 ШШЗ X 0 X ♥ — 85%
2 5 7 3 2 8 ЗMЗ 0 0 X — 90%
4 9 6 8 5 3 ШEM 0 X X — 95%
7 3 7 8 4 9 ШE X 0 0 — 100%

Der Abstand der Abbildung zum Auge sollte bei guter Beleuchtung ca 35 cm betragen.
Die Augen sollten getrennt voneinander und mit und ohne Sehhilfe untersuch werden.

Pupillendurchmesser (mm)
2 3 4 5 6 7 8 9

Fig. 437: Snellen chart

spasm muscle cramp

spasmolytic 1) able to relieve seizures; 2) drug used to relieve seizures

spasmophilia tendency to convulsions or tetany, e.g. due to rickets

spastic pert. to *spasticity*

spasticity state of increased muscle tension

spectr– combining form: image, appearance

speculum surgical or examination instrument for insertion into natural body orifices; shaped like a trough, tube, blade or funnel; used to visualize structures that are not directly visible to the eye, e.g. the *portio* (*vaginalis*); see also *rectal speculum, nasal speculum, vaginal speculum*

sperm mature male reproductive cell

spermatic cord cord that leads from the *epididymis* through the *inguinal canal* and into the abdominal cavity; contains the *spermatic duct*, vessels and *nerves*

spermatic duct (ductus/vas deferens) duct connecting the *testicle* and *urethra*

spermatocyte immature form of *sperm* cell in the testes

spermicide substance that kills *sperm*

spermiogenesis formation of *spermatozoa* in the *testes*

spermiogram *microscopic* examination of *semen* to determine the number, shape and motility of *sperm*

sphenoid bone wedge-shaped bone in the cranial base

spher– combining form: sphere ball

spherocytic anemia (hereditary spherocytosis) inherited *hemolytic anemia*

sphincter muscle circular muscle that constricts an orifice, e.g. *anus, pupils pylorus, urethra*

sphygmo– combining form: pulse

sphygmomanometer, aneroid device used for non*invasive* (indirect) measurement of *blood pressure*; consists of an inflatable cuff and a *manometer*, from which the values are read as determined via *stethoscope* (*systolic* and *diastolic* readings) or *palpation* (systolic only)

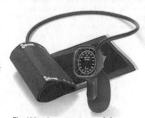

Fig. 438: sphygmomanometer [H]

sphygmos *pulse*

spider nevus star-shaped group of enlarged blood vessels around a central vascular node; classic external sign of *cirrhosis*

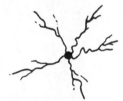

Fig. 439: spider nevus

spiderburst dilation of the smallest *veins*, most often on the inner ankle and thigh; see also *varicosis*

spina pointed bony prominence

spina bifida congenital defect in the posterior or anterior part of the *spinal column*, usually in the *lumbar* or *sacral spine*

spinal pert. to the *spinal column* or *spinal cord*

spinal anesthesia nerve block anesthesia for local numbing of the lower body, in which a *local anesthetic* is applied in the *subarachnoid space*, leading to a *reversible* conduction block of the *spinal nerve* roots; abbr. SPA

spinal column bony axis of the human body which carries the upper limbs, ribs and head; consists of the *cervical, thoracic* and *lumbar spine, sacrum* and *coccyx*

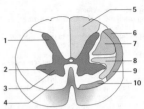

Fig. 441: spinal cord
1 Posterior horn 2 Anterior horn 3 Gray matter 4 White matter 5 Posterior funiculus 6 Posterior spinocerebellar tract 7 Lateral corticospinal tract 8 Lateral spinothalamic tract 9 Anterior spinocere-bellar tract 10 Anterior spinothalamic tract

spinal curvatures deformities characterized by abnormal curvature of the spine, e.g. kyphosis or scoliosis

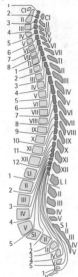

Fig. 440: spinal column

spinal cord cord running the length of the spinal canal, which contains important *motor* and *sensory nerve* pathways; extends from the *atlas* to the 2nd lumbar vertebra
spinal cord injury can be complete or incomplete, depending on how much of the cord is damaged; if complete, there is no feeling or movement below the injury point; if incomplete, the latter symptoms are less severe below the injury point

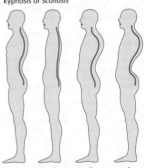

Fig. 442: spinal curvatures
1 Normal spine 2 Flatback 3 Humpback 4 Swayback

spinal ganglion *dorsal root ganglion*
spinal nerve *nerve* branching out from the *spinal cord*

spinal puncture *lumbar puncture*
spinal tap *lumbar puncture*
spiral fracture *torsion fracture*
spirochete screw-shaped spiral *microorganism*, e.g. *Treponema pallidum*
spirometry measurement of respiratory and pulmonary function; see also *total capacity, vital capacity, inspiratory capacity, functional residual capacity, inspiratory reserve volume, respiratory volume, residual volume*

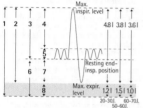

Fig. 443: spirometry values
1 Total capacity (TC) 2 Vital capacity (VC)
3 Inspiratory capacity (IC) 4 Inspiratory reserve volume (IRV) 5 Breath VT 6 Functional residual capacity (FRC) 7 Expiratory reserve volume (ERV) 8 Residual volume (RV)

splanch– combining form: viscera
splanchnic nerve *nerve* that innervates the pleural membrane, intestine, intestinal vessels and *kidneys*, et al.
splanchnon (viscera) internal *organs*, esp. the abdominal organs
spleen organ located in the left upper abdomen; function: production of *antibodies*, storage of blood, removal of spent blood cells
splen *spleen*
splenectomy *surgical* removal of the *spleen*
splenic vein *vein* that collects blood from the *spleen* and joins the *superior mesenteric* to form the *portal vein*
spleno– combining form: spleen

splenomegaly enlargement of the *spleen*
splinter forceps specialized *forceps*, e.g. according to Feilchenfeld, used for removal of small splinters from a wound

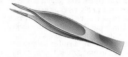

Fig. 444: splinter forceps [A]

spondylarthritis *inflammation* of the vertebral joints, e.g. in *Bechterew's disease*
spondylarthrosis (spondylosis) *degeneration* of the vertebral joints/spine
spondylitis *inflammation* of the *vertebrae*
spondylodiskitis *inflammation* of one or multiple *vertebrae* and the tissues of the corresponding *intervertebral disks*
spondylolisthesis displacement of the *vertebrae* from their normal position, usually occurring in the *lumbar* spine
spondylolysis degeneration of a *vertebra* due to congenital fissure formation in the vertebral arch
spondylosis spondylarthrosis
spondylus *vertebra*
spongio– combining form: spongy
spongiosa spongy layer inside a bone
spontaneous sudden, occurring without external interference
spontaneous fracture (pathological fracture) *fracture* involving little or no external force
spontaneous pneumothorax *pneumothorax* caused by a spontaneous tear in the *pleura*
spontaneous ventilation independent breathing
spor– combining form: seed; germ
sporadic occurring from time to time, irregular
spore resistant reproductive cell formed by *microorganisms* that reproduce asexually
spotting slight vaginal bleeding between *menstrual* periods or before labor begins

S

sprain (distortion) trauma to a *ligament*

Sprengel's deformity hereditary deformity in which the scapula is displaced upward

sprue *chronic* disease of the intestine marked by malabsorption, leading to *vitamin* deficiencies, weight loss, *anemia* and fatty stools; types include tropical and nontropical sprue (see *celiac disease*)

sputum (expectoration) mucus expelled from the *trachea* and *bronchi*; sputum culture identifies pathogens present in the sputum; first morning specimen collection is the best

squam- combining form: scales

squama flaking of the *epidermis*; one of the *secondary efflorescences*

squamous cell carcinoma antigen important *tumor marker* for *squamous cell carcinomas*, e.g. of the *cervix*, *lungs* and *esophagus*; abbr. SCCA

squamous epithelium tissue covering the skin and mucosa

squint *strabismus*

SS abbr. *Sjögren's syndrome*; Social Security

SSS abbr. *sick sinus syndrome*

ST segment complete depolarization of the ventricles, as seen in the *ECG*; begins in the QRS *complex* at the end of the *S* wave and ends at the beginning of the *T* wave

stable solid, lasting; opp. *labile*

stable disease treatment outcome that has either responded to therapy and is stable once treatment is stopped, or has not responded to therapy but has not progressed or gotten worse

stage 1 decubitus decubitus with sharply circumscribed skin redness and intact skin; darker-skinned people may exhibit skin discoloration; other signs may include edema, thickening or local hyperthermia of the skin

stage 2 decubitus decubitus with partial loss of the epidermis, including parts of the dermis; the surface damage is usually in the form of vesicles

stage 3 decubitus decubitus with damage to all three skin layers (epidermis, dermis and subcutis) down to the fasciae, which are not affected

stage 4 decubitus decubitus with loss of all skin layers, extensive tissue necrosis and damage to muscles, tendons and/or bones

stage 1) one part of the course of a disease; 2) platform of a *microscope*, on which the *slide* with the specimen with placed

staging classification of the *stage* of development of malignancies

standard bicarbonate binding potential of the body for *carbon dioxide*; measured as part of *blood gas analysis*; normal value for arterial blood: 22 to 26 mmol/l; abbr. SBC; chemical symbol: HCO_3

standard lead see *Einthoven*

standard of care the degree of care or competence that one is expected to exercise in a particular circumstance or role

standard therapy treatment that has been shown to be effective and safe in clinical studies and is adopted as a standard of practice outside of clinical trials

stapes (stirrup) one of the three ossicles in the middle ear, located between the *incus* and *cochlea*

Staphylococcus genus of spherical gram-positive *pyogenic bacteria* that form colonies resembling bunches of grapes; can cause numerous *infectious diseases*

staphyloderma collective term for purulent skin disease caused by *staphylococci*

startle reflex *Moro reflex*

-stasis combining form: stoppage, standstill

stasis stoppage or diminution of flow, e.g. of blood

status condition; state

status asthmaticus prolonged attack of *bronchial asthma*, or multiple attacks in rapid succession

status epilepticus continuous *epileptic seizure* without recovery of consciousness

steady state state of equilibrium in *physiological* functions

steal syndrome deviation of the bloodstream due to *hemodynamic* disorder, e.g. vascular occlusion; see also *subclavian steal syndrome*

steato- combining form: fat

S

steatocirrhosis *triglycerides* in more than 50% of the liver's cells; cf. *fatty liver*

steatorrhea fatty stool and/or diarrhea due to inadequate absorption of dietary fats by the intestine

steatosis fatty degeneration, e.g. of the *liver*

steatosis hepatis see *fatty liver*, *steatocirrhosis*

stellate block *injection* of a *local anesthetic* into a cervical nerve node (stellate ganglion) to treat *migraine* pain or other hemilateral headache

Stellwag's sign infrequent blinking; a symptom of *Graves' disease*

stem cells parent cells that grow and divide to produce RBCs, WBCs and platlets; found in the *bone marrow* and peripheral blood

stem cell transplant therapeutic procedure whereby bone marrow or perpherial blood stem cells are collected, stored and infused into a recipient to restore blood cell production following high-dose chemotherapy

Stemmer's sign rule stating that *lymphedema*, unlike *venous edemas*, does not involve the toes

steno– combining form: narrowing, narrow

stenocardia *angina pectoris*

stenosed narrowed

stenosis narrowing of a duct, canal, vessel or orifice in the body, e.g. *arteries*

stent metal mesh tube for holding a hollow structure or blood vessel open

Fig. 445: stent

stercus *feces*

stereo– combining form: stiff, solid, hard

stereoscopic creating the impression of depth

stereotaxis treatment procedure for precise spatial irradiation or *surgery*, usually used in the *brain* area

stereotypy persistently repeated actions

sterile 1) free of contaminants; 2) unable to reproduce

sterilization 1) hygienic measure taken to achieve sterile conditions; 2) rendering a male or female infertile

sterilize to perform a *sterilization*

sternal pert. to the *sternum*

sternal puncture *puncture* of the *sternum* in order to obtain *bone marrow*, usually for investigation of blood disease

sternoclavicular joint *joint* between the *sternum* and *clavicle*

sternocleidomastoid muscle muscle that turns and inclines the head; innervation: *accessory nerve* and *cervical plexus*

sternotomy *surgical* opening of the sternum, e.g. for heart surgery

sternum (breastbone) bone in the center of the anterior thorax, to which the *ribs* are attached

steroid short term for *corticosteroid*

steroidal pert. to *corticosteroids*

stethos ribcage; chest

stethoscope instrument for *auscultation* of auditory phenomena in the body

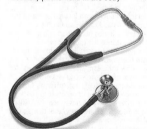

Fig. 446: stethoscope [H]

S

sthen- combining form: strong, powerful

-sthenia combining form: strength, power

stigma mark; sign

stillbirth any birth in which the newborn does not begin to breathe, the *heart* does not beat, or the *umbilical cord* does not pulsate, and birth weight is over 500 g; opp. *live birth*

stimulant 1) increasing activity or function; 2) a drug that increases activity or function

stimulate to provide a *stimulus*

stimulation frequency number of stimuli within a given time period

stimulus event that evokes a response from an organism

stirrup *stapes*

stitch cutter small surgical cutting instrument used for removal of sutures

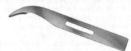

Fig. 447: stitch cutter [A]

Stokes-Adams syndrome (Adams-Stokes syndrome) inadequate blood supply to the brain caused by cardiac *dysrhythmias*, leading to unconsciousness

stoma mouth; natural or artificially created opening in a hollow organ

stomach hollow organ located between the *esophagus* and *duodenum* in the upper abdomen, which holds food and gradually releases it into the duodenum

stomach tube (gastric tube) tube introduced into the stomach, usually through the nose and down the *esophagus*; usually used for removal of *gastric secretions* or for nutrition in patients not suffering from stomach emptying disorders (e.g. *postoperatively*), or who have increased risk of *aspiration* (e.g. unconscious patients); see also *jejunostomy tube*

stomach ulcer *gastric ulcer*

stomachos *stomach*

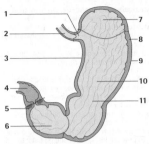

Fig. 448: stomach
1 Cardia 2 Esophagus (abdominal part)
3 Lesser curvature 4 Duodenum 5 Pyloric sphincter
6 Pylorus 7 Fundus 8 Stomach wall
9 Greater curvature 10 Body 11 Angular notch

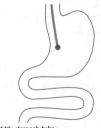

Fig. 449: stomach tube

stomatitis *inflammation* of the oral mucosa

-stomy combining form: formation of a hole; opening

strabismus (squint; crosseye) deviation of the optic axes from parallel position

strabotomy surgery to correct *strabismus*

strangulation 1) choking, throttling; 2) constriction or squeezing of hollow *organs*, e.g. the intestine

strangury strong spasmodic pain when emptying the *bladder*

strat- combining form: layer, stratum

stratum layer, coating

strawberry tongue classic mucosal rash seen in *scarlet fever*

Streptococcus genus of spherical *gram-positive bacteria* that form chains; can cause numerous *infectious diseases*, e.g. *scarlet fever* or *erysipelas*

streptodermatitis collective term for skin diseases caused by *Streptococci*

streptolysin toxin produced by *Streptococci* that causes *hemolysis*

stress fracture gradual development of a *fracture* under unusual weight-bearing, but without any detectable *trauma*

stress incontinence involuntary release of urine during stress, e.g. when coughing, laughing or sneezing; usually due to weakness of the pelvic floor muscles

stress reaction inability to cope with a *trauma* in the absence of a true psychic disorder; usually lasts a short time (hours to months)

striae stretch marks on the skin, e.g. due to *Cushing's syndrome* (reddish stretch marks), pregnancy or *obesity* (whitish stretch marks)

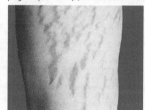

Fig. 450: striae

-strict, strict- combining form: narrowing

stricture extreme narrowing, e.g. of the *urethra* or *esophagus*, due to formation of scar *tissue*

stridor high-pitched breath sound during in- or expiration; inspiratory due e.g. to *laryngospasm* expiratory due e.g. to *bronchospasm*

stripping *surgical* removal of a pathologically altered *vein*, e.g. in *varicosis*

stroke (apoplexy) acute event with *neurological* deficit symptoms caused by *cerebral ischemia* or *hemorrhage*

stroke unit hospital unit devoted to treatment of *stroke* patients

stroke volume amount of blood ejected with one *contraction* of the heart

stroma supporting tissues of an *organ*

struma *goiter*

strumectomy *surgical* removal of a *goiter*

strumitis *inflammation* of a *goiter*

Stuart-Prower factor important blood *coagulation* factor (*Factor X*)

stump remaining portion of a body part that has been removed *surgically*

stupor type of altered mental status in which the patient cannot be roused by speaking, but reacts to painful stimuli

stuporous pert. to *stupor*

stye *hordeolum*

sub- combining form: under(neath); close by

subarachnoid pert. to the *subarachnoid space*

subarachnoid bleed bleeding in the *subarachnoid space*, usually due to *rupture* of a congenital *aneurysm*; abbr. *SAB*

subarachnoid space (CSF space) space between the *arachnoidea* and the *dura mater*, filled with *cerebrospinal fluid*

subcapital below the head of a *joint*

subcapital humerus fracture see *Neer III*

subclavian steal syndrome insufficient circulation triggered by arm movements, caused by obstruction of the *subclavian artery* proximal to the *vertebral artery*; this leads to impaired circulation in the *vertebral artery* at the expense of the *basilar artery*, with resultant dizziness and/or *syncope*

S

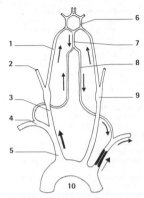

Fig. 451: subclavian steal syndrome
1 Internal carotid artery 2 External carotid artery
3 Common carotid artery 5 Brachiocephalic trunk
6 Circle of Willis 7 Basilar artery 8 Vertebral artery
9 Carotid sinus 10 Aortic arch

subclavian vein *vein* that transports blood from the shoulder and arm area; arises from the *axillary vein* at the level of the 1st rib and joins the *brachiocephalic* with the *internal jugular vein*

subconjunctival hemorrhage bleeding under the conjunctiva of the eye, e.g. due to *strangulation,* straining, or spontaneously due to *arteriosclerosis*

subcutaneous pert. to the skin layer below the dermis; abbr. s.c., SQ

subcutaneous emphysema *emphysema* in the subcutaneous tissue, e.g. in a *pneumothorax*

subcutis layer of fatty *tissue* below the *dermis*

subdural bleed (subdural hemorrhage) bleeding in the *subdural space* due to rupture of the bridging *veins,* leading to *subdural hematoma;* usually associated

with a *head injury* with immediate loss of consciousness

subdural hematoma *hematoma* in the *subdural space*

subdural hemorrhage *subdural bleed*

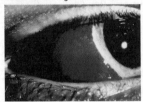

Fig. 452: subconjunctival hemorrhage

subdural space space between the *dura mater* and *arachnoidea*

subfebrile having a slightly elevated body temperature of 37-38° C

subglottic below the *glottis*

subicterus mild form of *jaundice,* marked by yellow discoloration of the normally white *sclera*

subileus incipient or incomplete *ileus*

subjective vertigo *vertigo* in which the patient has a feeling of spinning or rotating

sublimation direct transition of a substance from the solid state to the gaseous state

sublingual under the tongue; abbr. s.l.

sublingual gland salivary gland located under the tongue

subluxation incomplete *dislocation,* in which contact is maintained between the *articular* surfaces

subpoena the usual writ for summoning of witnesses or the submission of evidence, as records or documents, before a court or other deliberative body

substance material; mass

substantia adamantina *dental enamel*

substantial adj. of *substance*

substitute to replace or supplement

substitution replacement

substitutive transplantation
transplantation that replaces a defective *organ*; see also *auxiliary transplantation*

successive following in sequence

sucking reflex *pathological* polysynaptic *reflex* in adults in which stimulation of the oral cavity leads to sucking/swallowing motions; usually occurs with diffuse brain damage

suction catheter *catheter* in various calibers for aspiration of body fluids using a suction *pump*, e.g. to remove *secretions* from the *trachea* or *pharynx*

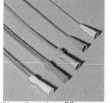

Fig. 453: suction catheter [H]

suction electrode *electrode* that is applied to the skin using a suction mechanism; likely to drop off if not monitored

suction pump device for aspiration of body secretions, e.g. using a *suction catheter* or through a *drain*

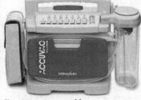

Fig. 454: suction pump [J]

Sudeck's atrophy (reflex sympathetic dystrophy) local growth disorder and *atrophy* of *tissues* following an injury, e.g. after prolonged manipulation of the injured area, premature aftercare or overly forceful *repositioning*

sudor sweat

sudoriferous gland *sweat gland*

sufficiency adequate function or performance; opp. *insufficiency*

sufficient performing or functioning adequately; opp. *insufficient*

suffusion extensive hematoma under the skin, occurring spontaneously or due to injury

suggestion influence over an individual's mind by another person

suggestive therapeutics therapeutic method that bypasses the rational part of the personality, e.g. hypnotism

sugillation milder form of *suffusion*

suicidal pert. to *suicide*

suicidality *suicidal* tendency

suicide causing one's own death

sulc- combining form: furrow, groove

sulcus furrow, groove

sunburn skin *burn* caused by excessive sun exposure

sunstroke irritation of the *meninges* caused by excessive sun exposure with the head uncovered

super- combining form: above

supercilium eyebrow

superficial on the surface

superficial flexor muscle of the fingers muscle that flexes the metacarpopha-langeal and middle phalanges of the finger; *innervation: median nerve*

superficial peroneal nerve *nerve* that innervates the *peroneal muscles*

superficial punctate keratitis punctate *erosions* of the corneal *epithelium*

superficialis *superficial*

superficies surface

superior upper, located above; opp. *inferior*

S

superior mesenteric vein upper *mesenteric vein*, which connects the *splenic vein* with the *portal vein*

superior oblique muscle of the eyeball oblique ocular muscle that pulls the eyeball downward and turns it to the side; innervation: *trochlear nerve*

superior ophthalmic vein *vein* that joins the *sinus cavernosus* from the upper orbit

superior rectus muscle straight ocular muscle that turns the eyeball upward; innervation: *oculomotor nerve*

superior vena cava *vein* that transports blood from the upper part of the body to the right atrium of the heart; abbr. SVC

supination *external* rotation of the hand and forearm, or rolling onto the outer edge of the foot; opp. *pronation*

supp abbr. *suppository*

supporting tissue tissue that has a supporting function in the body, e.g. connective tissue, fatty tissue, cartilage, bone and elastic tissue

supportive providing support, maintaining

suppository drug form intended for insertion into the rectum or vagina; abbr. supp

suppression 1) repression; 2) failure of a function

suppurate to form *pus*

suppuration formation of *pus*

supra– combining form: above; opp. *infra-*, *sub-*

supracondylar humerus portion of the *humerus* above the *condyle*

suprapubic above the *mons pubis*

suprascapular nerve *nerve* arising from the *cervical plexus* that innervates the *infraspinous* and *supraspinous muscles*

supraspinous muscle muscle that *abducts* the upper arm and tenses the shoulder joint capsule; innervation: *suprascapular nerve*

supraventricular extrasystole heart action occurring outside the normal *cardiac rhythm*, visible in an *ECG* and originating in the centers above the bundle of His; abbr. SVES

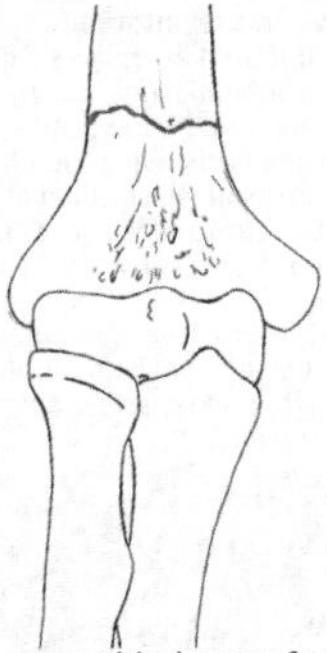

Fig. 455: supracondylar humerus fracture

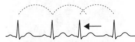

Fig. 456: supraventricular extrasystole

supraventricular tachycardia *paroxysmal supraventricular tachycardia*

sura calf of the leg

surfactant substance produced by the alveolar *epithelium* that reduces the surface tension of the *pulmonary alveoli* and thus prevents *atelectasis*

surgeon specialist in *surgery*

surgery treatment of disease through *surgical operations*

surgical pert. to *surgery*; opp. *conservative*

surgical basin small *sterilizable* metal bowl used to hold sterile liquids during *surgery* or for skin disinfectant

suspension 1) mixture of insoluble particles into a liquid; 2) hanging support for a body part

suspensory bandage bandage or sac designed to support a body part, e.g. the *scrotum* or female breast

suture 1) to stitch skin or other tissue; 2) thread or other material used for suturing; 3) (sutura) seam between fused bones, e.g. in the skull

suture dehiscence gap between the edges of a *wound* despite a surgical suture

SV abbr. *stroke volume*

SVC abbr. *superior vena cava*

SVES abbr. *supraventricular extrasystole*

SVR abbr. *systemic vascular resistance*

SVT abbr. *supraventricular tachycardia*

swab 1) piece of sterile cotton or gauze on the end of a stick or held with forceps, e.g. for applying disinfectant to the skin, or taking a *smear*; 2) to apply a swab

Swan–Ganz catheter *pulmonary artery catheter*

swan neck deformity classic malposition of the fingers in *rheumatoid arthritis*

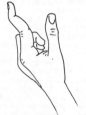

Fig. 457: swan neck deformity

swayback abnormal posture marked by *hyperkyphosis* of the *thoracic spine* and *hyperlordosis* of the *lumbar spine*

sweat gland (sudoriferous gland, glandula sudorifera) gland in the skin that produces sweat

sycosis inflammation of hair follicles caused by fungi or *bacteria*, often in the beard area in males

sym– combining form: with; together

symbiosis coexistence of different *organisms* with mutual benefits,

e.g. humans and *vitamin*-producing *colibacteria*

symbiotic pert. to *symbiosis*

symblepharon adhesion of the eyelid to the *cornea*, e.g. from a *chemical burn* to the eye

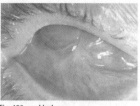

Fig. 458: symblepharon

symmetrical exhibiting *symmetry*; opp. *asymmetrical*

symmetry likeness, correspondence or equality of the opposite sides of a figure

sympath(ic)ectomy *surgical* removal of a part of the *sympathetic nervous system*, e.g. due to circulatory disorders

sympathetic nervous system part of the *autonomic nervous system* that controls the body's stress and flight reactions; counterpart: *parasympathetic nervous system*

sympathetic trunk part of the *sympathetic nervous system* that extends along the spinal column

sympathicolytic drug used to suppress the effects of *adrenaline* and *noradrenaline* on the body, e.g. *beta blockers*

sympathoblastoma malignant tumor originating in the sympathetic nerve cells

sympathomimetic drug used to stimulate the *sympathetic nervous system*, e.g. *adrenaline*

symphyseal rupture open book (pelvic) injury

symphysis connection between bones formed by fibrocartilage, e.g. between vertebrae or the pubic bones

S

symptom sign of disease

symptomatic pert. to a *symptom*; exhibiting symptoms; opp. *asymptomatic*

symptomatic transitory psychotic syndrome physically based acute confusion that subsides within a short period of time; usually an intermediate stage between occurrences of a mental disorder

syn- combining form: with, together

synap- combining form: contact point

synapse connection point between two *neurons* or between a neuron and a *cell*

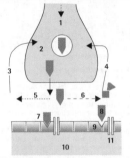

Fig. 459: synapse
1 Synthesis 2 Vesicle 3 Reuptake 4 Reuptake and resynthesis 5 Diffusion 6 Splitting 7 Complex formation 8 Transmitter (e.g. acetylcholine) 9 Receptor 10 Postsynaptic membrane 11 Membrane channel

synchronous simultaneous

syncope (fainting) sudden brief loss of consciousness due to inadequate blood supply to the *brain*

syndactyly disorder of *skeletal* development marked by development of bony or *connective tissue* connections between two fingers or toes

syndesmosis connection between bones formed by *connective tissue*, e.g. in the *pubic symphysis*

syndrome clinical picture characterized by various *symptoms*

systematic inflammatory response syndrome symptoms of *sepsis* without any detectable *pathogen*, e.g. due to *pancreatitis*; abbr. SIRS

synergistic acting together; supporting

synesthesia subjective sensation in a sense organ other than the one stimulated, e.g. sensation of taste under optical stimulation

syngeneic of the same species and *genetically* identical; see also *allogeneic*, *xenogeneic*

syngeneic graft *transplantation* in which the donor and recipient are genetically identical, e.g. between identical *twins*

syngeneic stem cell transplant procedure in which bone marrow or peripheral blood stem cells from an identical twin are collected, stored and infused into a patient

synovial chondromatosis *osteochondromatosis*

synovial fluid fluid that lubricates *joints*, produced by the *synovial membrane*

synovial membrane membrane lining the inner surface of a *joint*, which forms the *synovial fluid*

synthesis bringing together of individual parts to form a whole; opp. *analysis*

syphilis (lues) *infectious disease* caused by *Treponema pallidum* that progresses in stages over a period of years; leads to development of *ulcers* on the genitals (*hard chancre*), swollen *lymph nodes* and *organ* damage; transmitted by sexual contact or via the *placenta* during childbirth

syringe pump (Perfusor®) portable device for precise dosing of *injections*, which enables adjustment in milliliters per hour for administration of drugs via a *venous catheter*

sys- combining form: connected

systemic pert. to the entire body

systemic lupus erythematosus *autoimmune disease* affecting the entire body that leads to the formation of *antinuclear antibodies*; a classic symptom is the *butterfly rash*

systemic vascular resistance resistance in the vascular system that the left heart must work against in order to pump blood into the circulatory system; can be measured with a pulmonary artery catheter et al.; normal value: 800-1200 dyn x sec x cm[5]; elevated in *hypovolemia, cardiogenic shock, pulmonary embolism*; depressed in *sepsis, AV fistula, anemia* and *hyperthyroidism*; abbr. SVR

systole contraction phase of the cardiac muscle, in which the heart chambers empty; opp. *diastole*

systolic murmur auscultable heart sound during *systole*

systolic pert. to *systole*

T

T 1) symbol: trillion (10^{12}); prefix: tera-; 2) temperature; 3) thoracic segment of the spine

T wave repolarization wave as seen in the *ECG*; a sign of repolarization of the cardiac muscle *cells*

T-drain T-shaped *postoperative drain* used to support the *bile* duct and divert bile flow outside the body following *cholecystectomy*

T1, T2, etc. abbr. *thoracic vertebra* 1, 2, etc.

T3 abbr. *triiodothyronine*

T4 abbr. *thyroxin*

TAA abbr. *thoracic aortic aneurysm*

tabes wasting

tabes dorsalis (locomotor ataxia) *degeneration* of portions of the spinal cord in the late stages of syphilis, with impaired muscular coordination

table salt *sodium chloride*

tachy- combining form: rapid

tachyarrhythmia cardiac dysrhythmia in which the heart rate exceeds 100 beats per minute

tachycardia accelerated heart rate, over 100 beats per minute in adults; opp. *bradycardia*

tachycardic pert. to *tachycardia*; opp. *bradycardic*

tachyphylaxis diminished response to a drug resulting from repeated doses at short intervals

tachypnea increase in respiratory rate to more than 20 breaths per minute in adults; usually caused by excitement, exertion, fever or *lung* disorders; opp. *bradypnea*

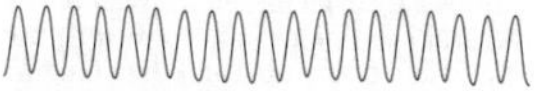

Fig. 460: tachypnea

tact- combining form: touch

tactile pert. to the sense of touch

tactile body *Meissner's corpuscle*

taenia collective term for *parasitic* tapeworms of the genus Taenia with ribbon- or band-like body; found in the large intestine; e.g.

Taenia saginata *beef tapeworm*

Takayasu's arteritis *aortic arch syndrome*

tal- combining form: anklebone

talar fracture *fracture* of the *talus*

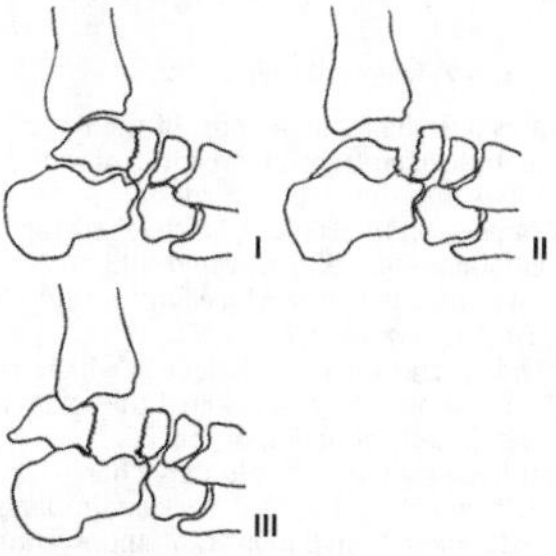

Fig. 461: talar fractures I - III

talaris pert. to the *talus*

talipes calcaneus deformity of the foot in *dorsal extension*

talipes cavus deformity of the foot with an excessively high longitudinal arch

talipes equinovarus (clubfoot) deformity of the foot with *plantar flexion, adduction* and *supination* of the entire sole

talipes equinus deformity of the foot in *plantar flexion*

talipes valgus deformity of the foot in which it forms a C shape turned outward

talipes varus deformity of the foot in which it forms a C shape turned inward

talocrural joint hinge joint formed by the articulation of the tibia and the fibula with the talus below

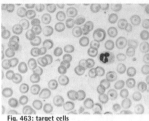

Fig. 463: target cells

tarry stool *melena*

tarsal glands (meibomian glands, palpebral glands) *sebaceous* glands at the margins of the eyelids

tarso– combining form: 1) flat of the foot; 2) edge of the eyelid

tarsus 1) ankle; 2) supporting structure of the eyelid

Tawara branch ramification of the *bundle of His* into right and left branches; see also *excitation* and *conduction system*

taxia combining form: movement, coordination

TB abbr. *tuberculosis*

TBG abbr. *thyroxin-binding globulin*

tbl. abbr. tablet

TC abbr. *total capacity*

TE abbr. *tennis elbow; tooth extraction*

TEA abbr. *thromboendarterectomy*

tear *lacrima*

tear duct passage leading downward from the lacrimal sac on each side of the nose

tect– (tegmen–) combining form: roof

TED hose abbr. antithrombosis stockings/hose (*medical elastic stockings*)

TEE abbr. *transesophageal echocardiography*

tegmen cover, roof, e.g. the tegmen tympani, which covers the *tympanic cavity* in the middle *ear*

telangiectasia (telangiectasis) visible dilation of small blood vessels in the skin, e.g. in *liver* disease or *collagenosis*

Fig. 462: talocrural joint

talus anklebone; uppermost of the *tarsal bones* which transfers weight from the *tibia* onto the arch of the foot

tampon roll of cellulose, gauze or cotton

tamponade packing a *wound* with a *tampon*, e.g. to arrest bleeding; but see also *cardiac tamponade*

tandem transplant technique in which patient receives two planned transplants within a short period of time

tardive dyskinesia involuntary chorea-like movements of the face, neck and/or limb after more than 6 months of antipsychotic drug treatment with dopamine blockers, e.g. antipsychotics

target cell altered form of *erythrocyte* occurring in *thalassemia*, post *splenectomy*, and in *liver* disease

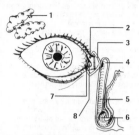

Fig. 464: tear ducts
1 Lacrimal gland 2 Superior lacrimal punctum
3 Lacrimal canaliculus 4 Lacrimal sac
5 Nasolacrimal duct 6 Inferior nasal meatus
7 Inferior lacrimal punctum 8 Caruncula lacrimalis

tele- combining form: distant
telemetric pert. to *telemetry*
telemetry remote transmission of measurements
telencephalon (endbrain) part of the brain from which the cerebral hemispheres et al. develop
teleological pert. to a goal or final purpose
telescopic crown *crown* that combines natural teeth with a removable denture
telo- combining form: end
telophase final phase of cell division
temp- combining form: time, temporal
temple *(os temporale)* temporal bone
tempora temple
temporal 1) pert. to the temple or *temporal bone*; 2) pert. to time
temporal bone temple bone between the *sphenoid* and *occipital* bones; contains the organs of hearing and equilibrium
temporal squama bone plate at the side of the head
temporomandibular arthritis *arthritis* in the temporomandibular joint, usually a consequence of *otitis media*

temporomandibular arthrosis *arthrosis* of the temporomandibular joint following damage to the joint cartilage from *habitual dislocation*, injury or *inflammation*; opening the jaw is hindered by joint clicking and deviation of the *mandible*
temporomandibular joint syndrome (Costen's syndrome) pain radiating from the temporomandibular joint into the ear, head and tongue, due to *dorsal* displacement of the head of the joint as a result of positional or bite anomalies or poorly fitting *dentures,* causing irritation to the surrounding nerves
ten(d)otomy *surgical* section of a *tendon*
tenalgia pain in a *tendon*
tendinitis *inflammation* of a *tendon*
tendinosis *degenerative* changes in *tendon tissue* caused by *inflammation* from overuse
tendo- *tendon*
tendon final portion of a muscle, consisting of connective tissue that anchors it to a bone
tendon sheath fibrous covering of a *tendon*
tendopathy collective term for noninflammatory *tendon* disease
tendovaginitis *tenosynovitis*
tenesmus persistent painful urge to empty the bladder or bowel due to spasms in the corresponding muscles
tennis elbow (lateral humeral epicondylitis) pain and muscular weakness in the forearm due to inflammation of the humeral *epicondyle* and associated tissues
tenon *tendon*
Tenon's capsule *connective tissue* capsule of the *eyeball*
tenosynovitis *inflammation* of a *tendon sheath*
TENS abbr. *transcutaneous electrical nerve stimulation*
-tension combining form: stretching pressure

tension banding *osteosynthesis* of a *fracture* in which the attempt is made to convert flexion force into axial force, e.g. in an *avulsion fracture*

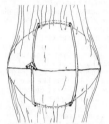

Fig. 465: tension banding

tension pneumothorax (valvular pneumothorax) *pneumothorax* in which a valvelike mechanism allows more and more air to enter the *pleural cavity* with each inhalation, which cannot escape on exhalation; this leads to increased pressure in the *mediastinum*, which can press against the *heart* and limit its motion

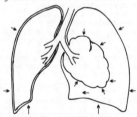

Fig. 466: tension pneumothorax during expiration

tentorial notch notch in the *tentorium* through which the *brain stem* passes

tentorium tent or tent-like structure; pl. tentoria

tentorium cerebelli process of the *dura mater* located between the *cerebrum* and cerebellum, which stretches over the cerebellum like a tent

TEP abbr. *total endoprosthesis*

tephr- combining form: ash-gray

tera- combining form: trillion (10^{12}); symbol T

terato- combining form: deformity

teratogenic able to cause birth defects

teratogenicity ability of a substance to cause birth defects

teratoma mixed tumor composed of *embryonic* components of several *organs*

teratospermia presence of malformed *sperm* in the *ejaculate*, accounting for more than 40% in a *spermiogram*

termin- combining form: boundary; end

terminal final; pert. to or located at an end

terminology study of specialized terms

tertiary third, in third place; see also *primary, secondary*

testicle *testis*

testicular pert. to the *testicles*

testicular torsion acute lengthwise twisting of the *testicle*, cutting off its blood supply

testis male gonad, which produces *sperm*; pl. testes

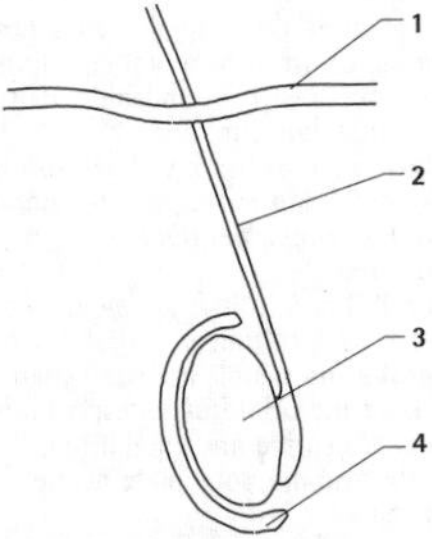

Fig. 467: testis (serous membranes)
1 Peritoneum 2 Vas deferens 3 Testis
4 Tunica vaginalis

testosterone most important male sex *hormone*, produced primarily in the *testes*, but also in the *ovaries* and *adrenal cortex*; regulates the development of male sexual characteristics

tetanus (lockjaw) 1) *infectious disease* caused by *Clostridium tetani*, leading to paralysis of the respiratory musculature; usually occurs via contaminated *wounds*; 2) muscle spasm, e.g. of the *uterus*

tetany *neurogenic* hyperexcitability due to lack of *calcium* in the blood, with intermittent spasms of certain muscle groups

tetra– combining form: four

tetrahydrocannabinol active component in marijuana; abbr. THC

tetraiodothyronine *thyroxine*

tetralogy disease with four cardinal signs, e.g. *tetralogy of Fallot*

tetralogy of Fallot congenital heart defect marked by *right-to-left shunt*; consists of 1) *pulmonary stenosis*, 2) *ventricular septal defect*, 3) right displacement of the *aorta* and 4) right-heart *hypertrophy*

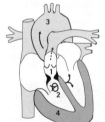

Fig. 468: tetralogy of Fallot
1 Pulmonary artery stenosis 2 Ventricular septal defect 3 Overriding aorta 4 Right ventricular hypertrophy

tetraplegia *quadriplegia*
Tg abbr. *thyroglobulin*
TG abbr. *triglycerides*

TGV abbr. *transposition of the great vessels*

TH abbr. *thyroid hormone*

thalamus large gray nuclear mass in the *diencephalon*

thalassemia (Cooley anemia) inherited disorder that causes decreased synthesis of *hemoglobin* and leads to *anemia*; usually occurs in children 5 to 18 months old

thalassotherapy therapy by sea bathing

thanato– combining form: death

thanatos death

THC abbr. *tetrahydrocannabinol*

thec– combining form: vessel

theca cells layer of *cells* in the ovarian *follicles*

thelarche initiation of female breast development due to *estrogenic* activity; usually occurs between age 10 and 11

thelitis *inflammation* of the nipples

thenar atrophy atrophy of the *thenar* muscle, e.g. in *carpal tunnel syndrome*

thenar eminence fleshy eminence at the base of the thumb

Ther abbr. *therapeutic*

therapeutic pert. to *therapy*; abbr. Ther

therapeutic range dose amounts for a drug, ranging from the lowest effective dose to the highest dose tolerated

therapy measures taken to treat a disease; abbr. Tx

therapy–refractory not responding to *therapy*

therapy–resistant *refeactory to therapy*

therm(o)– combining form: warmth, heat

–thermic combining form: warmth, heat

thermolabile able to be destroyed by heat; opp. *thermostable*

thermometer instrument for measuring temperature

thermostable able to withstand heat; opp. *thermolabile*

thiamine (*vitamin B₁*) water-soluble *vitamin* with an important function in *carbohydrate* metabolism; B₁ deficiency leads to *beriberi*

thiazide *diuretic* drug
thigh(bone) *femur*
thigm- combining form: touch
thio- combining form: sulfur
thoracentesis removal of fluid from the *pleural space*
thoracic pert. to the *thorax*
thoracic drain suction *drain* with suction rate of 15-20 cm H_2O, used for removing secretions from the *pleural cavity*

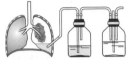

Fig. 469: thoracic drain

thoracic duct body's main *lymph* vessel; collects lymph from the legs, abdominal organs and upper left half of the body and drains it into the *left subclavian vein*
thoracic empyema accumulation of pus in the *pleural cavity*, e.g. due to a lung *infection*

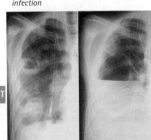

Fig. 470: thoracic empyema in chest x-ray

thoracic nerves nerves of the thorax; their ventral branches innervate the *greater pectoral muscle* et al.

thoracic outlet syndrome general term for *compression syndromes* in the upper *thorax* due to *anatomical* deformities or processes that cause narrowing such as *neoplasias*; see also *Adson's maneuver*
thoracic spine portion of the spine between the *cervical* and *lumbar spine*, consisting of 12 thoracic *vertebrae* (*vertebrae thoracicae*); abbr. TS
thoracic spine syndrome collective term for diseases involving pain in the *thoracic spine*
thoracic vertebrae see *thoracic spine*
thoracodorsal nerve *nerve* arising from the *brachial plexus* that innervates the *latissimus dorsi muscle*
thoracotomy *surgical* opening of the chest cavity
thorax chest; upper body
thought block disorder of the thought processes in which thoughts unexpectedly come to a halt, e.g. in *depression*
thought withdrawal disorder of thought processes characterized by the subjective belief that one's thoughts are being taken away from them by an outside force, e.g. in *schizophrenia*
three-way stopcock accessory for connecting an *infusion system* to a *venous catheter* with one *Luer* and two *Luer Lock* connectors; can be opened as needed by adjusting the lever, e.g. to administer multiple infusions through one *venous catheter*

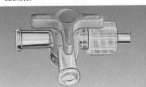

Fig. 471: three-way stopcock [J]

thrix hair
throat *pharynx*

thromb(o)– combining form: blood clot
thrombectomize to perform a *thrombectomy*
thrombectomy *surgical* removal of a blood clot from a vessel

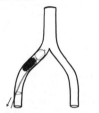

Fig. 472: thrombectomy with balloon catheter

thrombendangiitis obliterans (Buerger's disease) *inflammatory* vascular disease affecting the entire body
thrombin *coagulation factor* formed from *prothrombin*, which converts *fibrinogen* to *fibrin*
thrombin time end-phase blood coagulation test that measures the time required for conversion of *fibrin* to *fibrinogen*; important in suspected fibrinogen deficiency; e.g.; abbr. TT
thrombo abbr. *thrombocyte*
thrombocyte blood platelet made in the *bone marrow* that initiates blood coagulation; abbr. *thrombo*
thrombocyte aggregation clumping of *thrombocytes*
thrombocyte aggregation inhibitor drug used to prevent clumping of *thrombocytes*
thrombocythemia *thrombocytosis*
thrombocytic pert. to the *thrombocytes*
thrombocytopathy disease marked by normal thrombocyte count but deficient function
thrombocytopenia *thrombopenia*
thrombocytosis (thrombocythemia) pathological increase in *thrombocytes*; opp. *thrombopenia*

thromboembolism acute obstruction of an *artery* or *vein* caused by a detached *thrombus*
thromboendarterectomy (endarterectomy) *surgical* removal of a *thrombus* in a major artery, along with the *intima* of the vessel at the site; abbr. TEA
thrombokinase obsolete name for *Factor X*
thrombolysis dissolution of a blood clot, spontaneously or using a *thrombolytic agent*
thrombolytic pert. to *thrombolysis*
thrombolytic agent drug used to dissolve a blood clot
thrombopathy pathological disorder of *thrombocyte* function, resulting in defective coagulation
thrombopenia pathological decrease in *thrombocytes*; opp. *thrombocytosis*
thrombopenic pert. to *thrombopenia*
thrombophilia tendency to develop *thromboses* and *embolisms*
thrombophlebitic pert. to *thrombophlebitis*
thrombophlebitis *inflammation* of a superficial *vein*; see also *phlebothrombosis*
thromboplastin *Factor III*
thromboplastin time *Quick's test*
thrombopoiesis production of *thrombocytes*
thrombosed obstructed by a blood blot
thrombosis occlusion of a blood vessel by a blood clot; see *Virchow's triad* for causes
thrombosis stockings *medical elastic stockings*
thrombotic pert. to *thrombosis*
thrombus blood clot that can obstruct a blood vessel partially or completely, and can cause an *embolism* if it is carried along in the bloodstream
thrush fungal infection of the skin or mucous membranes, usually by Candida albicans
thumb pollex
thymectomy *surgical* removal of the *thymus*
–thymia combining form: state of mind
thymo– combining form: 1) state of mind; 2) thymus gland

thymus *organ* lying behind the upper sternum, which produces *lymphocytes* (T lymphocytes) in childhood and puberty and then shrinks

thyr(e)o- combining form: thyroid gland

thyrogenic originating in the *thyroid gland*

thyroglobulin *protein* made in the thyroid gland that plays an important role in the synthesis of the *hormones triiodothyronine* and *thyroxine*; abbr. Tg

thyroglobulin antibody *antibody* against *thyroglobulin*

thyroid cartilage (Adam's apple) large cartilage of the *larynx*, above the *cricoid cartilage*

thyroid gland gland located at the base of the throat that produces, stores and secretes the *hormones triiodothyronine* and *thyroxine*

thyroid hormone collective term for *thyroxine triiodothyronine* and *calcitonin*

thyroid inhibitor drug that inhibits the production and release of *thyroid hormones*

thyroid-stimulating hormone (thyrotropin) a *hormone* produced by the *adenohypophysis* that causes increased uptake of iodine by the thyroid gland and increased release of *thyroxine* and *triiodothyronine*; abbr. TSH

thyroiditis inflammation of the *thyroid gland*

thyrotoxicosis hyperthyroidism

thyrotropin thyroidstimulating hormone

thyrotropin-releasing hormone hormone produced by the *hypothalamus* that controls the release of *thyroid-stimulating hormone* in the *adenohypophysis*; abbr. TRH

thyroxine *hormone* produced by the thyroid gland; increases metabolism and facilitates growth and mental development; precursor of *triiodothyronine*; important parameter for testing *thyroid* function; abbr. T4

thyroxine-binding globulin transport *protein* for *thyroxie* in the blood; abbr. TBG

TIA abbr. transient ischemic attack

tibia (shinbone) anterior bone of the lower leg

tibial nerve nerve that innervates the *biceps femoris, gastrocnemius* and *posterior tibial muscles*

tic sudden, seemingly purposeful, involuntary, periodically occurring movement (motor tic) or utterance (vocal tic)

tick-borne encephalitis encephalitis transmitted by ticks, e.g. CEE

tidal volume amount of air inhaled in a normal breath; see illustration under *spirometry*; abbr. TV, V_T

Tiffeneau test (forced expiratory volume test) determination of the amount of air that can be expired within a second following maximal inspiration; abbr. FEV

tincture liquid extract of a medicinal substance, usually containing alcohol

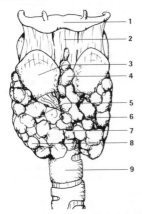

Fig. 473: anatomy of the thyroid gland
1 Hyoid bone 2 Thyrohyoid membrane 3 Thyroid cartilage 4 Pyramidal lobe 5 Right lobe 6 Left lobe 7 Isthmus 8 Lobules 9 Trachea

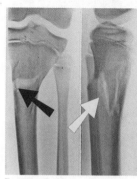

Fig. 474: proximal fracture of tibial head

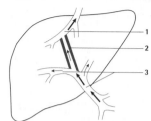

Fig. 475: TIPS
1 Efferent hepatic vein 2 TIPS 3 Portal vein (system)
Arrow = direction of blood flow

tine test (tuberculin skin test) *intracutaneous* test for previous immunization against *tuberculosis*, or for recent infection with the disease

tinea fungal skin disease caused by *dermatophytes*

tinea capitis (ringworm of the scalp) fungal disease affecting the scalp, causing patchy hair loss; usually occurs in children

tinnitus ringing in the *ears* due to disease of the ear, auditory nerve or blood vessels

TIPS abbr. *transjugular intrahepatic portosystemic stent/shunt*

tissue group of *cells* with shared function

titer 1) strength per volume of a solution; 2) number of *antigens* or *antibodies* that consitutates a positive reaction in a blood test

titrate to perform a *titration*

titration determination of the amount of a given substance in a solution

TIVA abbr. *total intravenous anesthesia*

TLC abbr. total lung capacity; see *total capacity*

TNM classification international classification of malignant neoplastic diseases according to 1) primary *tumor* (T), 2) local *lymph node* involvement (N), and 3) existing *metastases* (M)

tocogram *tocography*

tocography (tocogram) measurement of labor activity during childbirth; see also *cardiotocogram*

tocolysis inhibition of labor pains by administration of a *tocolytic*, e.g. to prevent premature delivery before the 36th week of gestation

tocolytic drug used to suppress *labor pains*

tocopherol (vitamin E) fat-soluble *vitamin* with unclear function

toe digitus pedis

Fig. 476: toes
1 D1 (hallux) 2 D2 3 D3 4 D4 5 D5

tolerance ability to digest or endure; opp. *intolerance*

tolerance stage stage of *general anesthesia* in which the defensive reflexes are disabled and *surgery* can begin

Tolosa–Hunt syndrome facial *neuralgia* with unilateral *retrobulbar* pain and *paresis* of one or more of the 3rd, 4th or 6th cranial nerves

-tome combining form: cutting instrument

tomogram *tomography*

tomography (tomogram) *radiological* examination in which planar images of the body are created, e.g. *computed tomography*

-tomy combining form: cut

tongue depressor instrument resembling a popsicle stick, used to inspect the oral cavity

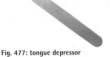

Fig. 477: tongue depressor

tongue lingua, glossa

-tonia combining form: state of tension

tonic 1) (roborant) drug with stimulating and strengthening properties, e.g. *iron preparations, vitamin preparations, glucose*; 2) pert. to *tonus*; opp. *clonic*

tonometry measurement of pressure, esp. of intraocular pressure to test for *glaucoma*

tonsil knife *surgical* knife used to open *tonsillar abscesses* or for *tonsillectomy*

tonsils almond-shaped *structures* in the oropharyngeal area; part of the *lymphatic system*

tonsill- combining form: tonsils

tonsillar pert. to the *tonsils*

tonsillectomy *surgical* removal of the *tonsils*

tonsillitis febrile *infectious disease* involving the *pharyngeal* and *palatine tonsils*, usually caused by *beta-hemolytic streptococci*

tonsillotomy *surgical* incision of the *tonsils*

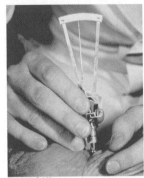

Fig. 478: Schiötz tonometer

tonus consistent state of muscular tension; opp. *clonus*

tooth (dens) natural mastication structure consisting of a *crown, neck* and *root*

tooth decay *caries*

tooth displacement displacement of a tooth out of its socket

tooth extraction removal of a tooth from its socket using instruments

tophaceous gout *gout* with development of tophi (nodes) consisting of *uric acid* crystals and reactive *granulation tissue*, usually in areas with poor circulation, e.g. cartilage or tendons

topical anesthesia local anesthesia of the skin or mucosa, e.g. using freezing spray prior to incising an *abscess*

topo- combining form: location, place

topography position of the *organs* within the body

torpid weak; sluggish

torsade de pointes (polymorphic ventricular tachycardia) special form of *ventricular tachycardia* with fluctuating amplitude of the *QRS complexes*

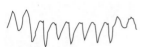

Fig. 479: torsade de pointes

-torsion combining form: twisting

torsion turning or rotating about the longitudinal axis, e.g. of the *testicles* in *testicular torsion*

torsion fracture (spiral fracture) *fracture* due to longitudinal twisting while one side of the bone is fixed, e.g. among skiers

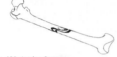

Fig. 480: torsion fracture

torso trunk

torticollis stiff neck with fixed malposition of the head, usually in lateral flexion and *rotation*; can be congenital or a relieving posture for muscle spasms or *disk prolapse*

Tossy classification classification system for *acromioclavicular joint* displacements

Tossy I sprain or contusion of the *acromioclavicular joint* with no damage to the capsule/ligament structures

Tossy II *subluxation* of the *clavicle* with rupture of the acromioclavicular ligament

Tossy III *dislocation* of the *clavicle* with rupture of the acromioclavicular and coracoclavicular ligaments

total body irradiation (TBI) application of radiation to the entire body for the purpose of killing tumor cells; done prior to stem cell transplant

total capacity amount of air in the lungs at the end of a maximal inspiration (*vital capacity* plus *residual volume*); abbr. TC, TLC; see illustration under *spirometry*

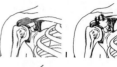

Fig. 481: Tossy I, II, III

total endoprosthesis joint *prosthesis* in which both the head of the joint and its socket are replaced, e.g. after a *femoral neck fracture*; abbr. *TEP*

total extirpation complete *surgical* removal of an *organ*

tourniquet rubber hose or elastic fabric strap used to constrict blood flow in a limb in order to make the veins more visible to facilitate *venipuncture*

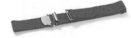

Fig. 482: tourniquet [H]

towel clamp Backhaus towel clamp

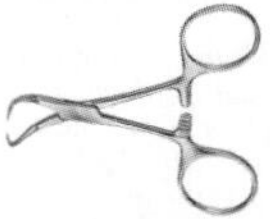

Fig. 483: Backhaus towel clamp [A]

tox(ico)- combining form: poison

toxemia presence of *toxins* in the blood

toxic poisonous

toxic epidermal necrolysis severe disease marked by widespread development of blisters on the skin and mucosa, usually due to an *allergic* reaction to a drug

toxicity degree of being poisonous

toxicology study of toxins and poisoning

toxin animal plant or *bacterial* poison

Toxoplasma gondii *parasite* that grows inside *cells*; causes *toxoplasmosis*

toxoplasmosis *infectious disease* caused by *Toxoplasma gondii* that leads primarily to *neurological* damage; transmitted mainly via cat feces, raw meat from infected animals or via the *placenta*

TPHA abbr. *Treponema pallidum hemagglutination test*

TPN abbr. total *parenteral* nutrition

TPT abbr. *thromboplastin time (Quick's test)*

TRAb abbr. *thyrotropin*-receptor antibody

trabecula supporting cord of tissue

trace element vital chemical element that exists in very tiny amounts in the body

trach- combining form: rough, uneven

trachea windpipe

tracheal pert. to the *trachea*

tracheal dilator instrument used to dilate the *trachea*, e.g. for introduction of a tracheal tube

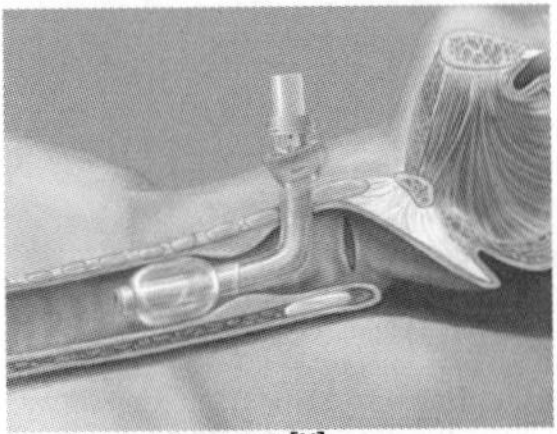

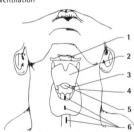

Fig. 485: tracheostomy [N]

tracheotomy *surgical* opening of the *trachea*, usually with direct attachment of the tracheal mucosa to the skin of the throat, e.g. under threat of asphyxia due to constriction of the *larynx* or long-term ventilation

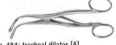

Fig. 484: tracheal dilator [A]

tracheitis *inflammation* of the *tracheal* mucosa

tracheo- combining form: *trachea*

tracheobronchitis *inflammation* of the *tracheal* and *bronchial* mucosa

tracheomalacia pathological softening of the tracheal cartilage

tracheostenosis narrowing of the *trachea*

tracheostomy airway created from the *trachea* to the outside via *tracheotomy*

tracheotomize to perform a *tracheotomy*

tracheotomized having undergone a *tracheotomy*

Fig. 486: tracheotomy, cricothyrotomy
1 Hyoid bone 2 Thyroid cartilage 3 Cricoid cartilage 4 Thyroid gland 5 Cricothyrotomy 6 Tracheotomy

trachoma tropical *infectious disease* caused by *Chlamydia trachomatis*, which leads to *inflammation* of the *cornea* with formation of vesicles and scar tissue; can result in blindness; transmitted mainly by flies or by *smear infection*

traction diverticulum diverticulum caused by external traction, e.g. in the *esophagus*

tractus path; tract

tragus projecting *cartilage* in front of the external meatus of the *ear*

tragus pain pain triggered by pressing a finger against the *tragus* as a diagnostic test; sign of *otitis media* or a *furuncle* of the external ear or external auditory canal

tranquilizer sedative

trans- combining form: through, across

transaminase collective term for *enzymes* that transfer *amino acid* groups from one substance to another; e.g. *glutamatic-pyruvic transaminase* or *glutamic-oxaloacetic transaminase*

transcutaneous electrical nerve stimulation stimulation of *nerves* by electrical impulses sent through adhesive electrodes on the skin, e.g. for pain therapy; abbr. TENS

transcutaneous through the skin

transdermal therapeutic system adhesive patch applied to the skin that contains a drug, which is released into the body gradually through the skin, e.g. strong *analgesics*; abbr. TTS

transesophageal echocardiogram *transesophageal echocardiography*

transesophageal echocardiography *(transesophageal echocardiogram)* form of *echocardiography* in which the *ultrasound* transducer is introduced through the *esophagus*; abbr. TEE

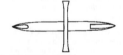

Fig. 487: transfer spike [C]

transfer spike plastic needle with points at both ends for transferring fluids from *infusion bottles* or *ampules*

transferrin *protein* produced by the *liver* that transports *iron* in the body

transformation conversion; changing form

transfuse to perform a *transfusion*

transfusion transfer of whole blood or blood components from a donor to a recipient, e.g. for *anemia*

transfusion device *transfusion system*

transfusion reaction acute incompatibility reaction triggered by a *transfusion*

transfusion system (transfusion device) tubing system for performing *transfusions*, with a filter that connects a unit of *stored blood* to a *venous catheter*

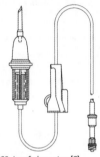

Fig. 488: transfusion system [C]

transient (transitory) temporary; opp. *persistent*

transient blindness amaurosis fugax

transient synovitis (coxitis fugax) *reactive* inflammation of the hip joint, usually occurring in children after a *cold*

transitory temporary, passing; opp. *permanent persistent*

transitory ischemic attack impaired blood supply to the *brain* in which the resulting functional impairments completely recede within 24 hours; abbr. TIA

transjugular intrahepatic portosystemic stent/shunt stent placed via the jugular vein for treatment of portal hypertension, which connects the portal with the hepatic vein through the liver tissues; abbr.: TIPSS

transmural through the wall of an *organ*

Transofix® trade name of a type of *transfer spike*

transparent not opaque, such that objects can be seen on the other side

transpiration secretion of sweat

transplantation *surgical* transfer of an *organ, cells* or *tissue* from a donor to a recipient, or from one area of the body to another; see also *autogeneic graft, syngeneic graft, allogeneic graft, xenogeneic graft, alloplastic graft, isotopic graft, orthotopic graft, heterotopic graft, substitutive transplantation, auxiliary transplantation*; abbr. Tx

transposition displacement of an *organ* to the opposite side

transposition of the great vessels congenital heart defect in which the *aorta* arises from the right ventricle and the *pulmonary artery* from the left ventricle; abbr. TGV

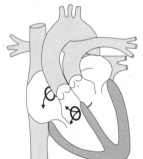

Fig. 489: transposition of the great vessels

transsexualism gender identification disorder in which an individual does not identify with his/her own sex and feels the need to assume the role of the other sex

transsphenoidal adenomectomy removal of a pituitary adenoma via the sphenoid sinus, e.g. in Cushing's syndrome

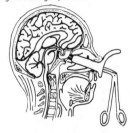

Fig. 490: transsphenoidal adenomectomy

transthoracic echocardiogram *transthoracic echocardiography*

transthoracic echocardiography (*transthoracic echocardiogram*) echocardiography in which the heart is examined through the outer wall of the thorax; abbr. TTE

transudate noninflammatory effusion into body cavities, containing small amounts of *protein*; opp. *exudate*

transudative pert. to *transudates*; opp. *exudative*

transurethral via the *urethra*

transurethral resection removal of tissue via the *urethra*, e.g. for *prostatic hyperplasia*; abbr. TUR

transverse crosswise

transverse lie abnormal position of the *fetus* in which it is tilted inside the mother's pelvis; danger of *umbilical cord prolapse* or of smaller body parts (arm, hand, foot) dropping into the birth canal

transverse plane plane extending horizontally through the upright body

transverse process process of a vertebra that extends sideways

transvest(it)ism *sexual* behavior marked by the tendency to dress like the opposite sex, but with no desire to change sexes

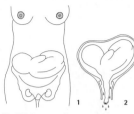

Fig. 491: transverse lie
1 Transverse lie 2 Transverse lie with prolapsed arm

trapezium bone larger of the multiangular *carpal bones*

trapezius muscle back muscle that raises and lowers the scapula and turns the head; innervation: *accessory nerve* and *cervical plexus*

trapezoid bone smaller of the multiangular *carpal bones*

trauma physical or mental injury

trauma(t)- combining form: injury

traumatic pert. to *trauma*

traumatic brain injury leading cause of death and disabilities for Americans under the age of 35; causes include motor vehicle accidents, falls, firearms and assaults; types are classified by mild, moderate and severe; severity is determined by scores from LOC assessment, Glascow Coma Scale totals, and the time interval from when a person regains consciousness until he/she is able to form memories for recent events, referred to as the length of post-traumatic amnesia (PTA)

trem- combining form: trembling

trema gap in the teeth between the upper incisors

tremor involuntary quivering of the muscles due to alternating *contractions* of *antagonistic* muscles, usually with uniform movements of particular body parts; usually occurs in hands and fingers, e.g. in *Parkinson's disease*

Trendelenburg position position in which the legs are elevated with the head lower, e.g. for *hypovolemic shock*

Trendelenburg sign sign of *paresis* or instability of the *gluteus medius muscle:* when the patient stands on one leg and lifts the other, the pelvis will drop on the side of the lifted leg, indicating weakness of the muscle on the other side

trepan hand drill, e.g. according to Hudson, for *trepanation*

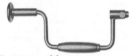

Fig. 492: trepan [A]

trepanation *surgical* opening of a medullary cavity or the skull, e.g. to perform *brain surgery*

Treponema genus of spiral *bacteria*

Treponema pallidum (Spirochaeta pallidum) spiral *gram-negative bacterium* that causes *syphilis*

Treponema pallidum hemagglutination test special blood test for *syphilis;* abbr. TPHA

-tresia combining form: opening

TRH abbr. *thyrotropin-releasing hormone*

tri- combining form: three

triad set of three *symptoms*

triage practice that originated in military medicine whereby the physician assigns patients to *triage groups* in the event of mass casualties in order to make the best use of limited personnel and/or material resources

triage groups categories for ranking treatment or transport priority of patients in the context of *triage;* group I = treatment priority, immediate treatment; group II = transport priority (IIa = immediate, IIb = urgent); group III = nursing care with later treatment; group IV = no therapy, can wait for treatment

triceps three-headed upper arm muscle that extends the forearm; see also *biceps*; innervation: *radial nerve*

triceps (tendon) reflex monosynaptic *reflex* in which percussion of the *triceps* tendon causes extension of the forearm; mapping: see C6/C7/C8 *dermatome*; abbr. TTR

trichiasis friction of the eyelashes against the *cornea*, e.g. due to inversion of the eyelid

Trichinella spiralis parasitic nematode that causes *trichinosis*

trichinosis *infectious disease* caused by *Trichinella spiralis*, leading to edema as well as intestinal and muscle pain (affecting respiratory, speech, mastication and swallowing muscles), with the danger of circulatory collapse; transmitted mainly via consumption of meat containing the *parasite*

tricho– combining form: hair

Trichomonas genus of pear-shaped flagellate protozoa that can infest the urinary tract or genitals as *parasites*

Trichophyton genus of parasitic fungi that can infest the skin, hair or nails, causing *trichophytosis*

trichophytosis *mycosis* of the skin, hair or nails, caused by *Trichophyton*

trichosis collective term for disorders involving the hair

trichosporia *mycosis* of the hair caused by *Trichosporon*

Trichosporon genus of *fungi* that infests the hair and causes *trichosporia*

trichotillomania urge to pull out one's own hair

tricuspid (valve) stenosis narrowing of the *tricuspid valve*

tricuspid atresia absence of the connection between the right *ventricle* and right atrium of the *heart*

tricuspid valve three-leaved heart valve between the right

trigeminal nerve 5th *cranial nerve*; contains sensory and motor fibers; mainly controls sensation in the face and movement of the mastication *muscles* (*masseter* and *temporal muscles*)

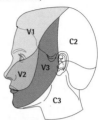

Fig. 493: trigeminal nerve

trigeminal neuralgia (facial tic, tic douloureux) lightning-like severe stabbing pain lasting a few seconds, occurring along one or several branches of the *trigeminal nerve* (usually V2 or V3)

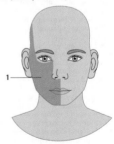

Fig. 494: trigeminal neuralgia
1 Pain

trigeminal pulse sequence of one normal heartbeat followed by two *extrasystoles*

trigeminus trigeminal nerve

trigger point injection treatment for temporary relief of nerve pain; marcaine and a steroid are used for the injection

triglyceride energy storage molecule consisting of one glycerol molecule and three fatty acids one of the dietary fats; abbr. TG

trigone (trigonum vesicae, vesical trigone) triangular space at the base of the *bladder*; common localization of *cystitis*

trigonum triangle

trigonum vesicae *trigone*

triiodothyronine *hormone* produced from *thyroxine*; has the same function as thyroxine, but a stronger effect; important parameter for testing *thyroid* function; abbr. T3

trimester period of three months; usually used in connection with *pregnancy*

−tripsy combining form: breakage, crushing

triquetral bone pyramidal bone; one of the *carpal bones*

trismus (lockjaw) *tonic* contraction of the mastication muscles, e.g. in *tetanus*

trisomy abnormal number of chromosomes, with three chromosomes occurring where normally there are two

trisomy 21 *Down syndrome*

tritanomalopia blue blindness

trocar tubular, typically pointed instrument for puncture of body cavities

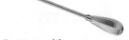

Fig. 495: trocar [A]

trochlear nerve 4th *cranial nerve*; contains motor fibers; controls eye movement, together with the *oculomotor* and *abducens* nerves

−trophic combining form: nourishment, nutrition

trophic pert. to *nutrition*

trophoblast outer layer of the *blastocyst*, which nourishes the *embryo* and adheres to the *endometrium* during *implantation*

−tropin combining form: stimulating effect

troponin important *protein* for muscular function; plays a prominent role in laboratory detection and monitoring of *myocardial infarctions*

Trypanosoma flagellate protozoa that can cause *sleeping sickness*

trypanosomiasis *sleeping sickness*

trypsin proteolytic *pancreatic enzyme*

TS abbr. *thoracic spine*

TSH abbr. thyroid-stimulating hormone

TT abbr. *thrombin time*

TTE abbr. transthoracic echocardiography

TTS abbr. transdermal therapeutic system

tuba (salpinx) tube

tubal abortion expulsion of a *tubal pregnancy* into the abdominal cavity due to *tubal rupture*

tubal pregnancy *ectopic* pregnancy located in the fallopian tube; see *extrauterine pregnancy*

tubal rupture *rupture* of the *fallopian tube* during a *tubal pregnancy*, resulting in a *tubal abortion*

tube narrow cylindrical device that is inserted into hollow structures, e.g. into the *esophagus* to maintain a passage for food in a patient with *stenosing esophageal carcinoma*; see also *endotracheal tube*

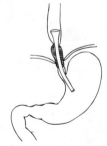

Fig. 496: plastic tube for esophageal carcinoma

tuber- combining form: bump, swelling

tubercle small lesion characteristic of *tuberculosis*, composed of *granulation tissue* and containing *Mycobacterium tuberculosis*; tending to degenerate into a caseous form

tuberculin *toxin* of *Mycobacterium tuberculosis*

tuberculin skin test *tine test*

tuberculoma *tubercular round lesion* surrounded by a membrane, with central tissue degeneration; usually appears in the *liver* or *lungs*

tuberculosis (consumption) *infectious disease* caused by *Mycobacterium tuberculosis*, which primarily affects the *lungs* but can involve other *organs*; transmitted mainly by *droplet infection*, food or via the *placenta* during birth; abbr. TB

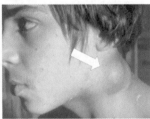

Fig. 497: lymph node tuberculosis

tuberculostatic *drug* used to inhibit growth of *Mycobacterium tuberculosis*

tuberculum knot; nodule

tuberous nodular

tubular cylindrical; tube-shaped

tubulus renalis *renal tubule*

tubulus tubule, small tube

tularemia (rabbit fever) febrile infectious disease caused by *Francisella tularensis*, which affects the skin *lymph nodes* and *lungs*; transmitted mainly by infected ticks, fleas, lice and mites, but also through direct contact with diseased animals or consumption of their meat

tumescence swelling

tumor nonspecific collective term for a swelling or growth; swelling; see also *signs of inflammation*

tumor marker laboratory value measured in body fluids for the detection and monitoring of neoplastic diseases

tumorous swollen

tunica covering layer, coat

tuning fork instrument used to test hearing, e.g. in the *Rinne test* or *Weber test*

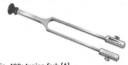

Fig. 498: tuning fork [A]

Tuohy needle *needle* used for *epidural anesthesia*

TUR abbr. *transurethral resection*

turgescence swelling or enlargement of tissues due to *hyperemia*

turgor *tissue* tension dependent upon fluid balance; reduced in *exsiccosis*, increased by development of *edema*

Turner's syndrome (monosomy X) nonhereditary *chromosomal* abnormality affecting only females, in which only one functioning X chromosome is present (rather than two), which results in short stature and infertility, among other things

turricephaly tower-shaped deformity of the skull

tussis coughing

TV abbr. *tidal volume*

twins two babies born from the same pregnancy; a) monozygotic (identical) twins: same sex and same genetic makeup; b) dizygotic (fraternal) twins: same or different sexes and different genetic makeup

Tx abbr. *transplant(ation); therapy*

tympan(o)- combining form: eardrum

tympanic cavity middle ear cavity

tympanometry determination of acoustic resistance of the *eardrum* and *middle ear* by measuring the amount of reflected sound

tympanoplasty *surgical* repair of the sound-transmitting apparatus in the *middle ear*

tympanum *eardrum*

tympany hollow drum-like resonance on *percussion* of bloated, air-filled *organs*, e.g. the abdomen in *meteorism*

Tyndall effect scattering of light due to an increased amount of *protein* in the aqueous humor of the *eye*

–type combining form: image, appearance

typhl- combining form: cecum

typhl(o)enteritis *typhlitis*

typhlitis (typhl(o)enteritis) *inflammation* of the *cecum* that may be associated with *appendicitis*

typhoid fever febrile *infectious disease* caused by *Salmonella typhi*, which leads to severe "pea soup" diarrhea, enlargement of the *liver* and *spleen*, as well as impaired consciousness; transmitted mainly via contaminated food and water, as well as *smear infection*

typhoid *typhus-like*

typhous pert. to *typhus*

typhus (exanthemicus) *epidemic typhus*

typus type

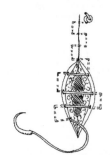

Fig. 499: U-suture

U

U abbr. unit

U-suture special *surgical* suturing technique for wound closure

U wave wave following the *T wave* in an *ECG*

UA abbr. *umbilical artery*; *upper arm*; *uric acid*; *urinalysis*

ubiquitous appearing everywhere; opp. *solitary*

ulcer lesion of skin or mucosa from various causes, e.g. erosion by stomach acid, defective circulation, etc.; pl. ulcera

ulcera pl. of *ulcer*

ulcerate to form an *ulcer*

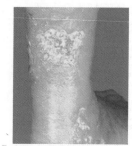

Fig. 500: venous leg ulcer

ulceration formation of *ulcers*

ulcerative colitis disease marked by *chronic inflammation* and *ulceration* of the lining of the *colon*

ulcerous pert. to an *ulcer*

ulcus ulcer

ulna small bone of the forearm on the little finger side, opposite the *radius*

ulnar toward the little finger; opp. *radial*

ulnar deviation classic deformity of the hand in *rheumatoid arthritis*, in which the fingers deviate towards the *ulna*

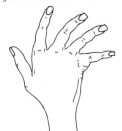

Fig. 501: ulnar deviation

ulnar extensor muscle of the wrist forearm muscle that extends and *adducts* the wrist; innervation: *deep radial nerve*

ulnar flexor muscle of the wrist forearm muscle that flexes the hand toward the ulna side of the arm; innervation: *ulnar nerve*

ulnar nerve *nerve* that supplies the ulnar finger muscles and several skin areas on the and fingers; damage leads to claw hand and *Froment's sign*; also innervates the following muscles: *adductor of the thumb, ulnar flexor of the wrist, deep flexor of the fingers and interosseous*

ulnaris, A. *arteria ulnaris*

ulnaris, N. *(nervus ulnaris)* ulnar nerve

ultima ratio last-resort measures for treatment of a health problem

ultra– combining form: beyond

ultrafiltration see *dialysis*

ultrasonic atomizer device for humidifying the air by atomizing *sterile* water, e.g. for patients who are mouth breathers or have other problems with dryness in the respiratory tract

ultrasonic lithotripsy *lithotripsy*

ultrasonography *ultrasound*

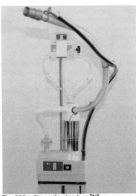

Fig. 502: ultrasonic atomizer [N]

ultrasound (sonography, sonogram, echography, echogram) examination procedure in which sound waves (beyond human hearing range) are measured through a transducer applied to the exam site; the sound is reflected off the "obstacles" to be examined (as in echolocation); from this information an ultrasound image is created (B scan), in which bones appear very bright and body fluids dark; other applications for ultrasound technology are *doppler sonography* and *duplex sonography*; abbr. sono, US

umbilical cord (funiculus umbilicalis) strand of blood vessels connecting the *placenta* to the unborn fetus, ca. 50 cm long and surrounded by Wharton's jelly

umbilical cord clamp instrument for clamping off the umbilical cord after birth

umbilical cord prolapse prolapse of the *umbilical cord* in front of the foremost part of the infant's body during birth, after rupture of the fetal membranes

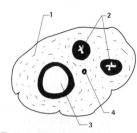

Fig. 503: umbilical cord
1 Wharton's jelly (connective tissue) 2 Umbilical arteries 3 Umbilical veins 4 Allantoic duct (vestige)

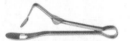

Fig. 504: umbilical cord clamp [A]

umbilical cord scissors curved scissors used to cut the umbilical cord after birth

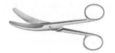

Fig. 505: umbilical cord scissors [A]

umbilical hernia (omphalocele) protrusion of intestine or omentum through the navel

umbilicus navel

UMN upper motor neuron

un- combining form: not

underweight reduction of body weight to a *body mass index* <19 in females or <20 in males; opp. *overweight*

undescended testicle cryptorchidism

undulating wave-shaped, e.g. the course of fever in *malaria*

ungu- combining form: nail

unguentum salve, ointment

unguis finger or toenail; pl. ungues

unguis hippocraticus hippocratic nail, watch-glass nail

unguis incarnatus ingrowing nail

uni- combining form: one

unilateral on one side; opp. *bilateral*

unilateral neglect unaware of one side of the body

unipolar having one pole

unmodified insulin (regular insulin) *injected insulin preparation* with rapid onset; opp. *depot insulin*

updraft treatment inhalation of medicated mist from a nebulizer, e.g. for *asthma*

upper arm brachium; abbr. UA

upper GI endoscopy special procedure done in an outpatient setting: a long, narrow, flexible endoscope is threaded down the esophagus to examine the upper GI tract

upper jaw maxilla

ur(in)- combining form: urine

ur(in)ometer instrument for measuring the specific gravity of urine

urea end product of *protein* breakdown in the *liver*; excreted via the *kidneys* in the urine

uremia strongly increased presence in the blood of substances normally found in urine

uremic pert. to *uremia*

uremic *coma* resulting from *uremia*

-uresis combining form: urination

ureter tube connecting the *kidney* to the *bladder*

ureter duplex duplicate *ureters* in cases of *renal duplication*, with each ureter having a separate *ostium* into the *bladder*

ureter fissus in cases of *renal duplication*, fusion of the duplicate *ureters* before they empty into the *bladder*

ureteral stricture narrowing of a *ureter*, e.g. following an *inflammation*

ureteritis inflammation of a *ureter*

ureterolithiasis presence of stones in a *ureter*

U

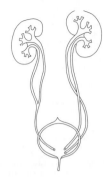

Fig. 506: renal duplication

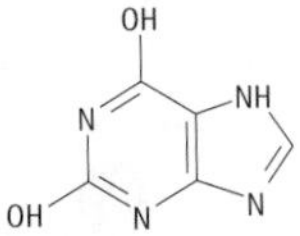

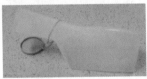

Fig. 507: uric acid

uricemia *hyperuricemia*
uricostatic drug used to reduce production of *uric acid*
uricosuric drug used to promote excretion of *uric acid*
urinal specialized receptacle used for urination by bedridden patients who cannot use a toilet

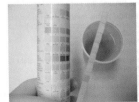

Fig. 508: urinal

ureterorenoscopy *endoscopy* of the *ureters* and *renal pelvis*
ureterosigmoidostomy *surgical* implantation of the *ureters* into the *sigmoid colon*
ureterostomy *surgical* relocation of a *ureter* into the *bladder* wall
ureterotomy *surgical* incision of a *ureter*
urethra tube that carries urine out of the body
urethral pert. to the *urethra*
urethritis *inflammation* of the *urethral* mucosa, e.g. due to *gonorrhea*
urethrocystoscopy *endoscopy* of the *urethra, prostate* and *bladder* using a *cystoscope*, usually for clarification of *hematuria*
urge incontinence involuntary release of urine with strong urge, e.g. in *cystitis*
-urgy combining form: handiwork
-uria combining form: condition of the urine
uric combining form: uric acid
uric acid end product of *purine* metabolism, excreted via the *kidneys* in the urine; important laboratory parameter for *gout*; abbr. UA

urinanalysis quick urine test with a test strip for detection and monitoring of *renal* and urinary tract diseases; the test screens for the following parameters: *leukocytes, nitrite, pH, protein, glucose, ketone, urobilinogen, bilirubin* and blood in the urine

Fig. 509: urinalysis

urinary bladder organ that collects urine from the *kidneys* via the *ureters* and releases it through the *urethra* when the vesical sphincter is relaxed

urinary catheter (Foley) *catheter* for withdrawal of urine from the *bladder*, to which a *collection bag* can be attached; types are disposable and *indwelling* catheters

urinary retention inability to empty a full *bladder*, e.g. due to *nerve* damage

urinary schistosomiasis see *schistosomiasis*

urinary sediment test *microscopic* examination of centrifuged urine sediment for detection and monitoring of *renal* and urinary tract diseases

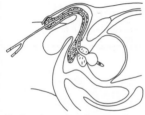

Fig. 510: urinary catheter (indwelling catheter)

urine fluid containing dissolved toxins filtered out by the *kidneys*

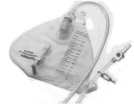

Fig. 511: urine bag [N]

urine bag bag for collecting urine, with a tubing system that can be connected to a *condom urinal* or bladder *catheter*

urine culture *microbiological* testing of urine using a coated *sterile slide* that is spread with urine and cultured in an incubator

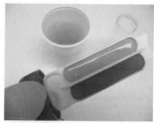

Fig. 512: urine culture

urine dipstick test strip for *urinalysis*

UROB abbr. *urobilinogen*

urobilin *oxidized urobilinogen*

urobilinogen *bilirubin* broken down by intestinal *bacteria*, which is reabsorbed by the intestine and then partially excreted renally with the urine, or back into the intestine with the *bile*; more plentiful in the urine in *liver* disease or *hemolysis*; abbr. UROB

urogenital diaphragm (urogenital trigone) wall consisting of muscle and connective tissue located between the inferior ischiopubic rami

urogenital pert. to the genital and urinary organs

urogenital organs collective term for the urinary and sexual *organs*

urogram *urography*

urography (descending urography, intravenous urography) *radiography* of the urinary tract using *contrast medium*; abbr. EU

U

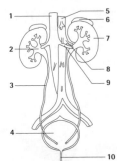

Fig. 513: urogenital tract
1 Inferior vena cava 2 Renal pelvis 3 Ureter
4 Bladder 5 Aorta 6 Adrenal gland 7 Kidney
8 Renal artery 9 Renal vein 10 Urethra

urolithiasis formation of kidney stones;
see also *nephrolithiasis*
urologic(al) pert. to *urology*
urologist specialist in *urology*
urology study of diseases of the *kidneys* and
urinary system
urosepsis *sepsis* originating in the *kidneys*
or urinary tract
urostomy artificially created diversion of
urine through the abdominal wall
urtica (wheal) skin eruption marked by
circumscribed *edema*; one of the *primary
effloerescences*
urticaria (hives, nettle rash) development of
areas of *urtica* on the skin, e.g. due to
allergies
US abbr. *ultrasound, ultrasonography*
usus habit
uter- combining form: womb
uterina, A. *arteria uterina*
uterine curette *curette* for scraping the
uterus, e.g. in *curettage*
uterine myoma tumor of the muscle in the
uterus

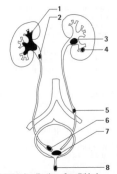

Fig. 514: localization of urolithiasis
1 Staghorn calculus 2 Ureteral calculus 3 Kidney
stone 4 Caliceal calculus 5 Ureteral calculus
6 Ureteral calculus 7 Urinary calculus
8 Urethral calculus

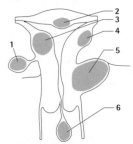

Fig. 515: uterine myoma
1 Pedunculated subserous 2 Submucous
3 Intramural 4 Subserous 5 Intraligamentary
6 Submucous polypoid

uterine tube *fallopian tube*
uterus pear-shaped muscular organ
ca. 8.5 cm long, located in the female

pelvis, in which the fetus and placenta are contained during *pregnancy*; viewed from the *vagina*, its parts are the mouth (portio vaginalis, os uteri), neck (cervix uteri) and body (corpus uteri)

uve- combining form: uvea

uvea middle layer of the eyeball, consisting of *choroid, ciliary body* and *iris*

uveitis *inflammation* of the *uvea*

uvula fleshy mass at the posterior edge of the soft palate, hanging down at the back of the throat

uvular deviation phenomenon seen in *vagus nerve* paresis: uvula pulls toward the unaffected side

V

V abbr. vision; *vitamin; volt*

V. abbr. *vein; vena*

V1–V6 designation for *Wilson* chest leads used for *ECG*
 V2 ICS left *parasternal*
 V3 between V2 and V4
 V4 ICS left *midclavicular*
 V5 ICS left anterior *axillary line*
 V6 ICS left medial *axillary line*

vaccination *immunization*

vaccine substance given for *vaccination*

vacuole fluid-filled cavity inside a *cell*

vacuum air-free space

vacuum extraction use of a *vacuum extractor* to end a difficult birth; extractor is attached to the fetal head and used to draw the infant out of the birth canal; abbr. VE

vacuum extractor obstetrical instrument used for *vacuum extraction*, which attaches to a baby's head by suction

vacuum mattress air cushion filled with tiny styrofoam pills that can be firmed up and shaped to the body by drawing out the air; used for transport of patients with suspected *cervical spine* injury

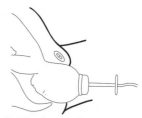

Fig. 516: vacuum extraction

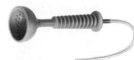

Fig. 517: vacuum extractor [A]

vacuum splint splint filled with tiny styrofoam pills that can be firmed up by drawing out the air and shaped around a limb, e.g. for transport of patients with suspected fracture in an extremity

vagina muscular tube ca. 10 cm long in the female genital region, leading to the internal genital organs

vaginal pert. to the *vagina*

vaginal carcinoma malignant tumor of the *vagina*

vaginal follicle aspiration puncture of the follicles by passing a needle through the wall at the back of the *vagina*

vaginal speculum *speculum*, e.g. according to Kallmorgen, used to dilate the *vagina* for *gynecological surgery* or examinations; enables visualization of the *cervix* et al.

vaginismus *reflexive* cramping of the pelvic floor muscles and *vagina*, leading to difficulties with sexual intercourse

vaginitis (colpitis) *inflammation* of the *vagina*

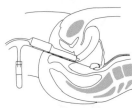

Fig. 518: vaginal follicle aspiration

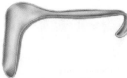

Fig. 519: vaginal speculum [A]

vagotomy *surgical* division of the *vagus nerve* to reduce production of stomach acid, e.g. for treatment of persistent *ulcers* in the *stomach* or *duodenum*; typically in the form of selective proximal vagotomy, in which only those branches of the nerve are severed that regulate stomach acid production

vagotonia hyperirritability of the *parasympathetic nervous system*

vagus nerve 10th *cranial nerve*; contains sensory, motor and parasympathetic fibers; mainly controls the *parasympathetic nervous system* and provides *motor* innvervation of the *pharynx*, *larynx* (together with the *glossopharyngeal nerve*) as well as the *sensory* innervation of the palate, pharynx and external auditory canal

vagus nerve stimulation implantation of a generator that stimulates the vagus nerve to reduce the incidence of seizures

vagus pulse *bradycardic heart rate*

vagus reflex (vagal reflex) *reflexive* reduction in *pulse* rate due to stimulation of the *vagus nerve*, e.g. from pressure on the *carotid artery* in the neck area

valerian herb with sedative properties

valgus bowed or bent inward, e.g. *genu valgum*; opp. *varus*

validity applicability; statistical term for the correctness of a parameter chosen and measured for the purpose of the study

vallate papilla taste bud at the back of the tongue, with receptors for bitterness

Valsalva's maneuver attempt to clear the *middle ear* by exhaling with the mouth and nose shut, or to increase intrathoracic pressure by exhaling with the *glottis* closed in order to slow the pulse, e.g. in *cardiac dysrhythmia*

valv(o)- combining form: valve

valva aortae *aortic valve*

valva atrioventricularis dextra *tricuspid valve*

valva atrioventricularis sinistra *mitral valve*

valva semilunaris (semilunar valve) collective term for the *aortic* and *pulmonary valves*

valva trunci pulmonalis *pulmonary valve*

valva venosa *venous valve*

valve membranous structure that can open or close, permitting passage of fluid through a hollow structure

valvotomy *valvulotomy*

valvular pneumothorax *tension pneumothorax*

valvulotomy (valvotomy) *surgical* opening of a stenosed heart valve

vanillyl mandelic acid main breakdown product of *catecholamine* metabolism; abbr. VMA

vapor steam

vaporizer device that converts liquid to vapor, e.g. for *anesthetic* gases

varia- combining form: change

variable changeable

variance distribution about a medan value

variation difference

varicella *chicken pox*

varicella virus (varicella-zoster virus) *DNA virus* that causes *chicken pox* or *shingles*; abbr. VZV

varices pl. *varix*

varicocele *varix*-like enlargement of the *veins* of the *spermatic cord*

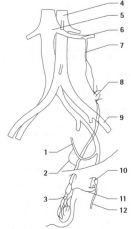

Fig. 520: varicocele
1 Inferior epigastric vein 2 External spermatic vein 3 Pampiniform plexus 4 Aorta 5 Inferior vena cava 6 Renal vein 7 Testicular vein 8 Ligature of varicocele 9 External iliac vein 10 Femoral vein 11 External pudendal vein 12 Great saphenous vein

varicophlebitis *thrombophlebitis* in a *varicose vein*; classic complication of *varicosis*

varicose vein stripping (stripping) removal of *varicose veins*

varicose veins *varicosis*

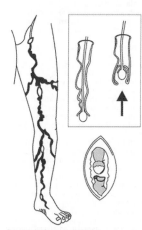

Fig. 521: varicose vein stripping acc. to Babcock

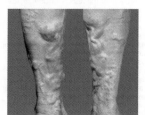

Fig. 522: pronounced varicose veins in leg

varicosis (varicose veins) dilation of *veins*, usually in the lower limbs or as *esophageal varices*

varicotomy *surgical* removal of *varices*

variola *smallpox*

variola virus *virus that causes smallpox*

varix pathologically dilated *vein*, usually in the lower limbs or as *esophageal varices*; *pl. varices*

varus bent or bowed outward, e.g. *genu varum*; opp. *valgus*

vas– combining form: vessel

vas deferens *spermatic duct*

vas lymphaticum *lymph vessel*

vasalgia vascular pain

vascular dementia *multi-infarct dementia*

vascular membrane (of the eye) *uvea*

vascular pert. to the blood vessels

vascularization formation of new blood vessels

vasculitis vascular *inflammation* that is triggered by an immune reaction

vasectomy *surgical* severing or removal of the *vas deferens*, e.g. for *sterilization*

vasoactive affecting the blood vessels

vasoconstriction narrowing of blood vessel due to contraction of the vascular smooth muscles; opp. *vasodilation*

vasoconstrictor drug used to constrict the blood vessels; opp. *vasodilator*

vasodepressor syncope *vasovagal syncope*

vasodilation dilation of blood vessels due to relaxation of the vascular smooth muscles; opp. *vasoconstriction*

vasodilator drug used to dilate the blood vessels; opp. *vasoconstrictor*

vasogenic originating in the blood vessels

vasography *radiography* of the vessels using a contrast medium, e.g. *phlebography*

vasomotion constriction and dilation of blood vessels by the vascular musculature

vasomotor headache sudden diffuse headache due to functional circulatory disorder

vasomotor nerves *nerves* that regulate vascular tone, including *vasodilation* and *vasoconstriction*, which are controlled by the *vasomotor center* in the *medulla oblongata*

vasomotor pert. to the *vasomotor nerves*

vasopathy nonspecific collective term for vascular disease

vasopressin *antidiuretic hormone*

vasopressor substance that constricts the blood vessels and increases *blood pressure*

vasospasm narrowing of vessels due to *spasms* of the vascular musculature

vasovagal syncope (vasodepressor syncope) *syncope* following unusual stress or emotional strain

VC abbr. *vital capacity*

VDRL lab test for *syphilis*

VE abbr. *vacuum extraction*

vegetarian 1) pert. to a plant-based diet; 2) person who has such a diet

vegetation proliferation; outgrowth

vegetative pert. to the *autonomic nervous system*

vein blood vessel, usually equipped with *venous valves*, which leads toward the heart; abbr. V.; opp. *artery*

velamentum covering

velum palatinum soft *palate*

vena vein

vena angularis origin of the *vena facialis*, between the bridge of the nose and the orbits

vena anonyma *(vena brachiocephalica)* *brachiocephalic vein*

vena axillaris (axillary vein) *vein* into which the arm veins and *basilic vein* empty; meets the *subclavian vein* at the level of the first rib

vena azygos *vein* that runs along the right side of the *spine* and joins the *superior vena cava*

vena cava one of the principal *veins* of the body; see *superior vena cava*, *inferior vena cava*

vena cutanea nonspecific collective term for a *vein* in the skin

vena mediana antebrachii *vein* that runs approximately through the center of the forearm between the *cephalic vein* and the *basilic vein*; see illustration under *basilic vein*

vena mediana cubiti (cubital vein) union of the *basilic vein* and *cephalic vein* in the elbow; see illustration under *basilic vein*

vena profunda nonspecific collective term for a deep vein; opp. *vena profunda*

vena renalis *renal vein*

vena retromandibularis *vein* running from the ear toward the lower jaw, which joins the facial vein

vena saphena magna *great saphenous vein*

vena saphena parva *small saphenous vein*

vena splenica *(vena lienalis) splenic vein*

vena subclavia *subclavian vein*

vena superficialis nonspecific collective term for a superficial *vein*; opp. *vena profunda*

venae pl. of *vena*; abbr. Vv.

venae cavernosae (penis) *veins* that run from the spongy bodies of the *penis* to its superficial and internal veins

venae cordis (coronary veins) *veins* of the heart that transport blood to the *coronary sinus*

venae dorsales linguae *veins* that transport blood from the back of the tongue to the *retromandibular vein*

venae emissariae valveless veins that mainly transport blood out of the interior of the skull, connecting the skull's internal and external veins

venae perforantes collective term for *veins* that connect the deep and superficial veins in the limbs

venae peronaeae veins in the calf that transport blood from the back of the lower leg to the posterior *tibial veins*

venectasia dilation of a *vein* due to slackening of its wall

veneer 1) thin ceramic shell that is bonded onto an intact *tooth* for cosmetic purposes; 2) to apply a *veneer* to a *tooth*

venereology (venerology) study of *sexually transmitted diseases*

venesection surgical exposure and opening of a vein, e.g. when *puncture* is not possible, for purposes of *infusion*

venography *phlebography*

venous pert. to the *veins*; opp. *arterial*

venous catheter see *central venous*

**catheter, peripheral venous catheter*

venous hum murmur *auscultable* over the *jugular vein*, indicative of increased blood flow velocity, e.g. in *anemia*

venous pulse visible pulsation of *veins* in the skin, usually due to *tricuspid valve insufficiency*

venous valve valve within a *vein* that prevents blood from flowing in the wrong direction and causing congestion

venovenous hemofiltration (continuous venovenous hemofiltration) procedure for removing urophanic substances and liquids from the blood in *renal failure*; technique: a membrane with a specific pore size is inserted between two *veins* and filters out a urine-like liquid via pump pressure, which is then substituted with electrolyte solution, depending on electrolyte balance status and need; abbr. CVVH

ventil- combining form: air, circulation

ventilate to cause air to circulate

ventilated having adequate air circulation

ventilation air circulation

ventilation bag *Ambu bag*

ventilation disorder impaired ventilation of the *lungs* due to *pulmonary restriction* or *pulmonary obstruction*

ventilation mask face mask for non*invasive* ventilation, e.g. with an *Ambu bag*, which is secured against the face using a *C-grip*; masks are available with an inflatable ring for a better seal, or without the ring for use with children (*Rendell-Baker mask*)

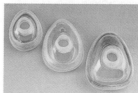

Fig. 523: ventilation masks [H]

ventral toward the abdomen, on the abdomen; opp. *dorsal*

ventricle chamber, esp. of the *heart* or *brain*

ventricul- combining form: chamber

ventricular pert. to a *ventricle*

ventricular drainage artificial internal or external drain to remove *CSF fluid* from the ventricles of the brain, e.g. in *hydrocephalus, subarachnoid bleed* or *brain edema*

ventricular extrasystole heart action occurring outside the normal *cardiac rhythm*, visible in an *ECG* and originating in the ventricular centers, e.g. the bundle of His; categorized according to the *Lown classification*; abbr. VES

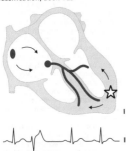

Fig. 524: ventricular extrasystole
1 Schematic 2 ECG

ventricular fibrillation life-threatening cardiac dysrhythmia visible in an *ECG*; usually caused by completely asynchronous cardiac muscle cell actions at a frequency of 350-500 per minute, which shows as rapid fibrillation waves in the ECG; can lead to complete circulatory collapse

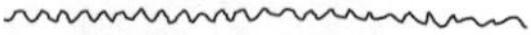

Fig. 525: ventricular fibrillation

ventricular flutter life-threatening cardiac dysrhythmia visible in an *ECG*; usually

caused by synchronous cardiac muscle cell actions at a frequency of 250-350 per minute, which shows as hairpin spikes in the ECG

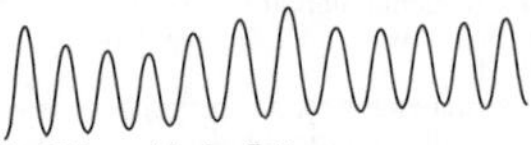

Fig. 526: ventricular flutter

ventricular septal defect congenital heart defect in which an opening exists between the left and right *ventricles*, leading to a left-to-right shunt; abbr. VSD

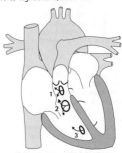

Fig. 527: ventricular septal defect
1 Infundibular VSD 2 Membranous VSD
3 Muscular VSD

ventricular tachycardia life-threatening cardiac dysrhythmia visible in an *ECG*; usually caused by re-entry in a ventricle with a frequency of 100-220 per minute; identifiable by the lengthened QRS complexes; abbr. VT

ventriculography *radiography* of the ventricles of the brain using a contrast medium

venule smallest type of *vein*, which leads out of the *capillaries*; opp. *arteriole*

VEP abbr. visual evoked potential; see *evoked potentials*

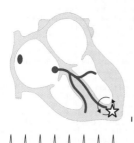

Fig. 528: ventricular tachycardia
1 Schematic 2 ECG

verbal oral, using speech; opp. *nonverbal*

verbigeration disorder of the thought processes in which words are meaningless or do not make sense, e.g. in *dementia*

verd– combining form: green

verm– combining form: worm

vermicide substance that kills worms

vermiform(is) worm-shaped

vermis worm

vernix caseosa *sebaceous* substance coating the skin of a *fetus* that enables easier passage through the birth canal

verruc– combining form: wart

verruca *wart*

verrucose *wart*-like

vers– combining form: turning

–version combining form: turning

vertebra (spondylus) bone of the spinal column; pl. vertebrae

vertebra– combining form: spinal (column)

vertebrae pl. of *vertebra*

vertebral pert. to the *vertebrae* or *spinal column*

vertebral foramen opening between the vertebral body and neural arch

vertex presentation normal presentation of a baby immediately before birth, with the crown of the head foremost in the birth canal

vertical mattress suture see *Allgöwer suture, Donati suture*

vertigo dizziness; disequilibrium; the perception that one's body or the environment is in motion, which is usually accompanied by nausea, vomiting, unsteady gait and sweating

verus true

VES abbr. *ventricular extrasystole*

vesica bladder

vesica fellea *gallbladder*

vesica seminalis *seminal vesicle*

vesicants intravenous chemotherapy drugs, e.g. vincristine; can produce skin blisters if they infiltrate during administration

vesicle small blister with a cavity measuring less than 0.5 cm; one of the *primary efflorescences*; see also *bulla*

vesicular resembling a blister; pert. to a *vesicle*

vesicular breathing normally *auscultable* breath sounds heard on inspiration

vesiculitis *inflammation* of the *seminal vesicle* vessels, e.g. in a *wound* or a *tissue*

vestibul– combining form: atrium, entry

vestibular pert. to a *vestibule*

vestibular organ organ of equilibrium located in the inner ear; includes the three semicircular canals

vestibule space or cavity at the entrance to a canal

vestibule of the vagina space between the *labia minora* into which the *vagina* opens, as well as the *urethra*

vestibulocochlear nerve 8th *cranial nerve* contains sensory fibers; mainly controls acoustic perception and sense of balance

via through, by way of

vial small bottle for solutions used for injections top of bottle has a rubber membrane for multiple withdrawals

vibration rapid back-and-forth movement

V

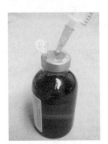

Fig. 529: vial

Vibrio cholerae *Vibrio* bacterium that causes *cholera*

Vibrio genus of motile rod-shaped *gram-negative bacteria*; pl. Vibriones

vigil coma semiconscious state of delirium; patient appears awake, sometimes makes verbal sounds, and stares with the eyes wide open

vigilance watchfulness; alertness

villus projection or protrusion of a mucous membrane, e.g. in the small intestine; pl. villi

vir man

vir(u)- combining form: virus

viral pert. to *viruses*

Virchow's triad complex of risk factors for *thrombosis:* changes in vessel walls, blood flow and blood composition

viremia presence of *viruses* in the blood

viri men

virid- combining form: green

virilization (masculinization) presence of masculine characteristics in a female, including development of secondary sexual characteristics (e.g. facial hair growth); caused by *androgens*, e.g. due to *adrenal cortex tumors*

virological pert. to *virology*

virology study of *viruses*

virucide substance that kills *viruses*

virulence degree of infective power of a pathogen

virulent pert. to virulence

virus pathogen that can reproduce only inside a host organism

virustatic agent drug used to inhibit multiplication of *viruses*

viscer- combining form: internal organs

viscera (splanchnon) *organs* located inside the body esp. the abdomen

visceral pert. to the *viscera*

visceral pleura *pleura* that covers the *lungs*

viscosity thickness (pert. to fluids)

viscous thick, sticky (pert. to fluids)

vision test test of *visual acuity* in each eye, using an eye chart; for the chart shown here, the distance between the eye and the chart should be 35 cm in good light

visual pert. to the sense of sight

visual acuity resolving power of the *eyes*

visual field area that the eye can view from a fixed position

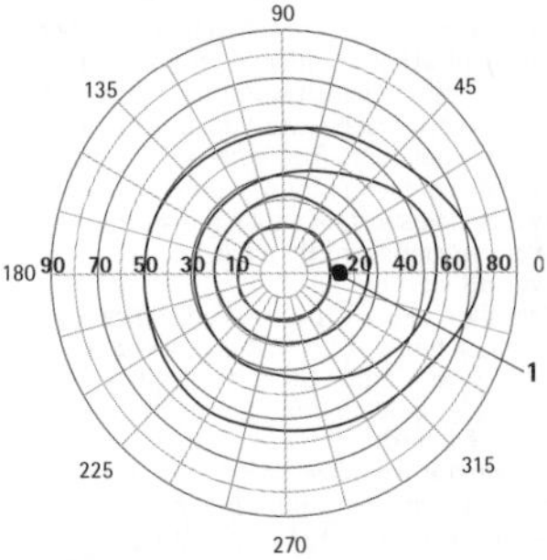

Fig. 530: visual field of right eye
1 Blind spot

visual field test *perimetry*

visual loss gradual or sudden failure of vision; if sudden, may be due to a stroke, which requires urgent testing and evaluation

vita life

vital having life

vital capacity volume of air present in the lungs at the end of a maximal inspiration, excluding the *residual volume*; abbr. VC, VT$_{max}$; see illustration under *spirometry*

vital functions collective term for respiration and circulation

vital signs collective term for measured values for respiratory and circulatory functions

vitality life force, animation

vitamin A *retinol*

vitamin B$_1$ *thiamine*

vitamin B$_{12}$ *cyanocobalamin*

vitamin B$_2$ *riboflavin*

vitamin B$_6$ *pyridoxine*

vitamin C *ascorbic acid*

vitamin D *calciferol*

vitamin E *tocopherol*

vitamin H *biotin*

vitamin K *phylloquinone*

vitamin substance essential to the body that must be acquired from food sources because the body cannot produce it in sufficient amounts; classified as fat-soluble (*E, D, K, A*) or water-soluble (*B$_1$, B$_2$, B$_6$, B$_{12}$, C, H, folic acid, niacin, pantothenic acid*)

vitiligo sharply defined white de*pigmented* patches on the skin

vitium defect; malformation

vitium cordis *heart defect*

vitrectomy *surgical* removal of the contents of the *vitreous body* of the *eye*

vitreous body gelatinous mass of *collagen* inside the *eye*, containing no blood vessels

vivi– combining form: living

VMA abbr. *vanillyl mandelic acid*

vocal cords (chordes vocales) mucous membrane-covered folds in the *larynx* necessary to vocal production

vocal fremitus *fremitus*

voiding cystourethrogram *voiding cystourethrography*

voiding cystourethrography reflux cystography with simultaneous visualization of the *urethra*, e.g. to detect narrowing of the bladder neck or urethral *stricture*

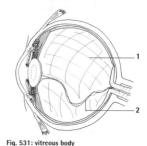

Fig. 531: vitreous body
1 Vitreous body 2 Hyaloid canal

vola palm of the hand

volar pert. to the palm of the hand

volatile easily evaporated or vaporized

–volemia combining form: blood volume

Volkmann's triangle triangular piece of bone at the posterior superior end of the *tibia*

volt electrical unit of pressure; abbr. V

volume deficiency shock *hypovolemic shock*

volume substitution replacement of body fluids via *infusion*, e.g. of *electrolyte* solutions or *plasma volume extenders*

volv– combining form: turning

volvulus twisting of the intestine about its own axis; can lead to mechanical *ileus*

vomer posterior inferior portion of the nasal septum

vomitus vomit

voussure bulging of the entire cardiac region due to a congenital heart defect

VRE abbr. vancomycin-resistant enterococcus; a gram-positive organism commonly found in the GI tract and female GU tract; infected patient must be isolated

VS abbr. *vital signs*

VSD abbr. *ventricular septal defect*

V$_T$ abbr. tidal volume

VT abbr. *ventricular tachycardia*

VT$_{max}$ abbr. maximal *tidal volume*; *vital capacity*

vulnerable able to be injured

vulnus *wound*

vulsellum forceps surgical instrument according to Czerny, resembling a forceps with sharp hooks; used to grasp tumors et al.

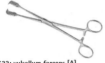

Fig. 532: vulsellum forceps [A]

vulva external female *genitalia*

vulvar carcinoma malignant tumor of the *vulva*, usually found in older women

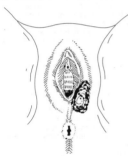

Fig. 533: vulvar carcinoma

vulvectomy removal of the *vulva*

vulvitis *inflammation* of the *vulva*

vulvovaginitis *inflammation* of the external female *genitalia* and *vagina*

Vv. abbr. *venae*

VZV abbr. *varizella-zoster virus*

W

W abbr. *watt*

Waldenström's macroglobulinemia disease marked by disorder of *protein* metabolism, resulting in abnormally large *globulins* in the blood

Wallace see *rule of nines*

wandering testicle retraction of the *testicle* out of the *scrotum*, caused by the *cremaster reflex*

wart benign circumscribed *viral* proliferation of *epithelial* cells

Wartenberg's disease (paresthetic nocturnal brachialgia) nighttime pain and paresthesias in the arm, occurring mainly in older women

watch–glass nails (hippocratic nails) excessive arching of the fingernails due to *chronic oxygen* deficiency; usually occurs in combination with *clubbing*

water on the brain *hydrocephalus*

Waterhouse–Friderichsen syndrome *septic infectious disease* caused by *meningococci*, with *shock* and *renal failure*

watt unit of electrical power, e.g. in *ergometry*; abbr. W

Weber A fracture fracture of the *lateral malleolus* at or distal to the joint space, or lateral *collateral ligament* tear, or avulsion of the ligament at the tip of the lateral malleolus

Weber B fracture oblique fracture of the lateral malleolus at the level of the *syndesmosis*, possibly with avulsion fracture of the medial malleolus

Weber C fracture *fracture* of the distal shaft of the fibula, proximal to the torn *syndesmosis*

Weber test hearing test for distinguishing between unilateral conduction deafness and nerve deafness; a *tuning fork* is placed on the midline of the *skull* and the patient indicates whether she perceives the sound as central or louder on one side

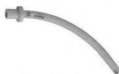

Fig. 535: Wendl tube [K]

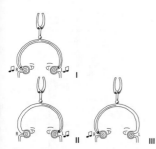

Fig. 534: Weber test
I Normal hearing, both ears II Perception deafness, right ear III Conduction deafness, right ear

wedge pressure (pulmonary capillary wedge pressure) pressure in the left atrium, which can be measured with a *pulmonary artery catheter* by inflating the balloon; mean pressure 8-12 mmHg; elevated in left-heart *infarction, cardiogenic shock, left heart failure, hypervolemia, mitral valve defect* and *cardiac tamponade*; depressed in *hypovolemia*; abbr. PCWP

Wegener's disease *Wegener's granulomatosis*

Wegener's granulomatosis (Wegener's syndrome) *granulomatous necrotizing vasculitis*, initially affecting the ear/ nose/ throat area and later the *joints, lungs* and *kidneys*

Wegener's syndrome *Wegener's granulomatosis*

Weil's disease *leptospirosis*

Wenckebach see *2nd-degree AV block*

Wendl tube (nasopharyngeal tube) short rubber tube inserted into the nasopharyngeal area; used for patients with altered mental state to prevent swallowing the tongue and blockage of the airway; see also *Guedel tube*

Werlhof's disease *idiopathic thrombocytopenic purpura*

Wernicke's encephalopathy (Wernicke's syndrome) genetically determined *brain* disease caused by a lack of *thiamine*, usually triggered by alcohol abuse; leads to severe *disorientation*, memory loss and visual hallucinations

Wernicke's syndrome *Wernicke's encephalopathy*

Westergren's blood test blood sedimentation test, using blood to which *sodium citrate* is added as an anticoagulant; blood sedimentation enables detection of changes in blood protein composition and thus is useful for monitoring *infections* and neoplastic diseases; see *erythrocyte sedimentation rate*

Western blot test technique used to check the validity of an ELISA test; can detect small amounts of antibiodies

wheal *urtica*

whiplash injury overextension of the *cervical spine* due to traction and shearing force, usually caused by a rear-impact car accident

Whipple's operation *operation* in which portions of the *stomach, pancreas, bile ducts* and *jejunum* are removed, along with the entire *duodenum* and *gallbladder*; usually performed in cases of malignant tumors of the bile ducts or pancreas

whisper test hearing test in which test words are spoken at normal volume and in a whisper at various distances

W

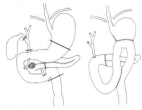

Fig. 536: partial duodenopancreatectomy
acc. to Whipple

WHO abbr. World Health Organization
whooping cough *pertussis*
Wilms' tumor (nephroblastoma) malignant
tumor of the *kidney*
Wilson block *right bundle branch block*
Wilson leads chest leads used for
electrocardiography, which branch into the
V1, V2, V3, V4, V5 and V6 leads; readings
are taken from these along with the *limb
leads*; see also *Einthoven* and *Goldberger*
leads; see Fig. 538 for *electrode* positions
for chest leads
Wilson's disease (hepatolenticular
degeneration) inherited disorder of copper
metabolism, with deposition of *copper* in
organs, e.g. the *brain*
windpipe *trachea*
Winterstein fracture metacarpal fracture
with no *joint* involvement; see also *Bennett
fracture*, *Rolando fracture*

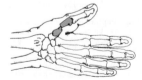

Fig. 537: Winterstein fracture

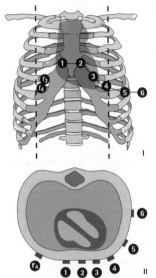

Fig. 538: Wilson leads
I Placement of unipolar Wilson precordial leads
II Mapping of electrodes to heart (cross section)

withdrawal bleeding *uterine* bleeding due
to decline in natural *hormone* production,
or from taking hormone preparations
Witzel's gastrostomy *surgically* created
connection of the skin of the abdomen to
the stomach for enteral nutrition in patients with impassable *esophageal carcinoma*
Wolff-Parkinson-White syndrome (pre-
excitation syndrome) premature excitation
of the heart chambers due to abnormal
congenital shunt between the atria and
ventricles, visible in an *ECG*; abbr. WPW

W

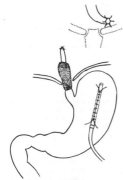

Fig. 539: Witzel's gastrostomy

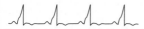

Fig. 540: Wolff-Parkinson-White syndrome with sinus rhythm

womb *uterus*

Woodbridge tube *endotracheal tube* with an integrated metal coil that prevents kinks from forming in the tube, e.g. during *operations* where the patient is in ventral position

workaholic person suffering from a form of *addiction* marked by excessive need to be working

wound open break in tissue, with or without loss of substance

wound dehiscence separation of the edges of a *wound*

wound healing healing process of a *wound* with 1) formation of a thin scar with no infection (healing by first intention), or 2) *infection* or impairment of the healing process (healing by second intention)

wound retractor sharp *surgical instrument* according to Volkmann, used to hold the edges of a wound apart and for various other holding tasks during surgery; may have one or several prongs

WPW abbr. *Wolff-Parkinson-White syndrome*

X

X chromosome sex *chromosome*, of which women have two and men only one, along with a *Y chromosome*

x-ray radiography (roentgenography) most commonly used imaging procedure; visualization of bones and calcified structures using brief bursts of electromagnetic waves (x-rays)

xantho- combining form: yellow

xanthelasma (palpebrarum) yellowish fatty plaques on the eyelids

xanthin substance that results from breakdown of *protein* bodies

xanthochromia yellowish discoloration of the *CSF fluid* caused by the presence of blood

xanthoderma yellowness of the skin, e.g. due to excessive consumption of carrots

xanthoma yellowish-brown nodules on the skin caused by *cholesterol* deposits

xanthomatosis presence of *xanthomas* in the skin due to disorders of fat metabolism

xanthopsia condition in which objects appear yellow, e.g. due to *digitalis* poisoning

xeno- combining form: foreign, strange

xenogene(t)ic of a different species; see also *allogene(t)ic, syngene(t)ic*

xenogeneic graft *transplantation* of *organs* or *tissue* from a different species, e.g. from human to animal; opp. *allogeneic graft*

xenoplasty *xenogeneic graft*

xero- combining form: dry

xerocheilia dry lips

xeroderma dry skin

X

xerophthalmia dryness of the *cornea* and *conjunctiva* of the eye, caused by reduced tear production, e.g. from *vitamin A* deficiency

xeroradiography *radiography* using selenium-coated *plates*

xerostomia dry mouth due to inadequate or absent secretion of saliva

xerotic dry

xiphoid process (processus xiphoideus) sword-shaped process of the *sternum*

xiphoiditis *inflammation* of the *xiphoid process*

XXX syndrome *trisomy* in which three *X*chromosomes are present

XXY syndrome *Klinefelter syndrome*

Y

Y chromosome sex *chromosome*, of which males have one plus an *X chromosome*, and women have none (having instead two X chromosomes)

Y-bypass Y-shaped vascular *prosthesis* placed between the *aorta* and *iliac artery*

Y-fracture *fracture* forming a Y-shaped fissure

Yamakawa drain *drain* that enables long-term diversion of *bile* into the *duodenum*, as well as through the abdominal wall to the outside, e.g. in *Klatskin tumor*

yellow body (of ovary) (corpus luteum) yellowish body that develops after ovulation and produces the *hormones progesterone* and *estrogen*

yellow fever febrile tropical *infectious disease* belonging to the *hemorrhagic fevers;* leads to swelling of the *liver, jaundice,* bleeding tendency, vomiting blood ("vomito negro"), *hematuria* and *renal failure;* the yellow fever *virus* is transmitted via the bite of the *Aedes aegypti* mosquito

yellow jaundice yellowish discoloration of the skin and *sclerae* due to buildup of *bilirubin* in the blood

Yersinia genus of motile non-*spore*-forming rod-shaped *gram-negative bacteria*

Yersinia pestis *Yersinia bacterium* that causes *plague*

yoga Indian teachings involving a system of poses and spiritual exercises

Young syndrome blockage of the *epididymis* by *secretions*

Z

Zangenmeister's maneuver obstetrical maneuver for determining the distance between the pubic *symphysis* and the head of the infant

Zeis' glands *sebaceous* glands near the eyelashes

Zeiss loop loop used to remove *distal* stones (< 10 mm) from the *ureter*

Zenker's diverticulum *esophageal diverticulum* in the lower pharyngeal area, usually occurring in older males

zinc important trace element required for numerous metabolic processes in the body; chemical symbol: Zn

Zn chemical symbol: *zinc*

Zollinger-Ellison syndrome *gastrinoma*

zon- combining form: zone, region

zoo- combining form: animal

zoonosis nonspecific general term for any disease that can be transmitted from animals to humans

zoster ophthalmicus *herpes zoster* affecting the 1st trigeminal branch, usually on one side only

zoster *shingles*

zyg- combining form: yoke; pair; joining

zygoma cheekbone

zygomatic bone yoke bone in the viscerocranium

zygomaticum os (os zygomaticum) zygomatic bone

zygote fertilized ovum

zymo- combining form: enzyme

Appendix
Medical Abbreviations

#	number; fracture; pounds
~	approximate; similar
@	at
+ve	positive
–ve	negative
↓ ; ↑	down, lowered; up, raised
↔	steady, normal, unchanged
? ...	query ...
2x, 3x ...	twice, three times ...
A	anemia
AA	African-American; Alcoholics Anonymous
AAA	abdominal aortic aneurysm
Ab	antibody; abortion
ABC	airway, breathing, circulation
abd	abdomen
ABG	arterial blood gases
Abn	abnormal(ity)
Abx	antibiotics
AC	air conduction; adrenal cortex; abdominal circumference
ac	before meals (Lat: ante cibum)
ACE(–I)	angiotensin-convert. enzy. (inhibitors)
A(C)LS	advanced (cardiac) life support
ACU	ambulatory (acute) care unit
ADD	attention deficit disorder
ADL	activities of daily living
adm	admission
AE	adverse effects/event
AF	atrial fibrillation; acid-fast
AFB	acid-fast bacilli
AG	antigen

AI	aortic insufficiency
aka	also known as
ALC	alternative level of care
Alk Phos	alkaline phosphatase
ALL	acute lymphocytic leukemia
ALS	amyotrophic lateral sclerosis
AMA	against medical advice; antimitochondrial Ab
AMI	acute myocardial infarction
AML	acute myelogenous leukemia
ANA	antinuclear antibody
ANCA	antineutrophil cytoplasmic antibodies
ANP	atrial natriuretic peptide
A&O	alert and oriented
AOB	alcohol on breath
AP	anteroposterior; angina pectoris
APB	atrial premature beat
APC	atrial premature contraction
ARDS	adult respiratory distress syndrome
ARF	acute renal/respiratory failure; acute rheumatic fever
AS	aortic stenosis; arteriosclerosis
ASA	acetylsalicylic acid (aspirin)
ASD	atrial septal defect
ASHD	arteriosclerotic heart disease
ASVD	arteriosclerotic vascular disease
AV	arteriovenous; atrioventricular; aortic valve
AVM	arteriovenous malformation
AVR	aortic valve replacement
AVRT	atrioventr. reentrant tachycardia
A&W	alive and well

AXR	abdominal x-ray
BAL	blood alcohol level; bronchoalveolar lavage
BBB	bundle branch block; blood-brain barrier
BC	blood culture; basal cell; birth control
BCG	bacillus Calmette-Guerin
BF	black female
bid	two times daily (Lat: bis in die)
biw	twice a week
BJ	biceps jerk; bone + joint
BJP	Bence Jones protein
BLS	basic life support
BM	black male; bowel movement; bone marrow
BMI	body mass index
BP	blood pressure; bullous pemphigoid
BPH	benign prostatic hypertrophy
BPM	beats/breaths per minute
BRBPR	bright red blood per rectum
BS	breath (or bowel) sounds; blood sugar
BUN	blood urea nitrogen
BW	black woman; birth weight
Bx	biopsy
c	with (Lat: cum)
C	Celsius; chlamydia; concentration; cyanosis
CA	cancer, carcinoma
CABG	coronary artery bypass graft (pron.: 'cabbage')
CAD	coronary artery disease
CAH	chronic active hepatitis
CAT	computed axial tomography
CBC	complete blood count

CBD	common bile duct
CC	chief complaint; creatinine clearance
CCB	calcium channel blocker
CCE	clubbing, cyanosis, edema
CCF	congestive cardiac failure
CCU	coronary (critical) care unit
CDC	Centers for Disease Control
CDH	congenital dislocation of hip
CEA	carcinoembryonic antigen
CF	complem. fixation; cystic fibrosis
CHD	congenital heart disease
CHF	congestive heart failure
CI	cardiac index; coronary insuff.
CIS	carcinoma in situ
CK(-MB)	creatine kinase (MB)
CLL	chronic lymphocytic leukemia
CMV	cytomegalovirus
CML	chronic myelogenous leukemia
CN	cranial nerve
CNS	central nervous system
CO	cardiac output
c/o	complains of
COPD	chronic obstructive pulmonary disease
CP	chest pain; cerebral palsy
CPAP	continuous positive airway pressure
CPK	creatinine phosphokinase
CPR	cardiopulmonary resuscitation
CRF	chronic renal failure
CRI	chronic renal insufficiency
CRP	C-reactive protein
C/S	Cesarean section
C&S	culture + sensitivity; conjunctiva + sclera

CSF	cerebrospinal fluid; colony-stimulating factor
CT	computed tomography
CV	cardiovascular; curriculum vitae
CVA	cerebral vascular accident, stroke; costovertebral angle
CVP	central venous pressure
CVS	cardiovascular system/surgery
c/w	consistent with
CXR	chest x-ray
d	days
DARF	dosage adjustment in renal failure
DAT	dementia of Alzheimer's type; diet as tolerated
D/C	discontinue; discharge
D&C	dilation and curettage
DD (Ddx)	differential diagnosis
D&E	dilation and evacuation
DHS	dynamic hip screw
DHx	drug history
DI	diabetes insipidus
DIC	disseminated intravascular coagulation
DJD	degenerative joint disease
DKA	diabetic ketoacidosis
DM	diabetes mellitus
DNKA	did not keep appointment
DNR	do not resuscitate
DO	disorder; Doctor of Osteopathy
DOA	date of admission; dead on arrival
DOB	date of birth
DOE	dyspnea on exertion
DPT	diphtheria, pertussis, tetanus
DSA	digital subtraction angiography

DSM	Diagnostic and Statistical Manual of Mental Disorders
DT	delirium tremens
DTR	deep tendon reflex
DU	duodenal ulcer; decubitus ulcer
DUB	dysfunctional uterine bleeding
D&V	diarrhea and vomiting
DVT	deep vein thrombosis
D5W	5% dextrose in water
Dx	diagnosis
EBL	estimated blood loss
EBV	Epstein-Barr virus
ECC	emergency cardiac care
ECF	extracellular fluid
ECG	electrocardiogram
ECT	electroconvulsive therapy
ED	emergency department; epidural
ED50	median effective dose
EDC	estimated date of confinement
EDD	estimated delivery date
EEG	electroencephalogram
EENT	eyes, ears, nose, throat
EF	ejection fraction
EGC	early gastric carcinoma
EGD	esophagogastroduodenoscopy
EKG	electrocardiogram
ELISA	enzyme-linked immunosorbent assay
EMD	electromechanical dissociation
EMG	electromyogram
EMS	emergency medical services
ENT	ear, nose and throat
EOM(I)	extraocular muscles (intact)
EOS	eosinophil(s)
ER	emergency room
ERCP	endoscopic retrograde cholangiopancreatography

ESR	erythrocyte sedimentation rate
ESRD	end stage renal disease
EtOH	ethanol
ETT	exercise tolerance test; endotrach. tube
EW	emergency ward
F	father; female; Fahrenheit
FB	foreign body
FBS	fasting blood sugar
FD	Forceps delivery; fully dilated
FEV	forced expiratory volume
FFP	fresh frozen plasma
FH(x)	family history
FMP	first menstrual period
FNA	fine-needle aspiration
FOBT	fecal occult blood testing
FOC	father of child
FRC	functional residual capacity
FT	full-term
FTND	full-term normal delivery
FTT	failure to thrive
F/U	follow up
FUO	fever of unknown origin
FVC	forced vital capacity
Fx	fracture
G	gravida
GA	general anesthesia; gestational age
GB	gall bladder
GBS	Guillain-Barré syndrome
GCS	Glasgow Coma Scale
GDM	gestational diabetes mellitus
GERD	gastroesophageal reflux disease
GFR	glomerular filtration rate
GI(T)	gastrointestinal (tract)
GIFT	gamete intrafallopian transfer
gluc	glucose

GN	glomerulonephritis
G6PD	glucose-6-phosphate dehydrog.
GSW	gun shot wound
GTT	glucose tolerance test
gtt	drops (Lat: guttae)
GU	gastric ulcer; genitourinary
GUS	genitourinary system
HA	headache; hemolytic anemia
HAV	hepatitis A virus
Hb	hemoglobin
HBP	high blood pressure
HBV	hepatitis B virus
Hct	hematocrit
HCV	hepatitis C virus
HDL	high-density lipoprotein
HDU	hemodialysis (high dependency) unit
HEENT	head, eyes, ears, nose and throat
HI	head injury; hepatic insufficiency
HIB	hemophilus influenzae type B
HIV	human immunodeficiency virus
HLA	human leukocyte antigen
HMO	health maintenance organization
h/o	history of
HOCM	hypertrophic obstructive cardiomyopathy (pron.: 'hocum')
H&P	history and physical examination
HPI	history of present illness
HPV	human papilloma virus
HR	heart rate
HS	heart sounds; herpes simplex
hs	at bedtime, hour of sleep (Lat: hora somni)

HSM	hepatosplenomegaly; holosystolic murmer
HSP	Henoch-Schönlein purpura
HSV	herpes simplex virus
HTN	hypertension
HUS	head ultrasound, hemolytic uremic syndrome
HVA	homovanillic acid
Hx	history; hospitalization
IA	intraarterial
IBD	inflammatory bowel disease
ICD-9	International Classification of Diseases, 9th Revision
ICH	intracerebral hemorrhage
ICP	intracranial pressure
ICS	intercostal space
ICU	intensive care unit
ID	infectious disease
I&D	incision and drainage
IDA	iron deficiency anemia
IDDM	insulin-dependent diabetes mell.
IFN	interferon
Ig	immunoglobulin
IHD	ischemic heart disease
IL	interleukin
IM	intramuscular
IMI	inferior myocardial infarction
imp	impression; important; improved
IMV	intermitt. mandatory ventilation
INR	international normalized ratio
I&O	intake and output
IP	inpatient
IPPB	intermitt. pos. pressure breathing
IRDS	infant resp. distress syndrome
ITP	idiopathic thrombocytopenic purpura

IUD	intrauterine contraceptive device
IUGR	intrauterine growth retardaton
IUP	intrauterine pregnancy
IV	intravenous
IVC	inferior vena cava
IVCD	intraventr. conduction defect
IVDU	intravenous drug user
IVF	intravenous fluids; in vitro fertilization
IVH	intraventricular hemorrhage
IVIG	inravenous immunoglobulin
IVP	intravenous pyelogram/push
IVU	intravenous urogram
JOD(M)	juvenile onset diabetes mellitus
JPC	junctional premature contraction
JRA	juvenile rheumatoid arthritis
JVC	jugular venous catheter
JVD	jugular venous distension
JVP	jugular venous pulse/pressure
KJ	knee jerk
KS	Kaposi sarcoma; kidney stone
KUB	kidneys, ureters, bladder (x-ray)
L	left
LA	left atrium; local anesthesia
Lab	laboratory
lac	laceration
LAD	left anterior descend. (coronary artery); left axis deviation
LAE	left atrial enlargement
LAFB	left anterior fascicular block
LAHB	left anterior hemiblock
LAP	leukocyte alkaline phosphatase; left atrial pressure
lap	laparoscopy
lapt	laparotomy

LBBB	left bundle branch block
LBP	lower back pain
LBW	low birth weight
LDH	lactate dehydrogenase
LDL	low-density lipoprotein
LE	lower extremity; lupus erythematosus
LFD	low fat diet
LFT	liver function test
LGA	large for gestational age
LGV	lymphogranuloma venerum
LKS	liver, kidney, spleen
LLE	left lower extremity
LLL	left lower lobe
LLQ	left lower quadrant
LMD	local medical doctor
LMN	lower motor neuron
LMP	last menstrual period
LN	lymph node
LOC	loss (level) of consciousness
LP	lumbar puncture
LPFB	left posterior fascicular block
LPHB	left posterior hemiblock
LPN	licensed practical nurse
LSB	left sternal border
LUE	left upper extremity
LUL	left upper lobe
LUQ	left upper quadrant
LV	left ventricle
LVEDP	left ventric. end-diast. pressure
LVF	left ventricular failure
LVH	left ventricular hypertrophy
M	mother; male
m	murmur
MAE	moves all extremities
MAO(I)	monoamine oxidase (inhibitor)
MAT	multifocal atrial tachycardia

MAP	mean arterial pressure
MCH(C)	mean corpuscular hemoglobin (concentration)
MCL	midclavicular line
MCTD	mixed connective tissue disease
MCV	mean corpuscular volume
MDD	max. daily dose, manic-depr. DO
MDI	metered-dose inhaler
MEA	multiple endocr. adenomatosis
meds	medication
MEN	multiple endocrine neoplasia
MGF	maternal grandfather
MGM	maternal grandmother
MHC	major histocompatib. complex
MI	myocardial infarction; mental illness; mitral insufficiency
MIC	minimal inhibitory concentration
MLC	mixed lymphocyte culture
M&M	morbidity and mortality
MMFR	maximal midexpiratory flow rate
MMPI	Minnesota Multiphasic Personality Inventory
MMR	measles, mumps, rubella
MOS	mitral opening snap
MPGN	membranoproliferative glomerulonephritis
MR	mitral regurgitation; mental retardation
MRA	magnetic resonance angiogr.
MRDD	max. recommended daily dose
MRI	magnetic resonance imaging
MRSA	methicillin-resistant Staphylococcus aureus
MRT	magnetic resonance tomography

MS	mitral stenosis; multiple sclerosis; mental status; medical student; morphine sulfate	noct	at night (Lat: nocte)
		NOS	not otherwise specified
		NP	nasopharyngeal
MSE	mental status examination	NPH	neutral protamine Hagedorn (regular insulin); normal pressure hydrocephalus
MSO4	morphine sulfate		
MV	mitral valve		
MVA	motor vehicle accident		
MVI	multiple vitamin injection	NPO	nothing by mouth (Lat: nihil per orem)
MVP	mitral valve prolapse		
MVR	mitral valve replacement	NQWMI	non-Q wave myocard. infarction
MVV	maximum voluntary ventilation	NS	normal saline; not specific
N	normal; nerve	NSAID	nonsteroidal anti-inflamm. drug
N/A	not applicable	NSR	normal sinus rhythm
NAD	no acute distress	NT	nasotracheal; not tested; not tender
NAI	nonaccidental injury		
NAS	no added salt	NTD	nothing to do; neur. tube defect
NB	note well (Lat: nota bene)	NTT	nasotracheal tube
NBN	newborn nursery	NTG	nitroglycerine
NC	no change; nasal cannula; normocephalic	N&V	nausea and vomiting
		NVD	nausea, vomiting, diarrhea
NC/AT	normocephalic, atraumatic	O	objective
ND	not detected/diagnosed/done	OA	osteoarthritis; occiput anterior
NDI	nephrogenic diabetes insipidus	OAF	osteoclast-activating factor
NE	norepinephrine	OB	obstetrics
NEC	necrotizing enterocolitis	OBS	organic brain syndrome
neg	negative	occ	occasionally
NG	nasogastric	OCG	oral cholecystogram
NGT	nasogastric tube	OCR	oculocephalic reflex
NH	nursing home	OCT	oral contraceptive therapy
NHL	non-Hodgkin's lymphoma	OD	overdose; once daily; right eye
NIDDM	noninsulin-dependent DM	OE	on examination
N/K	not known	OF	open fracture
NKA	no known allergies	OGTT	oral glucose tolerance test
NKDA	no known drug allergies	OM	otitis media
NL	normal limits	OOB	out of bed
NM	neuromuscular	OP	oropharynx; occiput posterior; opening pressure
NMS	neuroleptic malignant syndrome		
		O&P	ova and parasites

OPD	outpatient department
OPV	oral polio vaccine
OR	operating room
OREF	open reduction, external fixation
ORIF	open reduction, internal fixation
orth	orthopedic
OS	by mouth (Lat: os); left eye (Lat: oculus sinister); overall survival; opening snap (heart sound)
OSA	obstructive sleep apnea
osmo	osmolality
OT	occupational therapy
OTC	over the counter
OU	both eyes (Lat: oculus uterque)
P	after (post); parent; plan; pulse
P_2	second pulmonic heart sound
PA	patient; posteroanterior (x-ray); physician's assistant; pulmonary artery
PAC	premature atrial contraction
PAN	polyarteritis nodosa
PAP	pulmonary artery pressure
PAT	paroxysmal atrial tachycardia
PAWP	pulm. artery wedge pressure
PBC	primary biliary cirrhosis
PBP	penicillin-binding protein
PC	present complaint
pc	after meals (Lat: post cibum)
PCA	patient-controlled analgesia
PCB	postcoital bleeding
PCN	penicillin
PCO	polycystic ovaries
PCP	pneumocystis carinii pneumonia; primary care physician
PCR	polymerase chain reaction
PCV	packed cell volume
PCW	pulmonary capillary wedge
PD	peritoneal dialysis; Paget's disease; Parkinson's disease
PDA	patent ductus arteriosus
PDR	Physician's Desk Reference
PE	pulmonary embolism; physical examination
PEEP	positive end-expiratory pressure
PEF(R)	peak expiratory flow (rate)
PEG	percutaneous endoscopic gastrostomy
PERRLA	pupils equal, round, react to light and accommodation
PET	positron emission tomography
PFT	pulmonary function test
PG(E)	prostaglandin (E)
PGF	paternal grandfather
PGM	paternal grandmother
PH	past history; pulmonary HTN
PI	present illness
PICC	peripherally inserted central catheter
PICU	pediatric intensive care unit
PID	pelvic inflammatory disease
PKD	polycystic kidney disease
PKU	phenylketonuria
PLT	platelets
PM	postmortem; postmenopausal
PMB	postmenopausal bleeding
PMH	past medical history
PMI	point of maximal impulse; past medical illness
PMN	polymorphonuclear leukocyte
PMR	polymyalgia rheumatica; phys. medicine and rehabilitation
PMS	premenstrual syndrome
Pn	pneumonia

PND	paroxysmal nocturnal dyspnea
PNH	paroxysmal nocturnal hemoglobinuria
PNS	peripheral nervous system
PO	by mouth (Lat: per os); postoper.
POC	postoperative care; product of conception
POD	postoperative day
POP	plaster of Paris
PPD	purified protein derivative; packs per day
PPH	postpartum hemorrhage
PPHN	persistent pulmon. hypertension
PPN	peripheral parenteral nutrition
PPP	peripheral pulses present
PPS	peripheral pulmonary stenosis; postpartum sterilization
PPTL	postpartum tubal ligation
PR	per rectum; pulse rate
PR(B)C	packed red (blood) cells
prn	as required (Lat: pro re nata)
PROM	premature rupture of membrane
PS	pulmonary stenosis
PSA	polysubstance abuse
PSH	past surgical history
PSS	progressive systemic sclerosis
PSVT	paroxysmal supraventricular tachycardia
PT	prothrombin time; paroxysmal tachycardia; physical therapy
pt	patient
PTA	prior to admission
PTC	percutaneous transhepatic cholangiogram
PTCA	percutaneous transluminal coronary angioplasty
PTE	pulmonary thromboembolism

PTL	preterm labor
PTSD	posttraumatic stress disorder
PTT	partial thromboplastin time
PTX	pneumothorax
PU	passed urine; peptic ulcer
PUD	peptic ulcer disease
PUO	pyrexia of unknown origin
PUPPP	pruritic urticarial papules and plaques of pregnancy
PV	examination per vaginam; pemphigus vulgaris; polycythemia vera; portal vein
PVC	premature ventric. contraction
PVD	peripheral vascular disease
PVR	peripheral vascular resistance; pulse-volume recording
PVT	paroxysmal ventr. tachycardia
py	pack years (of cigarettes)
q	every, each (Lat: quaque)
qam	every morning
qd	every day, once a day (quaque die)
qh	every hour (Lat: quaque hora)
q2h	every two hours
qhs	every bedtime (Lat: hora somni)
qid	4 times daily (Lat: quater in die)
ql	as much as pleased (Lat: quantum libet)
qm	every morning (Lat: quaque mane)
qn	every night (Lat: quaque nocte)
QNS	quantity not sufficient
qod	every other day
qpm	every evening
QS	as much as will suffice (Lat: quantum suffict); quantity sufficient (Lat: quantum satis)

qv	as much as you like (Lat: quantum vis)	**RPR**	rapid plasma reagin (syphilis tx)
	right	**RR**	respiratory rate
RA	rheumatoid arthritis; right atrium; room air	**RRP**	relative refractory period
		RRR	regular rate and rhythm
RAD	reactive airway disease; right axis deviation	**RS**	right side; review of symptoms
		RSB	right sternal border
RAIU	radioactive iodine uptake	**RSV**	respiratory syncytial virus
RAST	radioallergosorbent test	**rt**	right
RBBB	right bundle branch block	**r/t**	related to
RBC	red blood (cell) count	**RTA**	renal tubular acidosis
RCA	right coronary artery	**RTC**	return to clinic
RDI	recommended daily intake	**RTS**	Revised Trauma Score
RDS	respiratory distress syndrome	**RUE**	right upper extremity
reg	regular(ly)	**RUL**	right upper lobe
REM	rapid eye movement	**RUQ**	right upper quadrant
RES	reticuloendothelial system	**RV**	right ventricle; residual volume
RF	rheumatic fever; rheumatoid factor; renal failure; risk factor	**RVH**	right ventricular hypertrophy
		Rx	drug; treatment; prescription (Lat: recipe)
r/g/m	rubs, gallops, murmurs	**Rxn**	reaction
RHD	rheumatic heart disease; renal hypertensive disease	**s**	without (Lat: sine)
		$S_1 ... S_4$	heart sounds, 1st to 4th
RIND	reversible ischemic neurol. deficit	**SA**	sinoatrial; salicylic acid; suicide attempt
RL	Ringer's lactate; right leg/lung	**SAB**	spontaneous abortion
RLE	right lower extremity	**SAD**	seasonal (schizo-) affective DO
RLL	right lower lobe	**SAH**	subarachnoid hemorrhage
RLQ	right lower quadrant	**SBE**	subacute bacterial endocarditis
RML	right middle lobe	**SBO**	small bowel obstruction
RN	registered nurse	**SBP**	systolic blood pressure
R/O	rule out	**SC**	subcutaneous
ROM	range of motion; rupture of membranes	**SD**	standard deviation
		SDH	subdural hematoma
ROS	review of systems/symptoms	**SEM**	systolic ejection murmur
RPF	renal plasma flow	**SEMI**	subendocardial MI
RPGN	rapidly progressive glomerulonephritis	**SES**	socioeconomic status
		SGA	small for gestational age

SGOT	serum glutamic oxaloacetic transaminase
SHx	social history
SIADH	synd. of inappropriate ADH secr.
sib	sibling
SICU	surgical intensive care unit
SIDS	sudden infant death syndrome
SK	streptokinase
SL	sublingual
SLE	systemic lupus erythematosus
SLR	straight leg raising (Lasègue)
SMA	sequential multiple analyzer
SNF	skilled nursing facility
SOB	shortness of breath
SP	suprapubic; systolic pressure
s/p	status post, no change
SPEP	serum protein electrophoresis
SQ	subcutaneous
SR	systems review; sustained release
SROM	spontaneous rupture of membrane
S&S	signs and symptoms
SSE	soapsuds enema
SSPE	subacute scleros. panencephalitis
SSS	sick sinus syndrome; scalded skin syndrome
ST	sinus tachycardia
stat	immediately (Lat: statim)
STD	sexually transmitted diseases
STS	serologic test for syphilis
SVC	superior vena cava
SVR	systemic vascular resistance
SVT	supraventricular tachycardia
SW	social worker
Sx	signs, symptoms

SZ	schizophrenia; seizure
T	temperature
T₃	T_3 triiodothyronine
T₄	T_4 thyroxine
T&A	tonsillectomy + adenoidectomy
tab	tablet
TAH	total abdominal hysterectomy
TAT	Thematic Apperception Test
TB	tuberculosis
T&C	type and cross-match (blood)
TCA	tricyclic antidepressant
TCI	to come in (hospital)
TD	tolerance dose
TEE	transesophageal echocardiogram
TEF	tracheoesophageal fistula
TFT	thyroid function test
TG	triglycerides
TGA	transient global amnesia
TGV	transposition of great vessels
T&H	type and hold
THC	transhepatic cholangiogram
THR	total hip replacement
TIA	transient ischemic attack
TIBC	total iron-binding capacity
tid	three times daily (Lat: ter in die)
TIG	tetanus immune globulin
TIPS	transjugular intrahepatic portosystemic shunt
tiw	three times a week
TLC	total lung capacity
TM	tympanic membrane
TMP	trimethoprim
TNM	tumor, node, metastasis
TO	telephone order
TOA	tubo-ovarian abscess
TOP	termination of pregnancy

TOS	thoracic outlet syndrome
TPA	tissue plasminogen activator
TPN	total parenteral nutrition
TPR	temperature, pulse, respirations; total peripheral resistance
TSH	thyroid-stimulating hormone
tsp	teaspoon
TSS	toxic shock syndrome
TT	tetanus toxoid; thrombin time
TTE	transthoracic echocardiogram
TTP	thrombotic thrombocytopenic purpura
TUR (P/BT)	transurethral resection (of prostate/bladder tumor)
TV	tidal volume
Tx	treatment
U	units
UA	urinalysis; uric acid
UC	ulcer. colitis; urinary catheter
UE	upper extremity
UGI	upper gastrointestinal (series)
UMN	upper motor neuron
UO	urinary output
unk	unknown
URI	upper respiratory infection
US	ultrasound
UTD	up to date
UTI	urinary tract infection
UV	ultraviolet
VA	Veterans Admin.; ventriculoatrial
VB	vaginal bleeding
VC	vital capacity
VCUG	voiding cystourethrogram
VD	venereal disease
VDRL	VD Research Lab (syphilis test)
VE	vaginal examination
VF	ventricular fibrillation

VH	vaginal hysterectomy
VIP	vasoactive intestinal peptide
VLDL	very low-density lipoprotein
VMA	vanillylmandelic acid
VNS	visiting nurse service
VO	verbal order
VPC	ventr. premature contraction
V/Q	ventilation-perfusion ratio
VS	vital signs
VSD	ventricular septal defect
VT	ventricular tachycardia
VZV	varicella-zoster virus
WB	whole blood
WBC	white blood (cell) count
WCC	white cell count
WD	ward; wound; well-developed
WF	white female
wk	week
WM	white male
WN	well-nourished
WNL	within normal limits
WPW	Wolff-Parkinson-White
wt	weight
X	times, except, cross
x/12	x number of months
x/24	x number of hours
x/40	x number of gestation weeks
x/52	x number of weeks
x/7	x number of days
XR	x-ray
XRT	(external) radiation therapy
y	year
yo	year(s) old
ZES	Zollinger-Ellison syndrome

Normal Values

Blood gases

	arterial	venous	Met. Ac.	Resp. Ac.	Met. Alk.	Resp. Alk.
pH	7.35–7.45	7.36–7.41	↓	↓	↑	↑
pCO_2	35–45 mmHg	44–48 mmHg	normal	↑*	normal	↓*
HCO_3^-	21–28 mEq/l	22–29 mEq/l	↓*	normal	↑*	normal
pO_2	80–100 mmHg	33–43 mmHg				
O_2-Saturation	95–99%	60–85%				
Base excess	**M:** –3.3 to +1.2, **F:** –2.4 to +2.3, **CH:** –4 to +2, **NB:** –10 to –2 (mEq/l)					

*= Primary change

Cerebrospinal Fluid

Albumin	10–30 mg/dl
Chloride	700–750 mg/dl
Protein, total	15–45 mg/dl
Glucose	50–75 mg/dl [2.4–4.0 mmol/l]
Immunglob. IgA	0.1–0.3 mg/dl
IgG	0.0–4.5 mg/dl
IgM	0.01–1.30 mg/dl
IgG, Synthesis rate	(–) 9.9 to (+) 3.3 mg/d
Lactate	10–25 mg/dl [1.1–2.6 mmol/l]
Leukocytes, total	< 4/mm³
Lymphocytes	60–70%
Monocytes	30–50%
Neutrophils	1–3%
Eosinophils	rare
Ependym. cells	rare
Pressure, CSF	<200 mmH₂O
Pyruvate	0.078–0.081 mEq/l
Cell count	<6/µl

Hematology

Hemoglobin	M: 14–18 F: 12–16 (g/dl)
Methemoglobin	<0.41–1.15% of total
Hematocrit	M: 42–52 F: 37–47 (%)
Erythrocyt. count	M: 4.5–5.7 F: 3.9–5.0 ($\times 10^6/\mu l$)
MCV	80–95 μm^3
MCH	27–31 pg/cell
MCHC	32–36 g/dl
Reticulocytes	Adults/Children: 0.5–2% Infants: 0.5–3.1%
Leukocytes, tot.	3.8–9.8 ($\times 10^3/\mu l$; **100%**)
Neutrophils	1.8–7.7 ($\times 10^3/\mu l$; **59%**)
Bands	0–0.7 ($\times 10^3/\mu l$; 3%)
Segmented	1.8–7.0 ($\times 10^3/\mu l$; 56%)
Eosinophils	0–0.45 ($\times 10^3/\mu l$; **2.7%**)
Basophils	0–0.2 ($\times 10^3/\mu l$; **0.5%**)
Lymphocytes	1.0–4.8 ($\times 10^3/\mu l$; **34%**)
B-cell	5–25%
T-cell	60–88%
T-Helper (CD4)	32–66%
T-Suppr. (CD8)	10–43%
CD4/CD8-rat.	1.0
Monocytes	0–0.8 ($\times 10^3/\mu l$); (**4%**)
Thrombocyt. cou.	150–400 ($\times 10^3/\mu l$)
AT III	functional: 80–120% immunologic: 17–30 mg/dl

Bleeding Time
   Duke:
   Ivy:
   Simplate:
	
	 1–4 min (<4 min)
	 2–7 min (5 mm wound <9min)
	 2.75–8.00 min

ESR Wintrobe	M: 0–9 mm/h F: 0–20 mm/h **CH:** 0–13 mm/h

Fibrinogen	200–400 mg/dl
Fibrin.degrad.pro.	<10 µg/ml
Prothrombin time	11–12.5 s
Part.Thro.pla.time	60–70 s
Thrombin time	11.3–18.5 s
Viscosity [P, S]	P: 1.7–2.1 (H_2O)
	S: 1.4–1.8 (H_2O)

Urine and Urinalysis

Albumin	50–80 mg/24h (at rest)
Ammonia Nitrog.	30–50 mEq/d (30–50 mmol/d)
Amylase	0.04–0.3 U/min; 60450 U/24h
Bilirubin	negative
Blood, occult	negative
Calcium	100–300 mg/d
Chloride	110–250 mmol/d
Copper	15–60 µg/d
Coproporphyrin	100–300µg/d[150–460nmol/d]
Cortisol, free	10–100 µg/d [27–276 nmol/d]
Creatinine	**M:** 0.8–1.8 g/d, **F:** 0.6–1.5 g/d
Cystine / Cysteine	10–100 mg/d
	[0.08–0.83 mmol/d]
δ-Aminolevulinic acid	1–7 mg/24h
	[0.1–0.6 mg/dl]
Dopamine	65–400 µg/d
Epinephrine	<0.5–20 µg/d [<275 nmol/d]
Fat	negative
Fructose	30–65 mg/h
Glomerular Filtration rate	125 ml/min (GFR)
Glucose	<0.5 g/d [<2.78 mmol/d]
5-HIAA	2–6 mg/d [10.4–31.2 µmol/d]
Hydroxyproli. tot	15–45 mg/d

Ketones total	negative
17-Ketos	M: 7–25 mg/d [24–88 µmol/d]
	F: 4–15 mg/d [14–52 µmol/d]
17-OCHS	M: 4.5–10 mg/d, F: 2.5–10 mg/d
Magnesium	6–8.5 mEq/d [3–4.3 mmol/d]
Metanephrine	24–96 µg/d
Norepinephrine	15–80 µg/d [88.5–472 nmol/d]
Osmolality	50–1400 mOsmol/kg
12h fluid rest	>850 mOsmol/kg/d
Oxalate	M: 7–44 mg/d [80–502 µmol/d]
	F: 4–31 mg/d [46–353 µmol/d]
Pentoses	2.0–5.0 mg/kg/24h
Phosphorus	0.4–1.3 g/d [13–42 mmol/d]
Porphobilinogen	0–2.0 mg/d [0–8.8 µmol/d]
Porphyrins	
Coproporphyrin	M: <97 µg/d, F: <61 µg/d
Uroporphyrin	M: <47 µg/d, F: <23 µg/d
Potassium	25–120 mEq/d
Protein, total	1–14 mg/dl [50–80 mg/d at rest]
Sodium	40–220 mEq/L/d
Spec. Gravit. rand.	1.005–1.030
U,12h fluid restric.	>1.025
U, 24	1.015–1.025
Urea-Nitrogen	6–17 g/24h [0.21–0.60 mol/d]
Uric acid	0.250.75 g/d [1.5–4.5 mmol/d]
Urobilinogen	1.0–3.5 mg/d
VMA	2.0–7.0 mg/d
Volume	600–2500 ml/d

Stool

Fat	<6 g/d (2.5–5.5 g/24h)
	(<30.4 % of dry weight)
Trypsin Activity	positive (2 + to 4 +)
Wet Weight	<197.5 g/d (74–155 g/d)
Dry Weight	<66.4 g/d (18–50 g/d)

Blood Chemistry

Acetoacetate [P]	0.2–1.0 mg/dl
ACTH, fasting [S]	<60 pg/ml [<13.2 pmol/l]
AFP [S]	0.0–8.5 ng/ml
Albumin [S]	3.5–5.0 g/dl
Aldolase [S]	0–8 U/l
Aldosterone	3–10 ng/dl (supine)
α_1-Antitryp. [S]	80–210 mg/dl [0.8–2.1 g/l]
Aluminum [S]	4–10 µg/l
Ammonia [P]	47–65 µmol/l
Amylase [S]	35–118 U/l [0.58–1.97 µkat/l]
Anion Gap	8–12 mEq/l
Base (total) [S]	145–155 mEq/l
Bile Acids, tot. [S]	0.3–2.3 µg/ml (fasting)
Bilirubin, tot. [S]	0.1–1.0 mg/dl [5.1–17 µmol/l]
Bilirubin, dir. [S]	0.1–0.3 mg/dl [1.7–5.1 µmol/l]
Bilirubin, ind. [S]	0.2–0.8 mg/dl [3.4–12 µmol/l]
CA 15-3 [S]	<22 U/ml
CA 125 [S]	0–35 U/ml
Calcitonin [P]	M: <20 pg/ml, F: <15 pg/ml
Calcium, ion. [S]	4.5–5.6 mg/dl
Calcium, tot. [S]	9–10.5 mg/dl
CEA [S]	0–2.5 ng/ml
Smoker	0–5.0 ng/ml
Ceruloplasm. [S]	23–43 mg/dl [1.5–2.8 µmol/l]
Chloride [S]	98–106 mmol/l
Cholest., tot. [S]	<200 mg/dl [<5,2 mmol/l]
LDL-Cholest.	<130 mg/dl [<3,37 mmol/l]
HDL-Cholest.	M: >45 mg/dl, F: >55 mg/dl
Cholinesterase [P]	0.5–1.5 mg/dl, 7–19 U/ml
Citrate [S+P]	1.7–3.0 mg/dl
CK [S]	M: 55–170 U/l
	F: 30–135 U/l
CK-MB (Heart) [S]	0–12 U/l (<5% of total)

Complem. C3 [S]	55–120 mg/dl
Complem. C4 [S]	20–50 mg/dl
Copper tot. [S]	70–160 µg/dl [11–25.1 µmol/l]
Cortisol, AM [P]	6–28 µg/dl [170–625 nmol/l]
Cortisol, PM [P]	2–12 µg/dl [80–413 nmol/l]
Creatinine [S]	0.5–1.2 mg/dl
Creatine kinase [S]	M: 55–170 U/l
	F: 30–135 U/l
MB fraction	0–12 U/l [0–0.20 µkat/l]
CRP [S]	<0.8 mg/dl
Ferritin, M [S]	12–300 ng/ml
F [S]	10–150 ng/ml
Fluoride	<0.05 mg/dl
Folate [P]	3.1–12.4 ng/ml [7–28 nmol/l]
Red cell	186–645 ng/ml
γ-GT [S]	M: 8–38 U/l, F: 5–27 U/l
Gastrin, fasting [S]	<200 pg/ml [<200 ng/l]
GH, fasting [P]	M: <5 ng/ml, F: <10ng/ml
Glucose [P]	45–96 mg/dl [2.5–5.3mmol/l]
Glutathione [vB]	24–37 mg/dl [0.77–1.2mmol/l]
SGOT [S]	11–47 U/l [0.18–0.78 µkat/l]
SGPT [S]	7–53 U/l [0.12–0.88 µkat/l]
Haptoglobin 1 [S]	100–150 mg/dl
HBDH, alpha [S]	140–350 U/l
Immungl. IgA [S]	85–385 mg/dl
IgD	0–8 mg/dl
IgE	<25 µg/dl
IgG	565–1765 mg/dl
IgM	55–375 mg/dl
Iron [S]	M: 45–160 µg/dl [8–31 µmol/l]
	F: 30–160µg/dl [5.4–31 µmol/l]
Iron bin. capac. [S]	25–420 µg/dl [45–73 µmol/l]
Ketones tot. [S]	0.5–1.5 mg/dl
Lactic Acid [P]	5–15 mg/dl [0.6–1.7 mmol/l]

LAP [S]	M: 80–200 U/ml
	F: 75–185 U/ml
LDH [S]	45–90 U/l [0.4–1.7 µmol/l]
Lead [vB]	<20 µg/dl [<1.0 µmol/l]
Lipase [S]	2.3–50.0 U/dl [0.4–8.34 µkat/l]
Magnesium [S]	1.3–2.2 mEq/l [0,65–1,1 mmol/l]
5'-Nucleotidase	2–16 U/l [0.03–0.27 µkat/l]
Osmolality [P]	285–295 mOsm/kg
Oxalate [S]	1.0–2.4 µg/ml [11–27 µmol/l]
Parathormon [P]	<2000 pg/ml
Pepsinogen [S]	25–100 ng/ml
Phenylalanine [S]	<2 mg/dl
Phosphatase, alk. [S]	38–126 U/l [0.63–2.1 µkat/l]
Phosphatase, acid. [S]	0–0.7 U/l [0–11.6 nkat/l]
Phosphate[S]	3–4.5 mg/dl [0.97–1.45 mmol/l]
Potassium [S]	3.5–5.0 mEq/l
Prealbumin [S]	10–40 mg/dl
Prolactin	**M:** 0–20 ng/ml
	F: 0–20 ng/ml
Protein, tot. [S]	6.4–8.3 g/dl
Albumin	3.5–5.0 g/dl (50–60%)
Globulins, tot	2.3–3.4 g/dl (40–50%)
α_1-Globulins	0.2–0.4 g/dl (4.2–7.2%)
α_2-Globulins	0.5–0.9 g/dl (6.8–12%)
β-Globulins	0.6–1.1 g/dl (9.3–15%)
γ-Globulins	0.7–1.7 g/dl (13–23%)
PSA [S]	<4 ng/ml
Renin activity [P]	0.9–3.3 ng/ml/h
Sodium [S]	135–145 mmol/l
T₄, tot. [S]	4.5–12 µg/dl [58–155 nmol/l]
free T₄ [S]	0.8–2.4 ng/dl [10–31 pmol/l]
T₃, tot. [S]	110–230 ng/dl [1.2–1.5 nmol/l]
T₃ uptake [S]	24–34%
Testostero. tot.[P]	**M:** 300–1000 ng/dl
	F: 20–75 ng/dl

Transferrin [S]	200–400 mg/dl [25–45 µmol/l]
Transferr. saturat.	30–40%
Triglycerides [S]	<250 mg/dl (fasting)
Troponin 1	
Normal	<0.7 ng/ml
Indeterminant	0.7–1.5 ng/ml
Abnormal	>1.5 ng/ml
TSH [S]	2–10 µU/ml
Urea [S]	17–42 mg/dl [6.0–15 mmol/l]
Urea Nitrogen [S]	10–20 mg/dl [3.6–7.1 mmol/l]
Uric Acid **M** [S]	2.1–8.5 mg/dl [150–480 µmol/l]
F [S]	2.0–6.6 mg/dl [90–360 µmol/l]
Vit. A [S]	20–100 µg/dl [0.7–3.5 µmol/l]
Vit. C [S]	0.6–2.0 mg/dl [23–57 µmol/l]
Vit. B_6	3.6–18 ng/ml [15–73 nmol/l]
Vit. B_{12} [S]	200–600 pg/ml [148–443 pmol/l]
Vit. D, 1,25-dihydr.	15–60 pg/ml [36–144 pmol/l]
Vit. D, 25-hydroxy	10–55 ng/ml [25–137 nmol/l]
Zinc	100–140 µg/dl [11.5–18 µmol/l]

Pleural Fluid

	Transudate	Exudate
Amylase		>500 U/ml
Erythrocytes	<10000/µl	>100000/µl
Proteins tot.	<3 g/dl	>3 g/dl
Pleura/Serum-rat.	<0.5	
Glucose	>60 mg/dl	<60 mg/dl
Leukocytes	<1000/µl	>1000/µl
LDH (Pl./Ser.-rat.)	<200U/l (<0.6)	>200U/l (>0.6)
pH	>7.3	<7.3
Specific Gravity	<1.016	>1.016

SI-Classification

The system of international units (Système International d' Unités "SI") is intended to supply standardized units of measurement for international use. Because many laboratories still use "old" units, here called conventional units, both will be given in the following section wherever possible, with conversion factor if needed.

SI Prefixes

Factor	SI Prefix	Abbreviation
1 000 000 000 000 000 000 (= 10^{18})	exa	E
1 000 000 000 000 000 (= 10^{15})	peta	P
1 000 000 000 000 (= 10^{12})	tera	T
1 000 000 000 (= 10^{9})	giga	G
1 000 000 (= 10^{6})	mega	M
1 000 (= 10^{3})	kilo	k
100 (= 10^{2})	hecto	h
10 (= 10^{1})	deca	de
1 (= 10^{0})		
0,1 (10^{-1})	deci	d
0,01 (10^{-2})	centi	c
0,001 (10^{-3})	milli	m
0,000 001 (10^{-6})	micro	µ
0,000 000 001 (10^{-9})	nano	n
0,000 000 000 001 (10^{-12})	pico	p
0,000 000 000 000 001 (10^{-15})	femto	f
0,000 000 000 000 000 001 (10^{-18})	atto	a

SI Base Units

Size	Symbol	Unit	Abbrev.	Conversion
Length	l	meter	m	1 inch = 0,0254 m 1 foot = 0,3048 m 1 yard = 0,9144 m 1 mile =1609,3 m
Mass	m	kilogramm	kg	1 pound = 454 g
Amount of substance	n	mole	mol	
Temperature	T	kelvin	K	$0 K = -273,15 °C$ $°F = (°C \times 9/5) + 32$ $°C = (°F - 32) \times 5/9$
Time	t	second	s	
Electric current	I	ampere	A	
Luminous intensity	I	candela	cd	

SI Derived Units

Size	Symbol	Unit	Abbrev.	Conversion
Area	A	square meter	m^2	
Volume	V	liter	l	$1 l = 10 cm^3$ 1 gallon = 3,785 l 1 fl.oz. = 29, 57 ml
Catalytic activity	ζ	katal	kat	$1 kat = 60 \cdot 10^6 U$
Velocity	v	meters per second	$m\,s^{-1}$	
Density	ρ	kilograms per cubic meter	$kg\,m^{-3}$	
Force	F	newton	N	$N = m\,kg\,s^{-2}$ $1 dyn = 10^{-5} N$ $1 pond = 9,8 \cdot 10^{-3} N$
Work	W	joule	J	$J = N\,m$ 1 kWh = 3600 kJ

SI Derived Units

Size	Symbol	Unit	Abbrev.	Conversion
Pressure	p	pascal	Pa	$Pa = N\ m^{-2}$ oder $kg\ m^{-1}s^{-2}$ $1\ cmH_2O = 98\ Pa$ $1\ mmHg = 133{,}3\ Pa$ $1\ bar = 100\ kPa$ $1\ atm = 101{,}324\ kPa$ $1\ dyn/cm^2 = 0{,}1\ Pa$ $1\ cmH_2O = 1{,}36\ x\ mmHg$ $1\ mmHg = 1\ Torr$
Energy	E	joule	J	$1\ kcal = 4{,}19\ 10^3\ J$
Electrical power	P	watt	W	$W = J\ s^{-1}$ $1\ PS = 735{,}5\ W$
Heat	Q	joule	J	$1\ kcal = 4{,}19\ 10^3\ J$
Mass concentration	C	grams per liter	g/l	$1g\% = 10g/l$ oder $1g/dl$
Molality	M	moles per kilogram	mol/kg	
Molarity	M	moles per liter	mol/l	$1\ M = mol/l$
Viscosity	η	pascal second	Pa s	$1\ Pa\ s = N\ s\ m^{-2}$
Frequency	ν	hertz	Hz	$1\ Hz = s^{-1}$
Halflife	$T_{1/2}$	second	s	
Resistance	R	ohm	Ω	$R = U/I$
Electromotive force	U	volt	V	
Luminous flux	Φ	lumen	lm	
Light	E	lux	lx	$lux = lm/m^{-2}$
Activity	A	becquerel	Bc	$1\ Ci\ (Curie) = 3{,}7\ 10^{10}\ Bc$
Ionization dose	I	coulombs per kilogram	C/kg	$1\ R\ (Röntgen) =$ $2{,}58\ 10^{-4}\ C/kg$
Absorbed dose	D	gray	Gy	$1\ Gy = 1\ J/kg$ $1\ rd\ (Rad) = 10^{-2}\ Gy$
Equivalent dose	D	sievert	Sv	$1\ Sv = 1\ J/kg$ $1\ rem\ (Rem) = 10^{-2}\ Sv$

Greek Letters

A	α	alpha	I	ι	jota	P	ρ	rho
B	β	beta	K	κ	kappa	Σ	σ	sigma
Γ	γ	gamma	Λ	λ	lambda	T	τ	tau
Δ	δ	delta	M	μ	my	Y	υ	ypsilon
E	ε	epsilon	N	ν	ny	Φ	ϕ	phi
Z	ζ	zeta	Ξ	ξ	xi	X	χ	chi
H	η	eta	O	o	omikron	Ψ	ψ	psi
Θ	θ	theta	Π	π	pi	Ω	ω	omega

List of illustrations and figures

[A] AESCULAP AG & CO. KG, 78532 Tuttlingen (Germany), http://www.aesculap.de
[B] AMBU DEUTSCHLAND GMBH, 62231 Bad Nauheim (Germany), http://www.ambu.de
[C] B. BRAUN MELSUNGEN AG, 34212 Melsungen (Germany), http://www.bbraun.de
[D] FRESENIUS AG, 61253 Bad Homburg v.d.H. (Germany), http://www.fresenius.de
[E] PAUL HARTMANN AG, 89552 Heidenheim (Germany), http://de.hartmann.info
[F] KARL STORZ GmbH & CO. KG, 78532 Tuttlingen (Germany), http://www.karlstorz.de
[G] LAERDAL MEDICAL GMBH, 82178 Puchheim (Germany), http://www.laerdal.de
[H] MEDISHOP, 71696 Möglingen (Germany), http://www.medishop.de
[I] OLYMPUS DEUTSCHLAND GMBH, 20097 Hamburg (Germany), http://www.olympus.de
[J] P & W MEDIZINTECHNIK GMBH, 13469 Berlin (Germany),
    http://www.medizintechnik-pw.de
[K] WILLY RÜSCH GMBH (TELEFLEX MEDICAL GMBH), 71394 Kernen (Germany),
    http://www.ruesch.de
[L] SARSTEDT AG & CO., 51582 Nümbrecht (Germany), http://www.sarstedt.com
[M] SCHILLER HANDELSGES.m.b.H, 4040 Linz (Austria), http://www.schiller.at
[N] TYCO HEATHCARE DEUTSCHLAND GMBH, 93333 Neustadt/Donau (Gemany),
    http://www.tycohealth.de

For students, residents and all other healthcare professionals

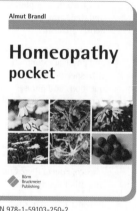

Almut Brandl

Homeopathy pocket

Börm
Bruckmeier
Publishing

ISBN 978-1-59103-250-2
US $ 14.95

- Aimed at physicians, medical students, practitioners, pharmacists and healthcare consumers

- Concise introduction to the holistic approach of homeopathic medicine

- Extensive descriptions of more than 100 homeopathic remedies

- Substantial list of diseases with references to the appropriate remedies

- Medical terms used in text are defined in a comprehensive glossary

*Vital communication tool for anyone
working with Spanish-speaking patients*

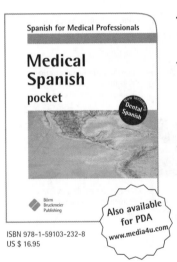

Spanish for Medical Professionals

Medical Spanish pocket

Now including Dental Spanish

Börm
Bruckmeier
Publishing

Also available for PDA
www.media4u.com

ISBN 978-1-59103-232-8
US $ 16.95

- **2nd edition, completely updated:** now including dental Spanish

- Clearly organized by history and physical examination with specific in-depth questions and phrases appropriate to each medical specialty

- Bilingual dictionary containing Spanish medical terminology specific to Mexico, Puerto Rico, Cuba, and other countries

- Provides hundreds of essential ready to use words and phrases

For students, residents and all other healthcare professionals

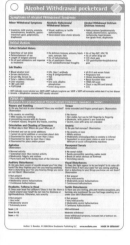

A concise reference guide for the assessment and treatment of acute alcohol withdrawal syndrome!

- Provides information on initial assessment, recommended lab studies, criteria for inpatient detoxification and discharge

- Contains the Clinical Institute Withdrawal Assessment - Alcohol revised scale (CIWA-Ar)

- Detailed treatment plan for acute alcohol withdrawal and its complications

ISBN 978-1-59103-031-7
US $ 3.95

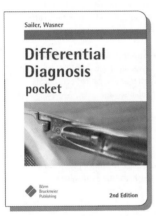

Börm Bruckmeier Products

pockets

Acupuncture pocket	ISBN 978-1-59103-248-9	US $ 16.95
Anatomy pocket	ISBN 978-1-59103-219-9	US $ 16.95
Canadian Drug pocket 2009	ISBN 978-1-59103-238-0	US $ 14.95
Differential Diagnosis pocket	ISBN 978-1-59103-216-8	US $ 14.95
Drug pocket 2008	ISBN 978-1-59103-240-3	US $ 12.95
Drug pocket plus 2008	ISBN 978-1-59103-241-0	US $ 19.95
ECG pocket	ISBN 978-1-59103-230-4	US $ 16.95
ECG Cases pocket	ISBN 978-1-59103-229-8	US $ 16.95
Homeopathy pocket	ISBN 978-1-59103-250-2	US $ 14.95
Medical Abbreviations pocket	ISBN 978-1-59103-221-2	US $ 16.95
Medical Classifications pocket	ISBN 978-1-59103-223-6	US $ 16.95
Medical Spanish pocket	ISBN 978-1-59103-232-8	US $ 16.95
Medical Spanish Dictionary pocket	ISBN 978-1-59103-231-1	US $ 16.95
Medical Spanish pocket plus	ISBN 978-1-59103-239-7	US $ 22.95
Medical Translator pocket	ISBN 978-1-59103-235-9	US $ 16.95
Normal Values pocket	ISBN 978-1-59103-205-2	US $ 12.95
Nursing Dictionary pocket	ISBN 978-1-59103-237-3	US $ 12.95
Respiratory pocket	ISBN 978-1-59103-228-1	US $ 16.95
Wards 101 pocket	ISBN 978-1-59103-253-3	US $ 19.95

pocketcards

Alcohol Withdrawal pocketcard	ISBN 978-1-59103-031-7	US $ 3.95
Anesthesiology pocketcard Set (3)	ISBN 978-1-59703-050-8	US $ 9.95
Antibiotics pocketcard 2008	ISBN 978-1-59103-041-6	US $ 3.95
Antifungals pocketcard	ISBN 978-1-59103-013-3	US $ 3.95
Asthma pocketcard Set (2)	ISBN 978-1-59103-046-1	US $ 6.95
COPD pocketcard Set (2)	ISBN 978-1-59103-047-8	US $ 6.95
Dementia pocketcard Set (3)	ISBN 978-1-59103-053-9	US $ 9.95
Diabetes pocketcard Set (3)	ISBN 978-1-59103-054-6	US $ 9.95
Dyslipidemia pocketcard Set (2)	ISBN 978-1-59103-055-3	US $ 6.95
ECG pocketcard	ISBN 978-1-59103-028-7	US $ 3.95
ECG Ruler pocketcard	ISBN 978-1-59103-002-7	US $ 3.95
ECG pocketcard Set (3)	ISBN 978-1-59103-003-4	US $ 9.95
Echocardiography pocketcard Set (2)	ISBN 978-1-59103-024-9	US $ 6.95

Börm Bruckmeier Products

pocketcards

Epilepsy pocketcard Set (2)	ISBN 978-1-59103-034-8	US $ 6.95
Geriatrics pocketcard Set (3)	ISBN 978-1-59103-037-9	US $ 9.95
History & Physical Exam pocketcard	ISBN 978-1-59103-022-5	US $ 3.95
Hypertension pocketcard	ISBN 978-1-59103-042-3	US $ 6.95
Immunization pocketcard	ISBN 978-1-59103-044-7	US $ 6.95
Medical Abbreviations pc Set (2)	ISBN 978-1-59103-010-2	US $ 6.95
Medical Spanish pocketcard	ISBN 978-1-59103-027-0	US $ 3.95
Medical Spanish pocketcard Set (2)	ISBN 978-1-59103-025-6	US $ 6.95
Neurology pocketcard (2)	ISBN 978-1-59103-021-8	US $ 6.95
Normal Values pocketcard	ISBN 978-1-59103-023-2	US $ 3.95
Parkinson pocketcard Set (2)	ISBN 978-1-59103-043-0	US $ 6.95
Periodic Table pocketcard	ISBN 978-1-59103-014-0	US $ 9.95
Psychiatry pocketcard Set (2)	ISBN 978-1-59103-033-1	US $ 6.95
Vision pocketcard	ISBN 978-1-59103-032-4	US $ 3.95
Wound Ruler pocketcard	ISBN 978-1-59103-051-5	US $ 3.95

pockettools

Asthma pockettool	ISBN 978-1-59103-802-3	US $ 9.95
DARF pockettool	ISBN 978-1-59103-803-0	US $ 9.95
ECG pockettool	ISBN 978-1-59103-800-9	US $ 9.95
ECG Ruler pockettool	ISBN 978-1-59103-805-4	US $ 9.95
Medical Spanish pockettool	ISBN 978-1-59103-804-7	US $ 9.95
Normal Values pockettool	ISBN 978-1-59103-801-6	US $ 9.95

PDA software

Differential Diagnosis pocket for PDA	ISBN 978-1-59103-600-5	US $ 16.95
Drug Therapy pocket for PDA	ISBN 978-1-59103-605-0	US $ 16.95
ECG pocket for PDA	ISBN 978-1-59103-601-2	US $ 16.95
Homeopathy pocket for PDA	ISBN 978-1-59103-650-0	US $ 16.95
ICD-9-CM 2005 for PDA	ISBN 978-1-59103-606-7	US $ 24.95
Medical Abbreviations pocket for PDA	ISBN 978-1-59103-603-6	US $ 16.95
Medical Calculator pocket for PDA	ISBN 978-1-59103-616-6	US $ 16.95
Medical Spanish pocket for PDA	ISBN 978-1-59103-602-9	US $ 16.95
Medical Spanish Dic. pocket for PDA	ISBN 978-1-59103-607-4	US $ 16.95
Medical Spanish pocket plus for PDA	ISBN 978-1-59103-608-1	US $ 24.95